CLINICAL DECISIONS IN
Neuro-Ophthalmology

CLINICAL DECISIONS IN
Neuro-Ophthalmology

Ronald M. Burde, M.D.

Professor of Ophthalmology, Neurology, and Neurological Surgery,
Washington University School of Medicine,
St. Louis, Missouri

Peter J. Savino, M.D.

Director, Neuro-Ophthalmology, Wills Eye Hospital,
Associate Clinical Professor of Ophthalmology and Neurology,
University of Pennsylvania,
Philadelphia, Pennsylvania

Jonathan D. Trobe, M.D.

Associate Professor of Ophthalmology,
University of Florida College of Medicine,
Gainesville, Florida

with 207 illustrations and 10 four-color plates

The C. V. Mosby Company

ST. LOUIS • TORONTO • PRINCETON   1985

MOSBY

A TRADITION OF PUBLISHING EXCELLENCE

Editor: Eugenia A. Klein
Manuscript editor: Mary Espenschied
Book design: Kay Michael Kramer
Cover design: Suzanne Oberholtzer
Production: Jeanne A. Gulledge, Mary Stueck
Cover art: Nadine B. Sokol

Printed in the United States of America

The C.V. Mosby Company
11830 Westline Industrial Drive, St. Louis, Missouri 63146

Library of Congress Cataloging in Publication Data

Burde, Ronald M.
   Clinical decisions in neuro-ophthalmology.

   Bibliography: p.
   Includes index.
      1.   Neuro-ophthalmology—Problems, exercises, etc.
I.   Savino, Peter J.   II.   Trobe, Jonathan D.   III.   Title.
[DNLM: 1.   Eye diseases—Diagnosis.   2.   Eye diseases—
Therapy.   3.   Nervous system diseases—Diagnosis.
4.   Nervous system diseases—Therapy.   WW 140 B949c]
RE725.B87 1985   617.7′3   84-3338
ISBN 0-8016-0891-0

GW/MV/MV   9 8 7 6 5 4 3 2   03/C/313

The inspiration for this book came to one of us
at the 60th birthday celebration of a revered teacher:

Jerome Y. Lettvin, M.D., Ph.D.

*Collectively, we would like to dedicate this book
to our loving families, without whose support
we could not have completed this task,
and to our teachers in ophthalmology and neuro-ophthalmology who,
we trust, will approve our efforts.*

R.M. Burde/P.J. Savino/J.D. Trobe

PREFACE

When physicians consult medical textbooks, they are usually seeking the answer to the question, "Given the disease, what are its symptoms and signs?" In evaluating patients, however, physicians search in the opposite direction, namely, "Given the symptoms and signs, what is the disease?" To answer that kind of question, they must combine textbook information with clinical experience to come up with the sensitivity and specificity of each indicator. With this estimate to guide them, they proceed deductively toward a diagnosis.

It is this subconscious deductive process that we have tried to simulate in *Clinical Decisions in Neuro-ophthalmology*. To the most common and puzzling signs and symptoms are applied, in stepwise fashion, the various inputs we use to arrive at a diagnosis. Since neither we, the authors, nor you, our readers, are usually explicit about this reasoning process, it was only after much gnashing of teeth and wringing of hands that we were able to agree on the uncoding of our collective intuitions.

The uncoding is in the form of the flow chart (decision tree or algorithm), which was first used by computer scientists but which has since been applied to human problem solving in many spheres, including clinical medicine.[3] In the charts, clinical symptoms or signs are contained in boxes (□), and inputs or maneuvers (history, examination, procedure) that elicit information that will start the diagnostic cascade are contained in ovals (○). The outcome of each maneuver determines the subsequent step until a diagnosis (□) is reached. We have tried to build a hierarchy that progresses from the broadest and most reliable determinant maneuvers to the narrowest and least reliable determinant maneuvers. For example, noting the presence or absence of lid retraction is an early step because lid retraction is a specific sign for a large diagnostic subgroup of proptosis, namely, dysthyroid orbitopathy. In many cases the chart does not follow the usual order of the patient workup. Indeed, we do not suggest that you necessarily alter the order in which you collect clinical data. But if you insert the data into the chart after they have been collected, you should be able to see clearly which diagnostic possibilities remain and which have been excluded and decide if further diagnostic steps are needed. In other words, the flow may not be chronological, but it is logical. When the charts extend beyond diagnosis to management, we do suggest a stepwise order of action.

Although the flow chart is succinct, graphic, and orderly, it can hardly be expected to cope with all the complexities of medical diagnosis or management. At the risk of further oversimplifying this process, we have reduced most steps to binary outcomes. The results, you will find, are excessively tall, slender decision trees with long branches. But studies of medical decision making[1] reveal that physicians often weigh a limited number of possibilities or outcomes at a time. More importantly, if the trees were built to encompass all possible alternatives, they would be so thick with arborizations they would be useless as teaching devices.

Perhaps a more severe indictment of algorithms in general is that new scientific developments can quickly cripple them. Consider, for example, the durability of neuro-ophthalmic algorithms designed before the advent of computerized tomography (CT). Advances in venous angiography and magnetic resonance imaging will doubtless have similar effects in the future. We have tried to build trees robust enough to survive at least until the next edition of this book!

Despite these drawbacks, we share the enthusiasm of Lewis and Pask,[2] who believe that algorithms "are optimal instruments for telling people how to cope with contingencies." In constructing them, we discovered how often the information we need to make sensible decisions is missing. In some instances we found that each of us had come to different conclusions about what the available information meant. Where we could come to agreement, we have presented a unified front; where we could not, we have indicated either that there is not enough information to provide clear guidelines, that controversy exists, or that several alternatives are considered acceptable. Even the most dramatic contortions did not permit us to fit the diagnosis of all the major neuro-ophthalmic symptoms and signs into the algorithmic mold (Gaze and Vergence Disorders; Lid Retraction; Headache and Facial Pain). These subjects are presented in the more conventional format.

The decision trees themselves would be very barren without foliage. The text is designed to explain each step in the diagnostic process and to amplify on the manifestations of each disease. The text is not intended to serve as a substitute for a comprehensive reference work, but we have endeavored to present up-to-date material with a special emphasis on the diagnostic specificity of particular signs and symptoms.

Ronald M. Burde, M.D.
Peter J. Savino, M.D.
Jonathan D. Trobe, M.D.

REFERENCES

1. Elstein, AS, Shulman, LS, and Sprafka, SA: Medical problem solving: an analysis of clinical reasoning, Cambridge, Mass, 1978, Harvard University Press.
2. Lewis, BN, and Pask, G: Case studies in the use of algorithms, London, 1967, Pergamon Press.
3. Margolis, CZ: Uses of clinical algorithms, JAMA 249:627, 1983.

CONTENTS

COLOR PLATES

CLINICAL DECISIONS IN
Neuro-Ophthalmology

CHAPTER 1

Unexplained visual loss

One of the most vexing diagnostic problems is visual loss that cannot be explained by obvious abnormalities of the eye. There are two variations to this problem: (1) the patient with subnormal best-corrected acuity without media or fundus abnormality (subnormal acuity; "normal" examination) and (2) the patient complaining of a visual disturbance in spite of "normal" acuity ("normal" acuity; symptoms of visual loss).

Having found no ocular lesions to account for the subnormal acuity or visual complaints, the examiner repeats the acuity and refractive measurements, confirms the initial result, and is perplexed. It is tempting to plunge into expensive laboratory and radiographic studies and consult a neurologist. Before doing so, one should be sure that the problem has been analyzed logically and that subtleties have not been overlooked. To be most effective, such an analysis should be used prospectively, from the moment the patient examination begins, and not retrospectively, after pupils have been dilated and the examination completed.

THE DECISION TREE: AN OVERVIEW

The recommended diagnostic approach involves a branching decision tree (Chart 1-1). Rather than being a recipe for the order of performing tests, it is a logical framework upon which to interpret these tests in arriving at a diagnosis. For example, history taking will precede ocular examination, but the data derived from it are not necessarily used as a diagnostic determinant until a later point in the decision tree.

In cases of unexplained visual loss the fundamental problem is separating visual loss caused by optical disturbances from visual loss caused by neuroretinal disturbances. Optical problems include refractive errors and abnormalities of the ocular media—tear film, cornea, lens, and vitreous. Neuroretinal disturbances involve the retina, optic nerve, chiasm, optic tract, optic radiations, and visual cortex.

The decision tree is built around these considerations. If a refraction establishes that subnormal acuity is present in one or both eyes, the pinhole test is used to separate optical from neuroretinal disease. Because the pinhole test is not fail-safe, the examiner must use additional tests that assess the transmission of light to the retina (biomicroscopy, keratometry, retinoscopy, ophthalmoscopy). If optical problems are not apparent, the swinging flashlight test is used to separate asymmetric optic nerve involvement (afferent defect present) from all other neuroretinal disease (no afferent defect present). If an afferent pupillary defect is present, the examiner follows the asymmetric neuroretinal disease branch of the decision tree and must differentiate retinal, optic nerve, and chiasmal lesions by means of visual fields, fundoscopy, and history. If there is no afferent pupillary

1

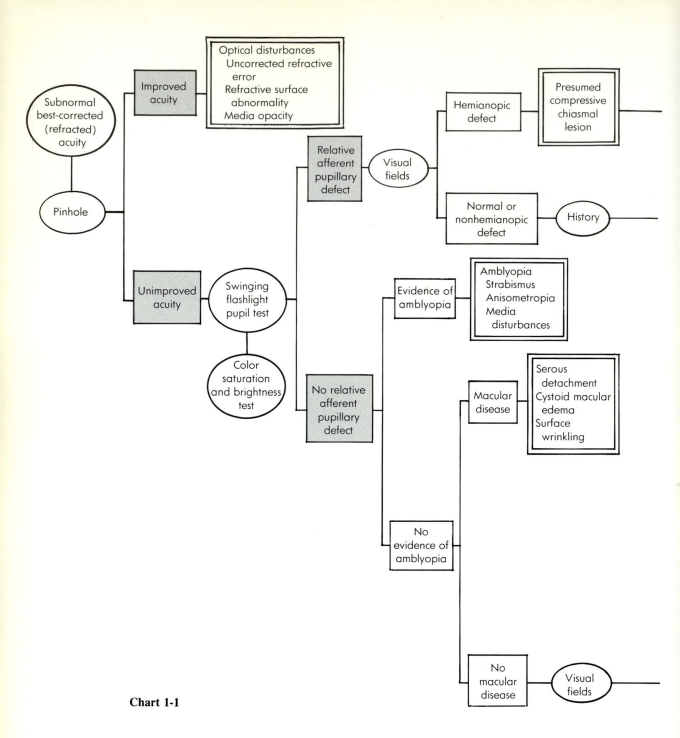

Chart 1-1

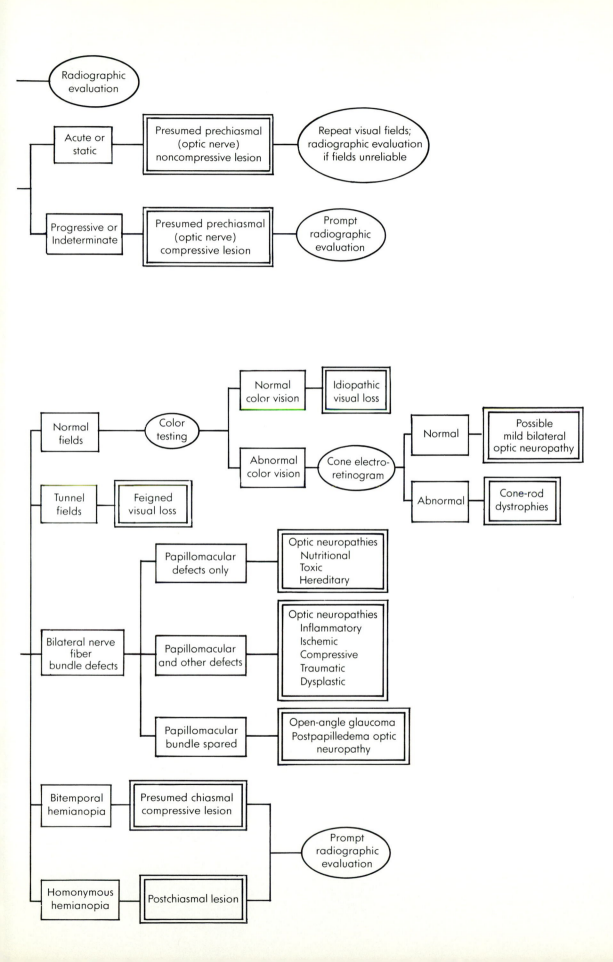

defect, the clinician follows the other branch of the decision tree, which includes the consideration of such entities as amblyopia, maculopathy, cone-rod dystrophy, symmetric optic neuropathies, chiasmal and postchiasmal disease, and feigned (''functional'') visual loss.

PART I

Diagnostic approach

○   **Best-corrected acuity.** The first determinant of the decision tree is the refraction. A punctilious refraction establishes the best-corrected acuity; no further improvement in acuity can be obtained with spectacles.

○   **Pinhole test.** The pinhole examination is an effective means of separating disturbances of refraction and ocular media from other causes of visual loss (Fig. 1-1). The pinhole will improve acuity in uncorrected refractive errors and in tear film, corneal, and lenticular abnormalities by selecting a narrow but choice viewing lane through uneven or unfocused optical terrain. Since some patients, particularly the elderly, are unable to use the pinhole, a negative result is not conclusive. We recommend the use of a multiple pinhole with hole diameters between 2.0 and 2.5 mm, which minimizes the degradation from diffraction (smaller than 2 mm) and surface aberrations (larger than 2.5 mm).[16]

▨ **Improved acuity: optical branch of decision tree** (Chart 1-1, *A*)

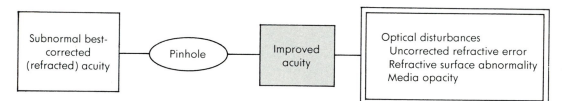

Chart 1-1, A

□   **Optical disturbances.** Of the subtle optical causes of subnormal vision, one must always first exclude an overlooked uncorrected refractive error. Of the remaining causes, it is the refractive surface abnormalities rather than the corneal or lenticular opacities that are likely to be at fault.

There are a variety of ocular adnexal diseases that disturb the precorneal tear film and show a paucity of signs in relation to symptoms. In tear-deficiency states the increased viscosity and mucous texture of the tears leads to visual distortion, a premature breakup of the tear layer, and to corneal drying. In milder cases, visual loss will be intermittent and clear with blinking. If the corneal epithelium becomes damaged, visual loss can become constant, even though very little staining of the cornea may be apparent with fluorescein. Rose bengal may be a more sensitive diagnostic agent since it stains devitalized epithelium, while fluorescein only stains areas of absent epithelium. It is also necessary to consider indolent inflammatory adnexal diseases, such as chronic blepharitis, vernal conjunctivitis, and dacryocystitis, as possible causes of a disturbed tear film. Diseases that produce poor apposition and coverage of the globe by the lids must be added to the

COLOR PLATE 1

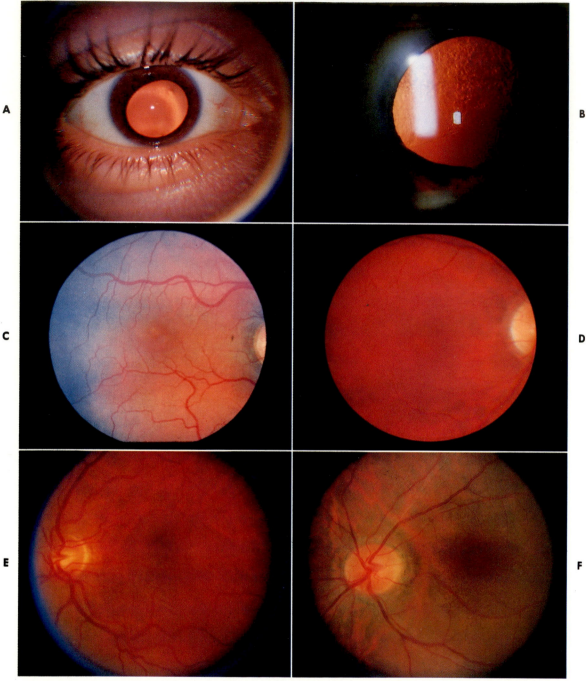

Plate 1. A, Keratoconus. Cone is seen inferotemporally by retroillumination. **B,** After cataract. Pearllike opacities are seen in pupillary space by retroillumination. **C,** Central serous choroido-maculopathy. **D,** Cystoid macular edema. **E,** Surface-wrinkling maculopathy. **F,** Cone dystrophy. Note subtle stippled depigmentation in macular area.

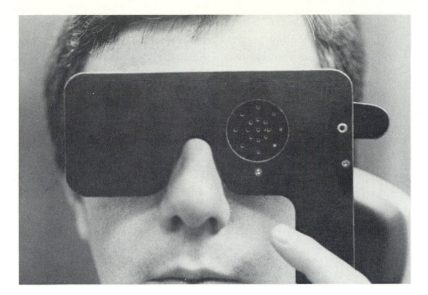

Fig. 1-1. Pinhole test. If acuity improves with viewing through a multiple pinhole, then either uncorrected refractive error or ocular media abnormalities contribute to subnormal vision.

list. Most clinicians readily think of seventh nerve palsy and senile ectropion but may overlook the decreased blinking characteristic of Parkinson's disease. The production of the tear film constituents may be perfectly normal in such cases, but the "windshield wiper" function of the lids has been lost.

Because the cornea is the first and most powerful refracting surface of the eye, minimal deformities will degrade vision. While clinicians are atune to abnormalities of corneal transparency, they may overlook the importance of irregularities of corneal curvature (Plate 1, *A*). All too often the irregular astigmatism of early keratoconus is diagnosed after neurologic studies are unrevealing. There is general agreement that the keratometer is the most sensitive device in the detection of an early cone,[5] although the irregular retinoscopic reflex should be a clue. Pinpoint biomicroscopic examination with oblique beam may illuminate a fine, brown horizontal epithelial line (Fleischer's ring) in the inferotemporal cornea. One may also observe vertical stretch lines deep in the stroma at the base of the cone. Significant corneal surface irregularities may also occur with chalazion, with pterygium, and anterior corneal scarring. If a contact lens placed on the affected eye produces improved acuity, the diagnosis of irregular astigmatism is confirmed.

The water clefts associated with early cataract or the Elschnig's pearls found on a residual lens capsule are other refractive surface abnormalities that commonly account for unexplained visual loss (Plate 1, *B*). With all optical surface irregularities, patients will frequently report a specific kind of blurred vision, a "ghosting" of images. Visual targets with sharp borders will be seen as having two borders—one clear, one fuzzy.

Unimproved acuity: neuroretinal branch of decision tree

Swinging flashlight pupil test. If the pinhole test is negative, the pupillary examination is performed. The relative size of the two pupils is interesting, but not critical in this context. Instead it is the relative reaction to direct light that is important. To maximize the diagnostic information the pupils hold about visual loss, perform this test carefully and according to the accepted protocol.

With the patient placed in a dimly illuminated environment and fixing at a distant target, a bright light is directed into one eye. The pupillary reaction is observed, and the light is briskly moved across the bridge of the nose and directed into the opposite eye. The pupillary reaction is compared in amplitude and direction with that of the first eye. In patients without visual pathway disease and with normal innervation and function of the iris sphincter muscle, the pupil will not constrict as the light is swung toward it. This is because the direct and consensual pupil reactions are equal in the normal case. (If the examiner moves the swinging light too slowly, there will be a temporary interruption of afferent input as the light dwells on the nasal bridge, so that when the light finally reaches the second eye, the pupil will be observed to constrict.) If proper technique is used and the swinging light produces dilatation of the pupil in the second eye, then that eye is said to show a relative afferent pupillary defect[11,19] (a Marcus Gunn pupil, Fig. 1-2). For the most part it indicates that unilateral or asymmetric bilateral optic nerve disease is present. Rarely, macular disease or optic tract disease may be responsible for a relative afferent pupillary defect.

The swinging flashlight test is so rapid, inexpensive, sensitive, reliable, and objective that its fine points deserve attention:

1. The patient must be seated in a room with the least amount of background illumination that permits observation of the unstimulated pupils.
2. The patient must be fixing at distance in order to provide maximal relaxation of the iris sphincter muscle.
3. The light stimulus must be bright, but not so bright as to produce photophobia, and should be directed from below the level of the eyes so as not to constitute a near target (and provoke the miosis associated with accommodation).
4. The light must be moved briskly and rhythmically from eye to eye several times. (The examiner should hold the light over each pupil for a fast count of three.) This is necessary to distinguish the consistent (although often minimal) differences in pupillary dynamics that characterize a true defect from the irregular movements unrelated to the light stimulus that characterize physiologic pupillary unrest.

In subtle cases the affected pupil may not show dilatation. Instead it may consistently show reduced amplitude of constriction and an accelerated recovery from contraction (escape) as compared to the "control" eye.

This test is still useful even if the iris of the affected eye has defective innervation or musculature. Look for constriction of the pupil in the control eye as the light is swung away from the affected side. Such a constriction would imply a relative afferent pupillary defect on the affected side.

The presence of a relative afferent pupillary defect means that the ipsilateral optic nerve conveys less pupillomotor power than does the fellow optic nerve. Since pupillomotor power derives principally from the fibers contained in the papillomacular bundle that subserves central vision, patients with diseases that affect this bundle may have obvious afferent pupillary defects with minimal acuity loss.[19] The papillomacular bundle fibers are most often damaged by optic nerve disease, although retinal artery occlusion may also involve these fibers. Macular disease will only cause an afferent pupillary defect

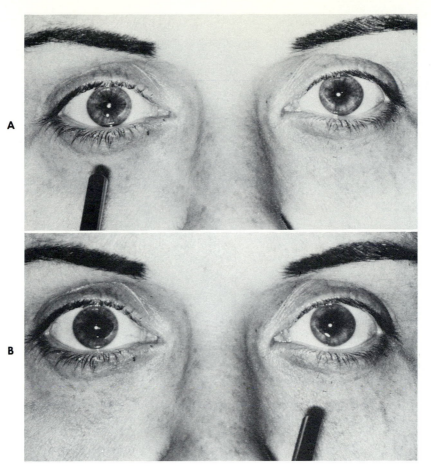

Fig. 1-2. Relative afferent pupillary defect (Marcus Gunn pupil). **A,** Strong light directed at right eye produces pupillary constriction in both eyes. **B,** Light directed at left eye causes dilatation of both pupils because of left optic nerve lesion.

if very extensive.[13,19] Whatever the cause, the involvement must be asymmetric in the two eyes in order to produce this pupillary defect.

If a relative afferent pupillary defect is observed after careful testing, the examiner may presume that asymmetric optic nerve (or extensive retinal) disease is likely to be responsible. If no defect is seen, then either there is no optic nerve disease or it is symmetric.

○ **Color saturation and brightness tests.**[3] The color saturation and brightness tests are helpful adjuncts to the swinging flashlight test. If the examiner has the impression that a relative afferent pupillary defect is present in one eye, he may present a red stimulus to each eye sequentially and ask the patient if there is any difference in the saturation or brightness of the red color (Fig. 1-3). If the patient says no and has clearly understood the question, then the result is interpreted as negative. If the patient replies that there is a difference, the examiner must ask the patient to describe the appearance of the red stimulus in each eye. On the side of the more defective optic nerve, the patient will report that the red appears either faded, orange, pink, gray, or brown. He is describing

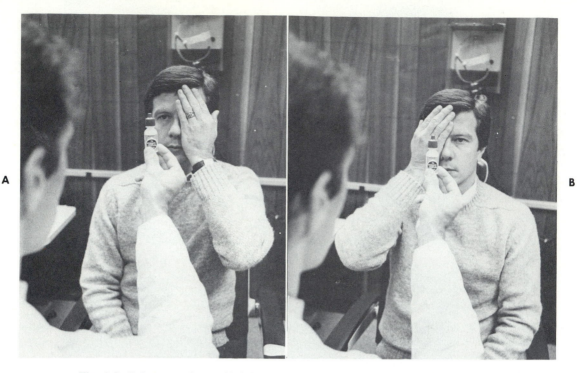

Fig. 1-3. Color saturation and brightness comparison test. As red-capped bottle is viewed first by right eye, **A,** and then left eye, **B,** patient is asked if there is any difference in color.

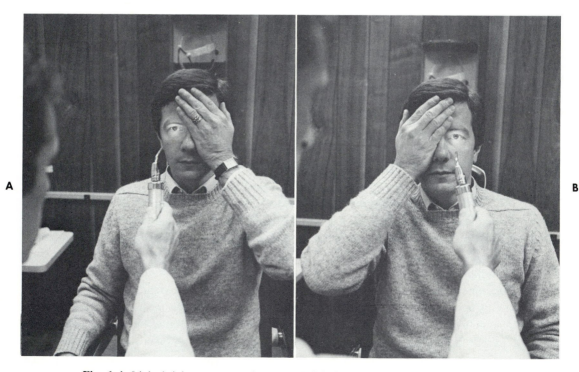

Fig. 1-4. Light brightness comparison test. Bright light is viewed first by right eye, **A,** and then by left eye, **B,** and patient is asked if there is any difference in brightness.

a relative reduction in the saturation or brightness of the color. A response of orange, pink, or faded implies reduced saturation; the color appears to contain less of its spectral hue and more white. A response of gray or brown indicates loss of brightness. If reproducible, this discrepancy in color perception implies asymmetric optic nerve disease. It is not noted in macular disease unless involvement is severe and therefore fundoscopically evident.

After completing the color comparison test, the examiner should shine a flashlight into each eye sequentially and ask a patient if there is any difference in the brightness of the light. Be certain that the patient is responding to the intensity rather than the clarity of the stimulus. If the patient notes a difference, this can be quantitated by giving the normal stimulus a value of unity and asking the patient what fraction he would assign to the brightness of the stimulus shown to the other eye (Fig. 1-4). This brightness comparison test is also highly specific for optic nerve disease. There is evidence that two different sets of ganglion cells subserve the sense of color and the sense of brightness.[8] However, to date there is no clear evidence that certain optic nerve diseases selectively affect one system or the other.

As subjective tests, the color saturation and brightness comparison tests are most helpful in corroborating rather than in establishing a diagnosis. They are most useful when the afferent defect is equivocal. Together with the pupil test, they form a battery that is highly specific in separating asymmetric optic nerve disease from all other causes of unexplained visual loss. They cannot, however, define the etiology or the location of the disease within the extent of the optic nerve.

☐ **Visual loss with afferent pupillary defect** (Chart 1-1, *B)*

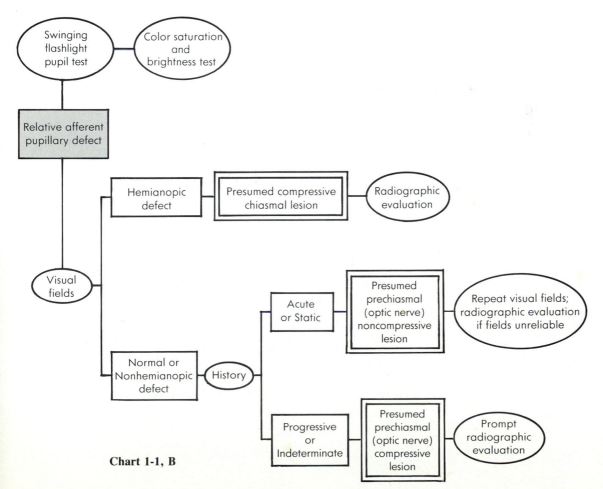

Chart 1-1, B

When an afferent pupillary defect accompanies visual loss, the clinician's approach depends upon the findings on visual field examination and the duration of the visual loss.

Visual field examination. The major purpose of visual field examination is to help localize the neuroretinal lesion, which in turn often suggests the nature of the lesion. If the field defect has a nerve fiber bundle configuration, the lesion may be in either the retinal nerve fiber layer or in that portion of the optic nerve that lies well in front of the chiasm (prechiasmal). Data from representative series indicate that if the field defect is of nerve fiber bundle type, there is less than a 3% chance that it will be a mass lesion.[1] That is, in at least 97% of cases the responsible disease will be congenital, inflammatory, ischemic, or traumatic. Only a small number of cases respond satisfactorily to treatment.

But if a temporal hemianopic defect is present in one or both eyes, the lesion is located either at the junction of the optic nerve and chiasm, at the chiasm, or in the optic tract. The probability of a compressive lesion in such cases is virtually 100%.[1] There are reported cases of inflammation involving the chiasm, but they are rare.[18] A majority of the mass lesions affecting the chiasm (pituitary tumor, meningioma, craniopharyngioma, aneurysm, mucocele) are treatable, and arriving at this diagnosis is a high priority. In the presence of an afferent pupillary defect the clinician's principal preoccupation, then, should be in differentiating nonhemianopic (nerve fiber bundle) from hemianopic (chiasmal) field defects.

Nonhemianopic (nerve fiber bundle) defects (Fig. 1-5). These defects correspond to the organization of the nerve fiber layer of the retina and have the following configurations:

1. Central scotoma, affecting those papillomacular fibers coming from the macular region
2. Centrocecal, affecting those fibers entering the optic nerve from the macula and the zone between the macula and the optic disc
3. Arcuate, affecting temporal retinal fibers that bend around the papillomacular bundle and course into the optic nerve
4. Wedge-shaped with apex at the blind spot, affecting nasal retinal fibers as they enter the optic nerve.

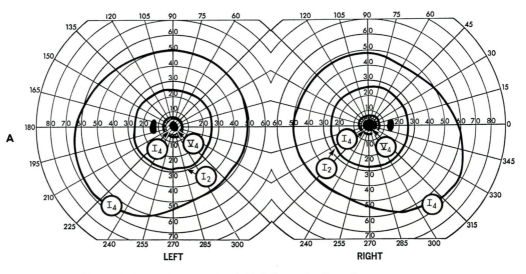

Fig. 1-5. Nerve fiber bundle field defects. **A,** Central scotomas.

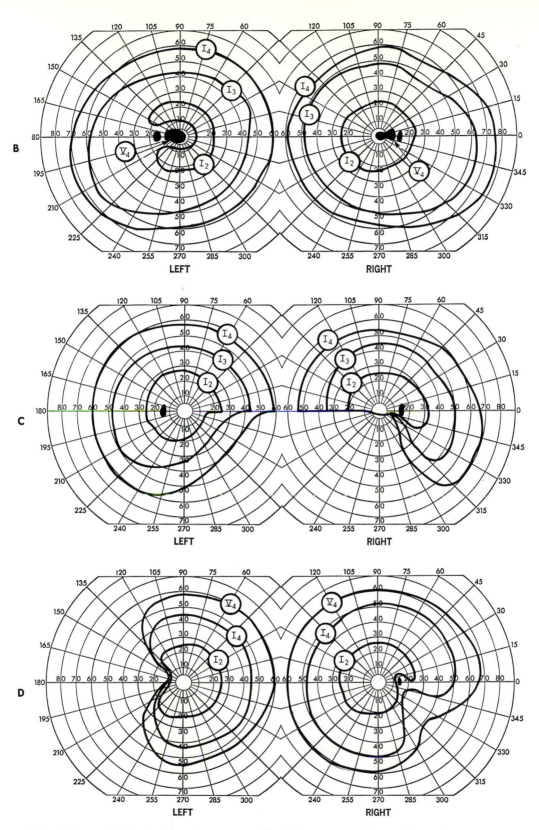

Fig. 1-5, cont'd. B, Centrocecal scotomas. **C,** Inferior arcuate defects with nasal steps. **D,** Temporal wedge defects.

Most nonhemianopic field defects consist of a combination of one or more of these configurations. In some cases the nerve fiber bundle field defect is so small that its configuration is nonlocalizing. In such instances it is usually called a paracentral scotoma or a nonspecific focal depression.

Hemianopic defects (Fig. 1-6). The hemianopic field defect is the hallmark of disease of the optic chiasm and postchiasmal visual pathways. Defined as any field defect with a border aligned to the vertical fixation meridian, a hemianopic defect need not involve the entire hemifield.

The classic pattern of visual field defects produced by compressive disease at the optic chiasm is the bitemporal hemianopia. However, the involvement of the fields of both eyes is rarely entirely symmetric (Fig. 1-6, *A*). Indeed the disease process usually affects one optic nerve as well as the chiasm, and sometimes both optic nerves, but asymmetrically. The result is that the patient will often have subnormal acuity in at least one eye and manifest a relative afferent pupillary defect on that side. In such cases, finding a bitemporal hemianopia means that the disease is at the junction of the optic

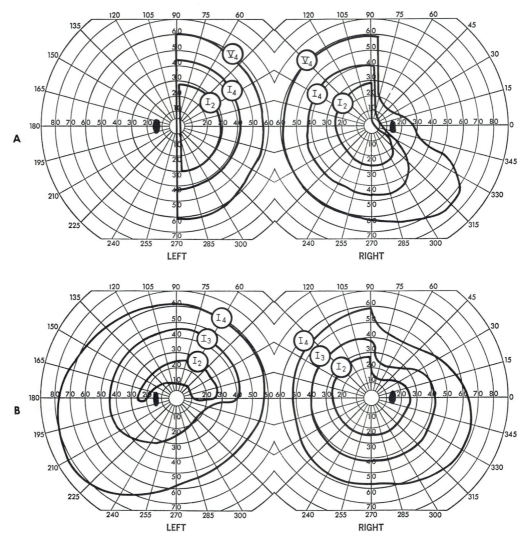

Fig. 1-6. For legend see opposite page.

nerve and chiasm. The temporal hemianopic defect may be present in one eye only (Fig. 1-6, *B*). In fact, it may be present in the eye opposite to that which has the subnormal acuity and which shows the relative afferent pupillary defect. In this "anterior junction syndrome," visual fields will reveal a nonhemianopic (nerve fiber bundle) defect in the eye with the subnormal vision and a supratemporal hemianopic defect on the opposite side. The supratemporal hemianopic defect in the opposite eye results from involvement of the fibers coming from the inferior nasal retina, which cross to the opposite side of the optic chiasm and loop anteriorly in the contralateral optic nerve before entering the optic tract. Perhaps one quarter of patients with compressive chiasmal disease will have the anterior junction syndrome.[25] Because of this fact and because the visual field may be so badly damaged in the affected eye, visual field examination in the unaffected eye

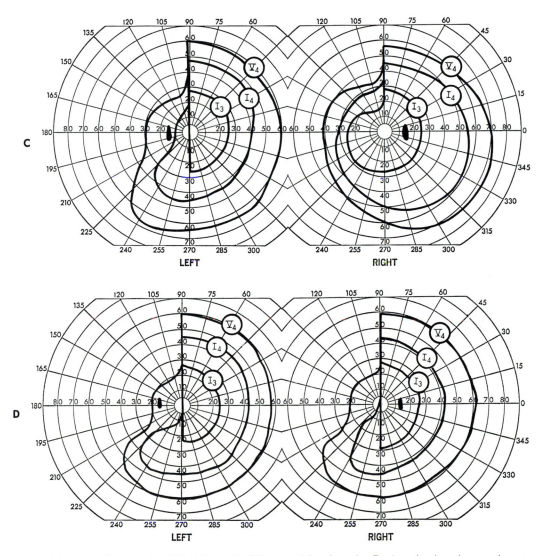

Fig. 1-6. Hemianopic field defects. **A,** Bitemporal hemianopia. **B,** Anterior junction syndrome, left. **C,** Incongruous homonymous hemianopia associated with optic tract disease. **D,** Congruous homonymous hemianopia associated with retrogeniculate disease of visual pathway. Such a field defect is not responsible for subnormal visual acuity.

must have a higher priority. The presence of a supratemporal hemianopic defect identifies the chiasmal location of the disease and demands the exclusion of a compressive lesion.

On rare occasions, patients with an afferent pupillary defect will prove to have homonymous hemianopic field defects (Fig. 1-6, *C*). These defects are usually caused by mass lesions that extend forward from the optic tract along the lateral border of the chiasm.[17] The afferent defect results either from the incongruity of the field defects in the two eyes or from compression of one optic nerve. Lesions that affect the visual pathway posterior to the optic tract do not produce afferent pupillary defects. Retrogeniculate lesions compromising the visual pathways produce congruous homonymous defects (Fig. 1-6, *D*).

○ **Visual field techniques.** Since the discovery of a hemianopic defect is so critical in the diagnosis and management of patients with unexplained visual loss, visual field techniques should be used with this objective in mind. Identifying a hemianopic border is more important than defining the extent and depth of the defect. Thus the ideal technique is one that identifies areas of differential visual sensitivity across a well-defined line.[22] Instead of comparing the two eyes, as was done in the swinging flashlight and brightness and color saturation tests, one compares the two halves of the visual field in each eye—with the vertical fixation meridian as the dividing line. Each hemifield is tested sequentially or simultaneously for sensitivity to brightness and color saturation.

Begin by presenting stationary fingers on either side of the vertical fixational meridian and asking the patient to count them (Fig. 1-7). (In examining children and illiterate, demented, or very poorly sighted adults, one may ask them to mimic the number of fingers presented, or look for eye movements elicited by the stimulus.) If all the fingers are counted correctly, present the two hands simultaneously and ask the patient to total the number of fingers presented. Then ask the patient to compare the brightness of single fingers or whole hands presented simultaneously across the vertical fixational meridian. In the same way, static red stimuli can be presented in both hemifields and the patient asked to compare saturation. If consistent differences are noted, attempt to confirm that a border lies at the vertical fixational meridian by moving the target from the relatively defective field perpendicularly toward the vertical fixational meridian and asking the patient if he notes a change in its appearance. If a true hemianopic defect exists, the patient will notice an abrupt change in brightness or color saturation at the vertical fixational meridian. Performed correctly, these tests are helpful predictors of the results of formal perimetry,[23] which may be performed on any instrument that allows the examiner to explore reliably the central 30° of field, where most field defects start.[21] For careful quantitation, however, fields must be performed under the controlled conditions of a bowl-type perimeter (Goldmann).

☐ **Hemianopic field defect present** (Chart 1-1, *C*)

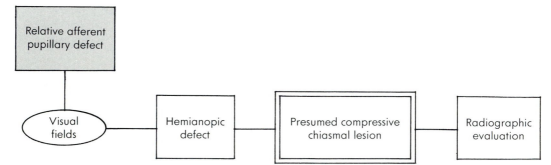

Chart 1-1, C

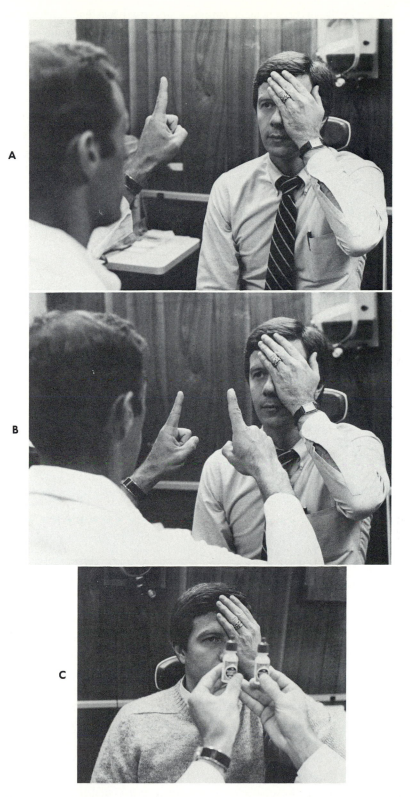

Fig. 1-7. Confrontation visual fields. Since this test is designed to detect gross defects and those with linear borders, examiner begins by exposing large static targets well within confines of normal visual fields. **A,** Single static finger presentation in each quadrant. **B,** Simultaneous finger presentation in two quadrants. **C,** Color comparison across relevant borders.

In the management of patients with visual loss and afferent pupillary defects the finding of a chiasmal hemianopic defect is paramount. If such a field defect is found, one must proceed to prompt radiographic identification and definition of the probable mass lesion, regardless of the time course of the visual loss. Adequate radiologic investigation includes high-resolution computerized tomography (CT) with the aid of metrizamide (Amipaque), a water-soluble dye infused in the subarachnoid space, as well as selective cerebral angiography, performed with percutaneous catheterization and viewed with magnification and subtraction films. If studies fail to reveal a lesion, one must suspect that (1) the studies are inadequate, (2) they have been misinterpreted, or (3) the lesion is too small for these detection methods and requires other maneuvers. In any event, one must continue to pursue vigorously the diagnosis of a mass lesion.

☐ **No hemianopic field defect present** (Chart 1-1, *D*)

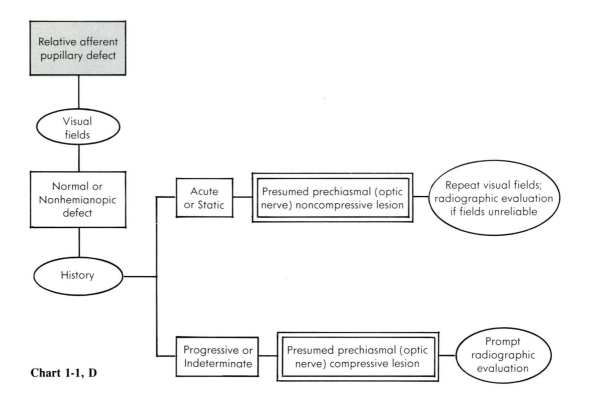

Chart 1-1, D

If reliable field examination fails to show a hemianopic field defect, these patients should be managed according to the time course of visual loss. If visual loss is acute (less than 2 weeks' duration), the odds are strongly against a compressive lesion. Despite the frequent publications highlighting tumors about the optic nerve, they are a rare (less than 5%) cause of optic neuropathy.[1] It is therefore prudent to wait and watch the patient without ordering diagnostic studies. Noncompressive disease should be nonprogressive. The visual loss of retrobulbar neuritis should stop progressing after 7 days and either remit or remain stationary thereafter. It may recrudesce, but there should be a stable interval. Similarly, a patient who is certain that visual loss has been present for at least several months without progression deserves to be watched for documented progression before being subjected to costly and probably unrevealing studies.

If these patients harbor a mass lesion, would delayed surgery result in increased deficits? Multiple studies have established that tumors of the anterior visual pathway grow slowly, and a diagnosis that is delayed by several weeks has not significantly altered mortality or postoperative visual or neurologic morbidity.[1]

On the other hand, if there is a history of chronic progressive visual loss, or if the history is unreliable, one must proceed with radiography even if the visual field defect is nonhemianopic in order to rule out a mass lesion of the orbit or cranioorbital junction. The likelihood of finding such a lesion remains low, since the vast majority of visual pathway masses produce hemianopic defects.

Visual loss without afferent pupillary defect

If no afferent pupillary defect accompanies visual loss, the examiner must be guided by a different set of possibilities: amblyopia, macular disease, cone-rod dystrophy, bilateral symmetric optic neuropathy, chiasmal and postchiasmal visual pathway disease, and feigned visual loss (see Chart 1-1).

Amblyopia (Chart 1-1, *E*)

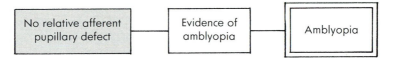

Chart 1-1, E

Amblyopia (or dim vision) is defined as subnormal vision that results from persistently unfocused imagery at the retina or suppression of the fovea in a deviating eye. Because it produces no objective signs of visual disturbance, amblyopia remains a presumptive cause of visual loss and should only be diagnosed if the precipitating circumstances are present and after other causes of visual loss have been excluded. Amblyopia usually arises in the setting of strabismus but may also be seen with anisometropia and with profound early childhood media opacities.

Strabismus. Large misalignments are difficult to overlook, but prismatic deviations of 10 diopters or less must be looked for carefully. Dense amblyopia (as much as 20/100 to 20/200) may be associated with microtropia in the nonfixating eye. A history of strabismus with corrective glasses, surgical alignment, or therapeutic occlusion of an eye is helpful information, but it is probably unsafe to make a diagnosis of strabismic amblyopia unless some deviation from normal alignment is detected. Be careful not to ascribe visual loss to amblyopia in the fixing eye, or in cases of obvious alternate fixation.

Anisometropia. The amblyopia associated with anisometropia is rarely seen in patients whose refractive errors differ by less than 2 diopters of sphere or cylinder. Moreover, it is more common to see amblyopia associated with hypermetropia than with myopia, since the myopic eye will be used preferentially for reading.

Media disturbances. Infants and young children with unilateral congenital or traumatic cataract or corneal or vitreal disease may never recover full visual potential even if the media problems are corrected. In each of these cases, subnormal vision due to amblyopia is typically monocular. Binocular amblyopia is rare and is only associated with media disturbances or high refractive errors in both eyes that are not corrected at an early age.

•   •   •

The difficult diagnostic problems occur when the examiner is not certain if a strabismus is present or if the difference in refractive error is believed to be insufficient to account for amblyopia. Under these circumstances the best policy is to consider amblyopia a diagnosis of exclusion. That is, be sure you have ruled out the other possible causes of unexplained visual loss before ascribing it to amblyopia. You may wish to try some additional tests, none of which, unfortunately, is very reliable or specific.

Crowding phenomenon. Patients with amblyopia are said to have a much higher acuity when they are asked to read single letters rather than an entire line of optotypes. While this is generally regarded as correct, your additional effort in isolating a single letter may eke out improved performance in nonamblyopes as well. For unknown reasons the crowding phenomenon cannot be demonstrated in adult strabismic amblyopia.

Neutral density filter. It is said that the amblyopic eye is in a relatively dark-adapted state and that the addition of a 2–log unit neutral density filter over this eye should have no effect on its acuity. By comparison, when the normal eye is similarly tested, it will show a fall in acuity of three to four lines.[24] In our experience this test is unreliable.

Monocular:binocular acuity differences. Since the amblyopic eye goes through a process of suppression first under binocular viewing conditions (facultative suppression) and later under monocular viewing conditions (obligatory suppression), its acuity under binocular conditions may be much poorer than under monocular conditions. Acuity may be tested binocularly with the Polaroid vector graph and then compared with the monocular Snellen acuity test. Again, this test is distinctly unreliable.

4-diopter prism test. With the patient fixing and both eyes open, a 4-diopter base-out prism is placed over the suspected amblyopic eye and then over the normal eye. The eye under the prism is observed for movement. The foveal region of an amblyopic eye is suppressed under binocular viewing conditions, and the eye will not move under the prism. A normal eye should show an inward deviation. However, lack of eye movement under the prism need not be due to amblyopia and may well be due to macular or optic nerve disease. In essence the 4-diopter prism test is an excellent means of separating organic from feigned central visual loss but cannot differentiate the various causes of organic central visual loss.

•   •   •

The presence of a relative afferent pupillary defect excludes amblyopia as the cause of visual loss. Even the densest amblyopia (counting fingers vision) does not produce a clinically apparent pupillary defect under conventional test conditions. The examiner must look for another explanation.

□ **No evidence of amblyopia—macular disease** (Chart 1-1, *F*)

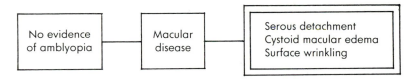

Chart 1-1, F

The diagnosis of subtle macular disease as the cause of subnormal acuity depends upon careful fundoscopy, photostress testing, and use of the Amsler grid.

The macular disturbances most frequently overlooked are (1) serous detachment (Plate 1, *C*), cystoid edema (Plate 1, *D*, and Fig. 1-8), and (3) surface wrinkling (Plate 1, *E*). Senile macular degeneration and other macular diseases affecting the pigment epithelium will usually disturb fundus color enough by the time acuity is degraded to be easily diagnosed with the ophthalmoscope. However, unless the macula is examined with the extra magnification of the Hruby or Goldmann lenses, the detachment of the sensory macula in idiopathic serous choroidoretinopathy, the spokelike edema of cystoid macular edema, and the internal limiting membrane irregularities of surface-wrinkling maculopathy will be overlooked.

The finding of a prolonged recovery of acuity after photostress and the report of metamorphopsia on the Amsler grid test are helpful in confirming the diagnosis of macular disease.

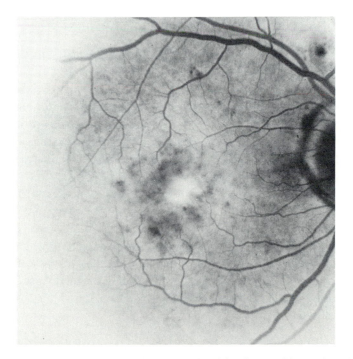

Fig. 1-8. Fluorescein demonstrating petaloid staining in cystoid macular edema.

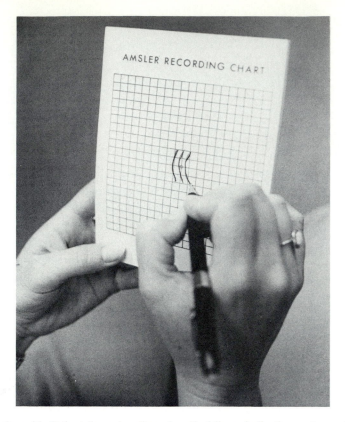

Fig. 1-9. Amsler grid. Patient draws bending of vertical lines, indicating metamorphopsia, a sign of macular disease.

Photostress test.[4] After the best-corrected visual acuity has been measured, a flashlight is directed into one eye for a 10-second period. The patient is then asked to read the next larger Snellen line. The latency between removal of the light stimulus and return of acuity to this level represents the regeneration time of photoreceptor pigments after bleaching with light. The test is most useful in comparing two eyes where one is believed to be normal. An eye that manifests a doubling of recovery time as compared to the normal is likely to have macular receptor disease. Prolonged recovery is not found in optic nerve disturbances.

Amsler grid (Fig. 1-9). A grid of black lines presented on a white background is held at reading distance. The patient is asked if he notes any bending or warping of the lines (metamorphopsia). One should also ask if the squares all appear equal in size (micropsia or macropsia). Again, interpreting these observations is much easier if disease is monocular and a control eye is available. Metamorphopsia and micropsia are diagnostic of macular disease. Unfortunately, significant macular disease can exist without producing either symptom.

☐ **No evidence of amblyopia—no macular disease** (Chart 1-1, *G*)

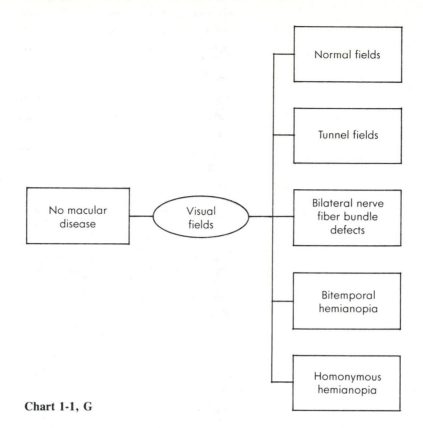

Chart 1-1, G

If there is no relative afferent pupillary defect and if amblyopia and macular disease have been excluded, one must turn to visual field testing. The visual field examination will yield one of five possible results:
1. Normal visual fields
2. Tunnel fields
3. Bilateral nerve fiber bundle defects
4. Bitemporal hemianopia
5. Homonymous hemianopia

☐ **Normal fields** (Chart 1-1, *H*). If visual fields are normal, then either the patient has no organic disease (and is anxious but not really malingering or hysterical), the chief complaint has been misunderstood, optic nerve disease is present but extremely subtle, or the patient has a cone-rod dystrophy. Color vision testing should separate optic nerve and cone diseases from the other possibilities. In optic neuropathies with acuities of 20/50 or better, the patient's performance on the standard color plates (Hardy-Rand-Ritter [H-R-R] or Ishihara) will be moderately poor. In cone-rod dystrophies, color vision will be absent or nearly absent, even in the face of relatively good acuity.[10]

In the majority of patients with the hereditary retinal receptor disorders the rods will be most severely affected; dark adaptation and peripheral field loss are the chief complaints, and pigmentary dispersion is often evident in the fundus. However, there exists an important subgroup of patients who present with failing central vision, sensitivity

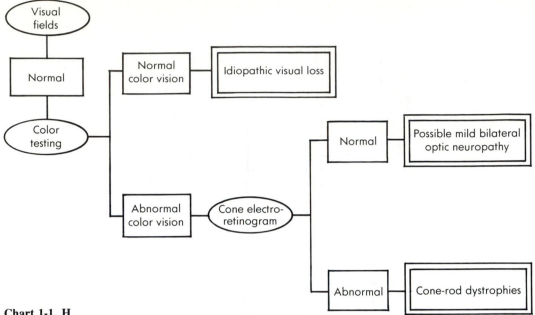

Chart 1-1, H

to bright light (day blindness or hemeralopia), and color disturbance.[10] These cases usually become evident in the second to fourth decade and reveal little funduscopic change in the early stages. Later, perifoveal pigment epithelial defects may be visible (Plate 1, *F*), and can be highlighted by fluorescein angiography (Fig. 1-10). Cone dysfunction is more prominent than rod dysfunction in these patients, and the diagnosis is made definitively by finding an abnormal cone electroretinogram (ERG) (Fig. 1-10). In later stages, failure of rod function may be signaled by a subnormal scotopic ERG and elevated dark-adaptation thresholds. The prevalence of these entities is not known. They are, however, important to recognize as the only examples of acquired color vision disturbances that are truly diagnostic. They are not treatable.

☐   **Tunnel fields** (Chart 1-1, *I*). The tunnel field, which is so characteristic of patients who feign visual loss, has two distinctive attributes: (1) it is contracted, and (2) its dimensions remain fixed regardless of the testing distance.

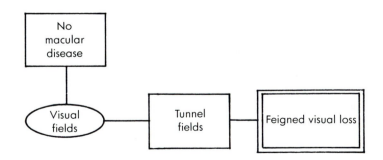

Chart 1-1, I

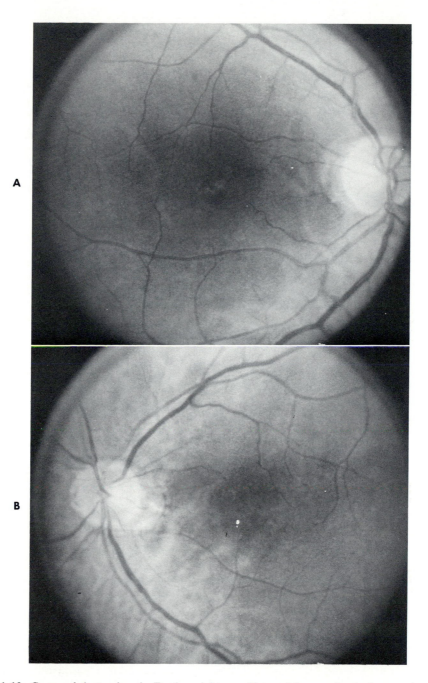

Fig. 1-10. Cone-rod dystrophy. **A,** Fundus, right eye. Note subtle macular depigmentation (also see Plate 1, *F*). **B,** Fundus, left eye. No macular defects are seen.   *Continued.*

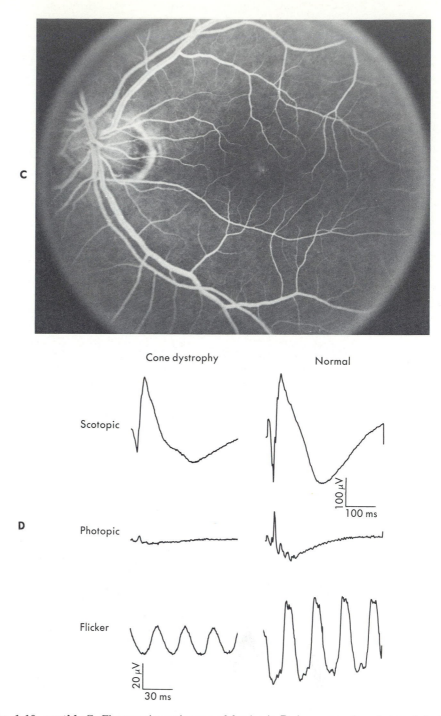

Fig. 1-10, cont'd. C, Fluorescein angiogram of fundus in **B** shows macular window defect. This study highlights pigment epithelial loss not visible on ophthalmoscopy. **D,** Electroretinogram. Note reduced B-wave amplitude most prominent under single-flash photopic conditions, and reduced amplitude to 30 Hz (flicker) stimulation.

Contraction of the visual field consists of inward displacement of the isopters. Opacification of the ocular media, uncorrected refractive errors, optic nerve disease, and generalized reduction of retinal sensitivity caused by age or myopia may all produce contraction of the field. However, this contracture will affect inner (within 20°) isopters somewhat more than outer isopters; the inner isopters will be displaced inward disproportionately (Fig. 1-11). The contracted field of feigned visual loss affects outer isopters, so that these appear collapsed upon relatively stable inner isopters. Although neuroretinal

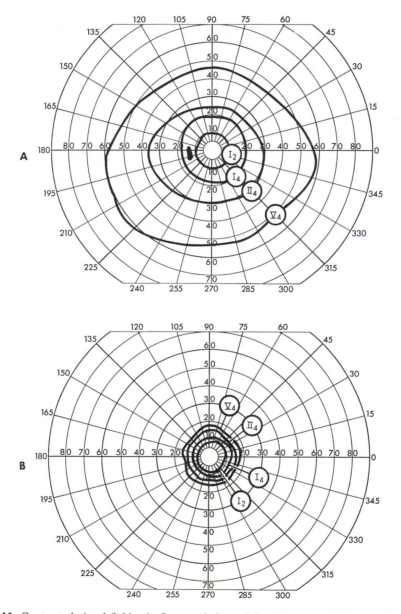

Fig. 1-11. Contracted visual fields. **A,** Symmetric inward displacement principally affecting inner isopters (aging, media opacity). **B,** Symmetric inward displacement of outer isopters, collapsing on inner isopter (feigned visual loss). *Continued.*

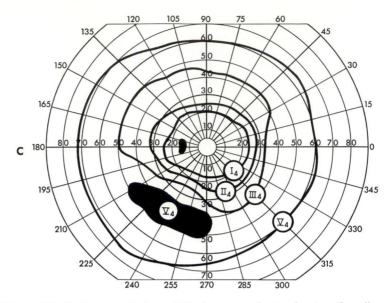

Fig. 1-11, cont'd. C, Asymmetric inward displacement of outer isopters (hereditary retinal degeneration).

diseases may also cause inward displacement of outer isopters, usually focal defects will also be evident. To further differentiate organic from feigned disease, note that when the testing distance and target size are doubled, the isopters do not change position in the malingerer or hysteric (tunnel field), while patients with organic defects will always show significant expansion of their field (funnel field; Fig. 1-12).

☐   **Feigned visual loss.** The broad category of feigned visual loss includes both malingerers and hysterics; distinguishing between them is difficult for ophthalmologists but is important, since psychotherapy is likely to benefit the latter and not the former group.

The diagnosis of feigned visual loss gained from the tunnel fields may be corroborated by observing inappropriate behavior or marked inconsistencies in the response to subjective tests of visual function. As a functional component often amplifies an underlying organic illness, one should be wary of overlooking this deeper element.

Mobility. Watching the patient enter the examining room and perform manual tasks during the examination may reveal the clue that visual loss is feigned. Patients with central visual loss but intact peripheral vision rarely have any difficulty with navigation. By contrast, those with peripheral visual loss move with great hesitancy but with a deliberation that results from an adaptation to their disability. Patients with feigned visual loss often appear paralyzed in one position, claiming that they cannot move or perform any manual tasks without assistance, lurching forward but rarely presenting any vulnerable parts of their body to hard obstacles. They always seem to be able to back away just in time to avoid any real injury. When asked to appose the index fingers of their two hands, they frequently have great difficulty and may be very hesitant about following a command to touch a part of their body. Even the most genuinely visually deprived patients can sign their names without extravagant sloppiness, while pretenders will frequently execute the wide flourishes of a disorganized signature.

Acuity testing. Patients with functional visual loss will frequently read to a certain level on the Snellen chart and be able to read no farther. It is as if they have established their own internal standard of how far they are willing to go. Fortunately the Snellen

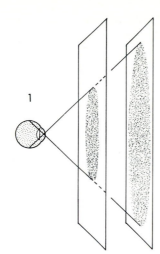

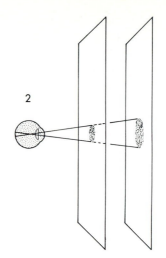

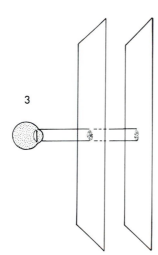

Fig. 1-12. Tunnel and funnel visual fields. *1*, Normal: normal-sized visual field (shaded area) expands as test distance is increased. *2*, Neuroretinal disease: contracted visual field expands as test distance is increased ("funnel field"). *3*, Feigned disease: contracted visual field does not expand as test distance is increased ("tunnel field").

chart has built-in checks against this deception. A patient who has successfully read all the letters on a given line will always be able to read at least one letter on the next smaller line, since at least one letter on the smaller line will be easier to resolve than a letter on the next larger line.

It is often difficult to recognize whether the patient's peculiar pattern of reading the Snellen letters represents an organic or functional disturbance. For example, a patient who consistently omits letters on one side of the Snellen chart may have a field defect involving the paracentral visual field on that side. A patient who reports that he must cock his head in a particular direction or move it around in order to see the letters may also be describing paracentral defects that impinge upon fixation. Some patients report that the letters appear clearer one moment and then they disappear. Be certain that this is not related to subtle shifts in head position. Otherwise the symptom is most likely to be functional. It is rare for visual acuity to fluctuate profoundly from moment to moment, although patients with demyelinating optic neuropathy report significant fluctuations from day to day. The patient who reports that the Snellen letters are gradually fading with exposure is describing a symptom with no proven physiologic correlates.

Any patient who is found to have subnormal best-corrected vision at distance should also be tested at near. With the appropriate presbyopic correction in place and the near card held at the correct distance, the recorded acuity should correspond closely with the distance acuity. If not, there are several possible explanations:

1. One of the measurements is inaccurate.
2. The refraction is incorrect.
3. A lens opacity has been overlooked that affects the near vision more than the distance vision.
4. The patient's level of arousal is depressed, such that he did not pay attention to the distance letters; he is much more interested in the near letters and performs better on these. This is frequently the case in the elderly, especially those with chronic neurologic disease or mild dementia. This near-far discordance may also be seen in children, who tend to be more interested in near stimuli. Unfortunately the near visual acuity is much less accurate, since an error in the testing distance (14 inches [35 cm]) will greatly alter the visual angle subtended by the optotypes.
5. The visual loss is functional.

Even if the examiner is convinced that a patient's subnormal acuity is nonorganic, it is much more satisfying to "trick" the patient into revealing that he sees much better than he admits.[19] The patient who admits to bare or no-light perception can be tested to threat, or with an optokinetic tape. However, visual threat is frequently ineffective, and patients can override the optokinetic stimulus unless it totally fills their visual environment. An effective device is to move a stock page of a newspaper in front of the tested eye or to place a large mirror close to the face and tilt it to-and-fro. It is difficult for the patient to resist the urge to follow the reflection of his eye as it changes position with the tilting of the mirror.

Several other maneuvers are available to test patients whose alleged subnormal vision is binocular and within the range of the Snellen chart. First, test their stereopsis. Patients with 60 arc seconds of stereo acuity must have 20/20 acuity in one eye and at least 20/40 in the other eye.[12] Second, test the near acuity, and if this is either consistent or worse than the distance acuity, then place a $+6.00$-diopter sphere in front of the tested eye, holding the near card at the appropriate distance. With the magnification and closer test distance the acuity should show significant improvement. If it does not, chances are the patient is feigning visual loss.

The patient with monocular subnormal vision is easier to test because a "normal" eye is available for comparison. Dissociate the two eyes so that the patient is unaware which eye is reading the Snellen chart. This can be done by fogging one eye surreptitiously with plus spheres, by placing a vertical prism in front of one eye, or by using the Polaroid vectograph slide. In each case the patient can defeat the test by closing one eye at a time. Sadly, these tests fail on the hard-core dissembler.

Manipulations of acuity and stereo testing will leave the examiner without a firm diagnosis in many patients. If the fields are normal in these cases, the diagnosis may be established only by excluding organic causes for the visual loss.

☐ **Bilateral nerve fiber bundle defects** (Chart 1-1, *J*). These defects indicate optic nerve disease or retinal artery occlusion. Based on the location of the nerve fiber bundle defects, there are three diagnostic categories to consider (Table 1-1): (1) defects that affect only the papillomacular bundle, (2) defects that affect all nerve fiber bundles, and (3) defects that relatively spare the papillomacular bundle. In the first group are the toxic, nutritional, and hereditary optic neuropathies, which produce only central and centrocecal scotomas. In the second group are the inflammatory, ischemic, compressive, traumatic, and dysplastic optic neuropathies and acute glaucoma, and in the third group are chronic open-angle glaucoma and postpapilledema optic neuropathy. The second and third groups produce both papillomacular and nonpapillomacular nerve fiber bundle defects, but the optic neuropathies of the third group typically spare the central 3° of field, including visual acuity, unless the disease has virtually obliterated the peripheral field.

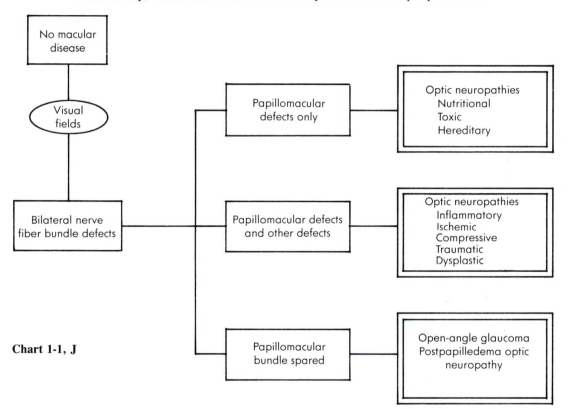

Chart 1-1, J

Table 1-1. Nerve fiber bundle field defects

Papillomacular only	Papillomacular or other nerve fiber bundles	Nonpapillomacular nerve fiber bundles predominantly
Hereditary optic neuropathies	Optic neuritis	Primary open-angle glaucoma
Toxic optic neuropathies	Ischemic optic neuropathy	Postpapilledema optic atrophy
Nutritional optic neuropathies	Compressive optic neuropathy	
Leber's optic neuropathy	Traumatic optic neuropathy	
Maculopathy (central but not centrocecal scotomas)	Acute glaucoma	
	Optic nerve dysplasias	
	Ischemic retinopathy (branch artery occlusion)	

Because differential diagnosis of these neuropathies depends upon the precise configuration of the field defect, careful plotting of the central 10° to 20° is critical. Any patient who has subnormal acuity with clear media, an appropriate refraction, and an intact peripheral field must either have central scotoma or be malingering. Unfortunately, even the most experienced perimetrists have difficulty plotting defects within the central 10° of field, especially in patients whose acuity is better than 20/60. One should recall that the central 3° of field are obliterated in the bowl perimeter by the examiner's viewing ''porthole.'' The detection of these scotomas may be improved by using a special fixation device provided with the bowl perimeter, by using colored targets, and by projecting static spots whose luminance is just above the normal threshold in the paracentral area. Such ''suprathreshold static'' presentation has become incorporated in the standard glaucoma screening protocol[2]; it has been very effective in detecting small paracentral scotomas regardless of etiology.

The management of patients with optic nerve disease without a relative afferent pupillary defect depends upon the history and the visual field result. If the fundus examination is normal or the discs are pale and the visual field shows bilateral central or centrocecal scotomas, the likelihood is great that the cause is either toxic, nutritional, or hereditary. Radiographic studies are not indicated. On the other hand, if there is one or more nerve fiber bundle defects not restricted to the papillomacular area, the lesion is likely to be inflammatory, ischemic, traumatic, or compressive. If the visual loss is nonprogressive, no radiographic studies are recommended. But a history of chronic progression suggests compression and justifies the performance of radiographic studies. Optic nerves may be compressed by the swollen extraocular muscles of dysthyroidism or infiltrated by meningeal spread of neoplastic cells. Other possibilities include a midline cranioorbital junction lesion, such as a meningioma of the planum sphenoidale, tuberculum sellae, olfactory groove, or anterior clinoid process. Such meningiomas may arise intracranially and then extend through both optic foramina. With such compression, all types of prechiasmal, as well as chiasmal, defects are possible.

☐   **Bitemporal hemianopia** (Chart 1-1, *K*). Bitemporal hemianopia indicates a lesion of the optic chiasm. At least 70% of patients with such lesions will have a relative afferent pupillary defect, but that leaves about 30% who have symmetric disease without pupillary defects. Such patients require prompt and thorough radiologic examination.

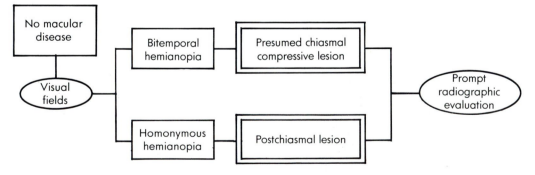

Chart 1-1, K

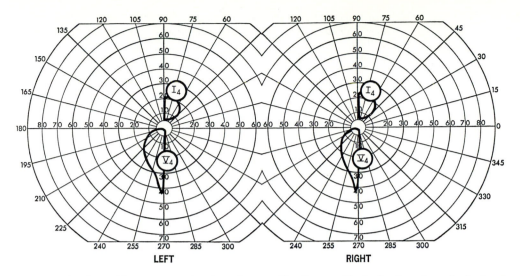

Fig. 1-13. Bilateral homonymous hemianopia caused by disease of both visual cortices. Such visual field defects, affecting both fixational areas, could explain subnormal acuity.

☐ **Homonymous hemianopia** (Chart 1-1, *K*). Patients with visual loss and no afferent defect may have the causative lesion in the postchiasmal visual pathway (Fig. 1-13). Although stroke is often implicated, neoplasms must be ruled out by radiologic evaluation. It is important to remember that a unilateral optic radiation or visual cortex lesion is never the cause of subnormal acuity, even if the macular projection area is involved. The uninvolved opposite visual cortex is sufficient to guarantee normal acuity, although the patient may have to hunt for the Snellen letters. Bilateral visual cortical disease may produce subnormal acuity if the large macular projection areas (posterior portion) are involved on both sides. In these cases, bilateral homonymous hemianopic defects will be found.

CLINICAL OR LABORATORY TESTS

If you have followed this strategy logically, you will have pigeonholed most causes of visual loss. In doing so, you have relied entirely on clinical tests with the one exception of using the ERG to confirm cone-rod dystrophies. Indeed, electrophysiologic and psychophysical tests of retinal function are rarely of diagnostic value in the patient with unexplained visual loss except in the receptor dystrophies. The ERG, electro-oculogram (EOG), and dark-adaptation and color-vision tests measure mass responses of retinal elements; abnormal results require widespread disease. Most maculopathies causing subnormal visual acuity are not associated with diffuse retinal damage and will therefore not affect these tests. Where macular disorders form part of the diffuse receptor dystrophies, decreased color vision should be evident. If color vision is normal, further testing is not advised, except in infants and young children.

The role of the visual-evoked cortical potential (VEP or VER, visual-evoked response) in the workup of unexplained visual loss has been a source of confusion. In the present state of the art, two aspects of the VEP signal are measured: the amplitude and the latency.[71] The intersubject variability of VEP amplitude is so great that it can only

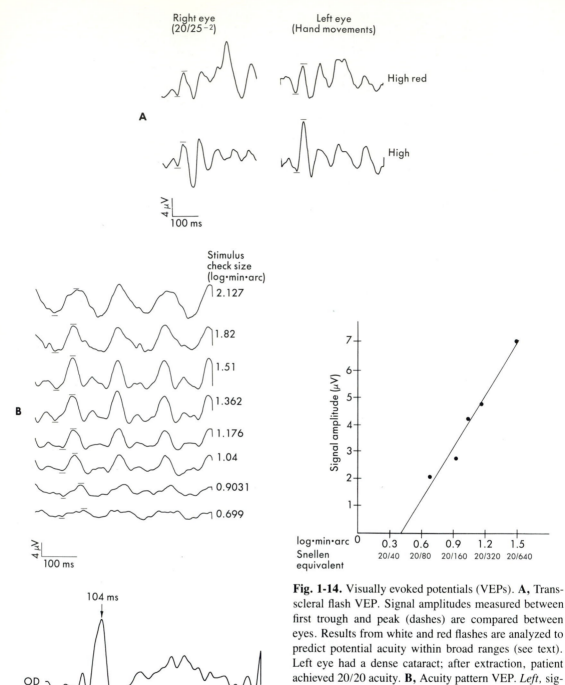

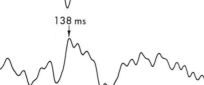

Fig. 1-14. Visually evoked potentials (VEPs). **A,** Transscleral flash VEP. Signal amplitudes measured between first trough and peak (dashes) are compared between eyes. Results from white and red flashes are analyzed to predict potential acuity within broad ranges (see text). Left eye had a dense cataract; after extraction, patient achieved 20/20 acuity. **B,** Acuity pattern VEP. *Left,* signal amplitudes measured between first trough and peak (dashes) are noted for different stimulus check sizes. *Right,* data are entered on graph and regression line drawn to intercept abscissa. This VEP measures an estimated acuity of 20/50. **C,** Latency pattern VEP. In right eye, latency of first major peak is in normal range, whereas in left eye, latency is prolonged beyond two standard deviations of normal. Findings are indicative of conduction delay in left eye associated with any optic neuropathy.

be used as a gross measure of central visual function. However, since intrasubject (interocular) differences are small, amplitude measures are helpful in comparing eyes, especially if one is known to be normal. Thus it may be used in estimating visual potential in an eye with opaque media (transscleral flash stimulus presentation, Fig. 1-14, *A*). Amplitude norms correlate reasonably well with broad acuity categories (better than 20/100, 20/100 to 20/200, 20/300 to 20/400, counts fingers–hand movements, light perception–no light perception).[15]

The pattern-reversal VEP is used to measure acuity objectively in patients with clear ocular media. This is done by noting the effect of varying stimulus size or clarity upon signal amplitude. Regression lines are drawn, and a VEP acuity is extrapolated to within reasonably narrow categories[20] (Fig. 1-14, *B*). This test is frequently effective in ruling out suspected feigned visual loss, but patients who fixate poorly (deliberately?) will produce false-positive abnormalities. In most cases it should be possible to make the diagnosis of feigned visual loss without resorting to the VEP.

The latency of the VEP signal shows less intersubject variability than does amplitude and has become a reliable and sensitive indicator of optic nerve disease[7] (Fig. 1-14, *C*). A prolonged latency results largely from delayed signal conduction, which is in turn most affected by demyelination of the nerve sheaths. Demyelination occurs in all optic nerve diseases but is relatively more extensive in the immunoinflammatory reaction associated with optic neuritis and multiple sclerosis. As expected, the greatest prolongation of latency does occur in optic neuritis and may be seen even in up to 97% of multiple sclerosis patients who have no historical or clinical evidence of optic neuritis ("subclinical optic neuritis").[7] However, because some degree of demyelination accompanies all optic neuropathies, a prolonged latency (unless extreme) in a patient with unexplained visual loss is, by itself, not diagnostically specific. Therefore, in patients with subnormal acuity and a relative afferent pupillary defect the VEP can only confirm the clinical impression of optic neuropathy; it cannot determine the cause. In the patient with optic neuritis the diagnosis of MS will not usually be aided by a VEP, since the uninvolved fellow eye usually demonstrates a normal VEP.[6,14]

What, then, is the clinical value of VEP latency data? It is helpful in the patient with possible MS without clinical optic neuropathy in whom the diagnosis could be established with more certainty if another central nervous system lesion were to be defined by finding a prolonged latency in one or both eyes. The VEP has now been partially displaced in this context by the brain stem auditory evoked response (BAER), which measures brain stem demyelination and is reported to have a comparable accuracy. It is our impression, however, that the results of VEPs and BAERs are rarely used to convert the diagnosis from possible to probable MS. We have yet to encounter a case of isolated transverse myelitis where the myelogram has been canceled because of abnormal evoked potential latencies!

Although the VEP has been used to study patients with chiasmal and postchiasmal lesions, bona fide clinical utility in this area has not yet been demonstrated.

REFERENCES

1. Acosta, PC, Trobe, JD, Shuster, JJ, and Krischer, JP: Diagnostic strategies in the management of unexplained visual loss. A cost-benefit analysis, J Med Decision-Making 1(2):125, 1981.
2. Drance, SM, Wheeler, C, and Pattullo M: The use of static perimetry in the early detection of glaucoma, Can J Ophthalmol 2:249, 1967.
3. Glaser, JS: Neuro-ophthalmology, Hagerstown, Md, 1978, Harper & Row, Publishers, p 10.
4. Glaser, JS, Savino, PJ, Sumers, KD, McDonald, SA, and Knighton, RW: The photostress recovery test: A practical adjunct in the clinical assessment of visual function, Am J Ophthalmol 83:255, 1977.
5. Grayson, M: Diseases of the cornea, St Louis, 1979, The CV Mosby Co, p 257.
6. Halliday, AM, McDonald, WI, and Mushin, J: Delayed visual evoked response in optic neuritis, Lancet 1:982, 1972.
7. Halliday, AM, and Mushin, J: The visual evoked potential in neuroophthalmology. In Sokol, S, editor: Electrophysiology and psychophysics: their use in ophthalmic diagnosis, Int Ophthalmol Clin 20(1):155,1980.
8. King-Smith, PE, Kranda, K, and Wood, JCJ: An acquired color defect of the opponent-color system, Invest Ophthalmol 15:584, 1976.
9. Kramer, KK, LaPiana, FG, and Appleton, B: Ocular malingering and hysteria: diagnosis and management, Surv Ophthalmol 24:89, 1979.
10. Krill, AE, Deutman, AF, and Fishman G: The cone degenerations, Doc Ophthalmol 35:1, 1973.
11. Levatin, P: Pupillary escape in disease of the retina or optic nerve, Arch Ophthalmol 62:768, 1959.
12. Levy, NS, and Glick, EB: Stereoscopic perception and Snellen visual acuity, Am J Ophthalmol 78:722, 1974.
13. Newsome, DA, and Milton, RC: Afferent pupillary defect in macular degeneration, Am J Ophthalmol 92:396 1981.
14. Regan, D, Milner, BA, and Heron, JR: Delayed visual perception and delayed visual evoked potentials in the spinal form of multiple sclerosis and in retrobulbar neuritis, Brain 99:43, 1976.
15. Rubin, ML, and Dawson, WW: The transscleral VER: prediction of postoperative acuity, Invest Ophthalmol 17:71, 1978.
16. Rubin, ML: Optics for clinicians, Gainesville, Fla, 1971, Triad Publishers, p 185.
17. Savino, PJ, Paris, M, Schatz, NJ, Orr, LS, and Corbett, JJ: Optic tract syndrome, Arch Ophthalmol 96:656, 1978.
18. Schatz, NJ, and Schlezinger, NS: Noncompressive causes of chiasmal disease. In Symposium on neuro-ophthalmology. Transactions of the New Orleans Academy of Ophthalmology, St. Louis, 1976, The CV Mosby Co, p 90.
19. Thompson, HS, Montague, P, Cox, TA, and Corbett, JJ: The relationship between visual acuity, pupillary defect, and visual field loss, Am J Ophthalmol 93:681, 1982.
20. Towle, VL, and Harter, MR: Objective determination of human visual acuity: pattern evoked potentials, Invest Ophthalmol 16:1073, 1977.
21. Traquair, HM: Clinical detection of early changes in the visual field, Arch Ophthalmol 22:947, 1939.
22. Trobe, JD, and Acosta, PC: An algorithm for visual fields, Surv Ophthalmol 24:665, 1980.
23. Trobe, JD, Acosta, PC, Krischer, JP, and Trick, GL: Confrontation visual field techniques in the detection of anterior visual pathway lesions, Ann Neurol 10:28, 1981.
24. von Noorden, GK, and Burian, HM: Visual acuity in normal and amblyopic patients under reduced illumination. I. Behavior of visual acuity with and without neutral density filter, Arch Ophthalmol 61:533, 1959.
25. Wilson, P, and Falconer, MA: Patterns of visual failure with pituitary tumors. Clinical and radiological correlation, Br J Ophthalmol 52:94, 1968.

PART II

Prechiasmal visual loss

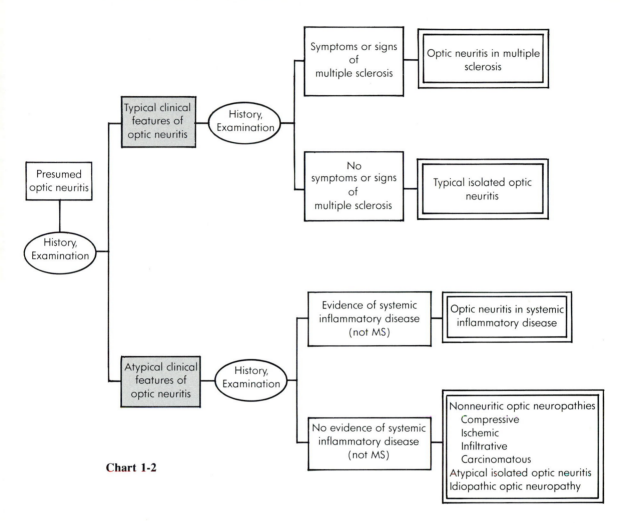

Chart 1-2

Diseases that affect the prechiasmal visual pathway include those that damage the retina and optic nerve. The diagnosis of these conditions was briefly discussed in Part I. In this part, we present more detailed management considerations of some of these entities.

OPTIC NEURITIS (Chart 1-2)

Optic neuritis is defined as an acute loss of vision caused by focal demyelination in the optic nerve without a known etiologic agent. The disease makes its appearance in two clinical forms, typical and atypical.

☐ **Typical optic neuritis**

The typical form of optic neuritis consists of monocular loss of vision in a patient between 20 and 50 years of age, which may or may not be accompanied by pain on movement of the globe. The patient may have a past history or present evidence of MS.

Examination reveals subnormal visual function in the affected eye, often but not necessarily accompanied by a measurable depression in acuity and a nerve fiber bundle visual field defect. A relative afferent pupillary defect is usually present on the affected side and the fundus examination may reveal a swollen disc (papillitis), especially in children[55] (Plate 2, A to C), but will commonly be normal in adults.[9,66] Systemic history and examination will be noncontributory, except for the possible evidence of MS.

The disease should run a typical clinical course in which visual loss reaches its nadir within 7 days after the onset of symptoms.[66] Visual acuity will begin to improve over the next several weeks and may or may not recover fully; in some cases there is no recovery at all. Little recovery occurs after 6 months.[23]

If optic neuritis conforms to these clinical criteria, then the patient has a disease for which the efficacy of treatment has not been established,[7] and the physician's only task is one of prognosis. He will be relatively safe if he predicts that visual function will recover to some degree after several weeks to months. Among 253 eyes with optic neuritis reexamined after an average of 7 years, visual acuity was 20/30 or better in 66%, finger counting or worse in 17%.[65]

The more serious question is the relationship between optic neuritis ("monoscle-rosis") and MS. MS may already be present in occult form. To detect its presence, the clinician should inquire about what may have seemed like short-lived and innocent past episodes of disequilibrium, numbness or tingling of an extremity, double vision, or blurred vision in one eye. The most helpful subtle signs to look for on examination are mild internuclear ophthalmoplegia, gait ataxia, and incoordinated rapid alternating movements performed by the arms.

If MS is not clinically detectable, epidemiologic data offer very vague guidelines about the chance of its developing later. The chance of developing definite MS after monosymptomatic optic neuritis varies from 11.5% to 85%,[18] depending on the definition of the disease, the care with which already-present MS is identified, the geographic domain, and the length of follow-up.

Two prospective studies of monosymptomatic optic neuritis, one involving 60 patients in the New England area,[18] the other involving 61 Scandinavian patients,[74] found, respectively, a 28% and 20% incidence of definite MS after 7 years. Most studies agree that most MS cases will be evident within 2 years of the onset of optic neuritis, but some cases will continue to appear after many years. The series with MS frequencies of greater than 50% all derive from the United Kingdom and Finland, which may be geographically predisposed regions. In other areas, approximately 25% to 33% of patients with typical optic neuritis will develop definite MS if observed long enough.[18]

Are there any factors that help narrow this prognostic range? Several studies report a twofold or threefold greater risk for women than for men, but one large retrospective study found no sex difference.[18] Recurrent episodes of optic neuritis increase the risk for MS; in one study the risk after multiple attacks was increased fourfold.[18] Compston et al.[19] found a fourfold greater risk of developing MS in optic neuritis patients possessing histocompatibility antigen BT 101, suggesting a genetic susceptibility. Age, the presence of pain, the appearance of the optic disc, and the visual outcome have not been helpful predictors.

When the history and physical examination of optic neuritis patients yield no clear evidence of MS, the examiner is likely to turn to evoked potentials—visual, auditory, and somatosensory—and spinal fluid examination. Evoked potentials will be of little value. Spinal fluid examination may provide evidence that MS is already present sub-clinically but offers no help in predicting the future severity of the disease.

Visual evoked potentials (VEPs) may be produced by nonpatterned and pattern-reversal stimuli.[40] The use of a patterned stimulus has become the preferred technique because it produces more consistent results in normals. The VEP became a popular diagnostic tool when Halliday et al.[41] reported in 1973 that 96% of MS patients without a history or clinical evidence of optic neuropathy showed prolonged signal latencies. Others have shown that a range of 78% to 97% of definite MS patients will have delayed latencies.[40] These results established the VEP as a valuable adjunct in patients with nonvisual neurologic presentations that suggested MS but could be accounted for by a single lesion. Prolonged latencies would suggest a second, subclinical lesion and fortify the diagnosis of MS.

The VEP has substantial drawbacks in the diagnosis of optic neuritis. The VEP signal from involved eyes is often badly deformed and indecipherable.[76] If readable, it will be prolonged in virtually all cases, a nonspecific finding of any optic neuropathy.[38] But because the search is for a second CNS lesion, it is the result in the asymptomatic fellow eye that is important. Thus far, in patients with uniocular optic neuritis and no prior history or evidence of MS, the latencies of the signals recorded from the fellow eye have always been normal.[39,71] Therefore, at this time the VEP may be of value in the workup of patients with suspected MS and no previous history of optic nerve involvement but essentially is of no value in the workup of patients with optic neuritis.

Nor are other evoked potential tests helpful in diagnosing MS in these patients. In one study, brain stem auditory evoked respones (BAERs) and somatosensory evoked responses (SERs) were normal in all 18 patients with typical optic neuritis.[15] Evidently these patients do not (yet?) have a disseminated central nervous system (CNS) disease.

The spinal fluid examination is more useful than evoked potentials in the workup of patients with typical optic neuritis but also has important limitations in its diagnostic value. The spinal fluid studies used in the diagnosis of MS are (1) the CSF IgG (gamma globulin) level, (2) the IgG/albumin ratio, (3) the IgG index (CSF IgG/CSF albumin)/ (serum IgG/serum albumin), (4) the IgG synthetic rate, and (5) oligoclonal bands. There is some dispute as to which of these tests offers the greatest accuracy, but one or more of them will be abnormal in more than 90% of patients with definite MS.[46,52] However, these abnormalities may be expected in approximately 51% or fewer cases of optic neuritis.[63,67] Evidently many cases of optic neuritis produce too small an inflammatory focus to affect the spinal fluid. In two prospective studies,[67,73] elevated CSF IgG and oligoclonal bands were significantly related to the eventual development of MS. However, over 50% of patients with normal CSF in these series also developed MS. A further caution in interperting results of CSF studies is that other diseases can produce similar spinal fluid abnormalities—including CNS infections, neurosyphilis, immunologic diseases such as lupus erythematosus, subacute sclerosing panencephalitis, and acute vasculomyelinopathies such as the Guillain-Barré syndrome and acute labyrinthitis.

Other examinations such as CT scanning, psychophysical tests, eye movement tests, and the blink reflex test have not yielded more sensitive and specific findings in documented MS patients, and none has been studied in monosymptomatic optic neuritis.[69]

If the clinician is satisfied that the patient deserves the diagnosis of typical optic neuritis, the judicious course of action is to delay any laboratory studies for at least 1 week in order to determine the clinical course. By that time the patient may have begun to have visual improvement or stabilization. Reexamination will confirm that no new findings have appeared. If the visual field result is reliable and if it reveals no hemianopic defects, then the chances of a compressive lesion are so remote that radiologic studies, including a CT scan, are not indicated. Similarly, it is not worthwhile to perform evoked potentials, examine spinal fluid, or draw blood for hematologic, metabolic, or connective tissue disease or vasculitis profiles.

The form of MS ushered in by optic neuritis is likely to be relatively benign. In one series only 43% of MS patients presenting with optic neuritis were functionally restricted, as compared to 73% who had other initial presentations.[64]

▪ Atypical optic neuritis (Chart 1-2, A)

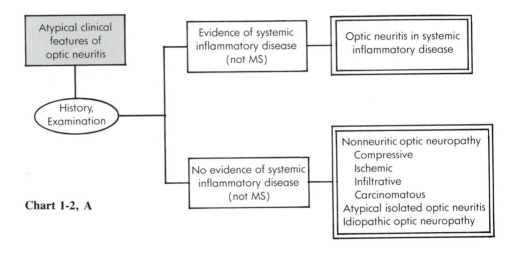

Chart 1-2, A

Optic neuritis qualifies as atypical if it occurs in a patient outside the 20- to 50-year age span, continues to show worsening vision beyond 7 days after onset, or shows other possibly contributory abnormalities in the ocular or systemic examination that are not ascribable to MS. There are four possibilities: (1) optic neuritis in the context of a systemic disease other than MS, (2) a nonneuritic optic neuropathy that has been misdiagnosed as optic neuritis, (3) an atypical, isolated form of optic neuritis, and (4) an idiopathic optic neuropathy. The clinician must direct his efforts at making the distinction between these four choices.

☐ Optic neuritis as part of a systemic disease other than MS

Optic neuritis may be a manifestation of either a collagen vascular disease,[37] a parainfectious syndrome,[29] or viral, bacterial, or fungal disease. The importance of recognizing these cases is that the underlying disease may need to be treated, and the optic neuritis itself may respond to treatment.

In these atypical cases, optic neuritis may be accompanied by anterior and posterior uveitis, including pars planitis, vitritis, and retinitis[22] (Plate 2, A to C). Whether these additional signs are merely a rare variant of MS is uncertain. Sheathing of retinal veins has been reported in 11% of a series of MS patients.[88] On the other hand, these inflammatory ocular signs may be part of a systemic infection, such as may be caused by cytomegalovirus, syphilis, or *Candida,* or may be part of a vasculitis such as Behcet's or lupus erythematosus.[22] In some cases the optic neuritis is a manifestation of a meningoencephalitis believed to be an immune reaction to a preceding, often trivial, viral illness.[69]

☐ Nonneuritic optic neuropathies: mimickers of optic neuritis

☐ **Ischemic optic neuropathy.** The distinction between optic neuritis and other optic neuropathies is made primarily on clinical grounds. The swollen disc of inflammatory optic neuritis may not be readily distinguished from the swollen disc of ischemic optic neuropathy, but a patient older than 50 years, a history of multiple risk factors for cerebrovascular disease, and a nonprogressive clinical course favor nonarteritic ischemic optic neuropathy. A patient over the age of 60 with symptoms of polymyalgia rheumatica (PMR), headache, or scalp tenderness suggests a diagnosis of arteritic ischemic optic neuropathy.

☐ **Compressive optic neuropathy.** Compressive optic neuropathy, as with cyst, tumor, sinus mucocoele, or aneurysm, usually progresses slowly but may have an explosive onset. These lesions usually produce progressive loss of vision that continues to worsen after 7 days. In addition, compressive optic neuropathy most commonly occurs at the junction of the optic nerve and chiasm, so that the visual fields will reveal a hemianopic defect in one or both eyes. Finely tuned radiography will be essential for diagnosis (see Part III of this chapter).

Dysthyroid optic neuropathy[82] may consist of an acute or subacute presentation with or without a swollen disc (Plate 2, *E* and *F*). The disc swelling is believed to result from axoplasmic stasis as the optic nerve is compressed at the orbital apex by swollen extraocular muscles. Generally patients will have the congestive adnexal features of dysthyroidism, including chemosis, conjunctival injection, lid retraction and lag, and ductional deficits. Proptosis need not be marked.

☐ **Infiltrative optic neuropathy.** It may be difficult to distinguish infiltrative optic neuropathy from optic neuritis. Infiltrative optic neuropathy may present with acute loss of vision and a swollen disc with hemorrhages and exudates because of infiltration of the optic nerve by a sarcoid granuloma,[51] lymphoma, leukemia[25] (Plate 2, *D*), or plasmacytoma.[36] Other granulomatous and neoplastic infiltrates are less common. There will almost always be evidence of systemic involvement.

☐ **Carcinomatous optic neuropathy.** It may be difficult to distinguish optic neuritis from carcinomatous optic neuropathy,[2] an entity that produces a sudden and devastating loss of vision in one or both eyes. Fundus examination is typically normal. Visual field deficits may be prechiasmal or chiasmal, and the patient will have a history of a known malignancy, which may, however, have been quiescent for several years. Other manifestions of intraparenchymal CNS or subarachnoid seeding may be present. Unless large intraparenchymal CNS spread has occurred, radiologic studies will be negative, since the damage is produced by microscopic cuffing of nerves. The visual loss is exquisitely responsive to systemic steroid therapy.

☐ **Atypical isolated optic neuritis**

If concurrent systemic diseases and nonneuritic mimickers have been excluded and the disease features fall outside the typical range, then the patient may have an unusual form of optic neuritis and must be observed carefully or possibly treated (see below).

One atypical group deserves special segregation—children. Relative to adults, optic neuritis in children is more likely to affect both eyes at the same time, involve the nerve head (papillitis and inner retinal edema with macular star figure), follow by 1 to 2 weeks a viral illness or a vaccination, resolve without permanent visual loss, and uncommonly lead to MS. Yet in one study,[55] 8 (27%) of 30 children developed MS after a mean of 8 years.

☐ **Idiopathic optic neuropathy**

In some cases a specific diagnosis cannot be made at the onset of visual loss ascribable to optic nerve disease. Atypical features mandate careful investigation. If this is negative, the patient may be diagnosed as having atypical optic neuritis or observed for the appearance of definite signs of another disease.

Management of optic neuritis

Whether typical or atypical, optic neuritis is clinically and pathologically an inflammatory disease with lymphocytic migration and edema. Clinical trials have failed to show a convincing effect of corticosteroid treatment in typical cases[7]—those that are monosymptomatic or part of established MS. Treatment may shorten the course of the acute illness but will not influence final visual outcome in these cases. The use of corticosteroids is therefore controversial. There is consensus that they should not be prescribed for prolonged periods.

In treating presumed optic neuritis with corticosteroids the physician must be aware that the therapy may obscure an important diagnostic indicator: the natural course of the disease. Continued worsening beyond 7 days after onset casts doubt on the diagnosis of typical optic neuritis and demands a careful workup. Neoplastic, infectious, and inflammatory conditions causing optic neuropathy may be exquisitely sensitive to steroids. In fact a sudden dramatic improvement (within 48 hours) in visual function after starting steroids is unlikely in typical optic neuritis and suggests one of these other entities! In effect, the use of steroids demands more careful preliminary diagnostic work, which is ordinarily unnecessary in typical optic neuritis.

The management of atypical cases falls outside these guidelines. First, one must attempt to diagnose a systemic illness and direct management at it. If, as often happens, no definite disease entity emerges, high-dose but short-term corticosteroids may be used. The protective effect of high steroid doses in cranial arteritis and a therapeutic effect in lupus nephritis support the use of prednisone in doses of greater than 100 mg per day; one report[22] documents dramatic improvement with daily intravenous doses of 500 mg of methyl prednisolone.

Experience with cytotoxic agents, especially azathioprine and cyclophosphamide, has given mixed results, none in controlled trials. Antilymphocyte serum, thoracic duct drainage, and plasmapheresis continue to be investigated in MS and in vasculitides, but no meaningful results are yet available.[26]

ISCHEMIC OPTIC NEUROPATHY

Ischemic optic neuropathy (ION) is characterized by sudden, painless, irreversible and nonprogressive loss of vision, accompanied by nerve fiber bundle field defects, an afferent pupillary defect, and disc edema (Plate 3, *A*) in patients between 45 and 80 years of age.[8] As such, ION shares many clinical characteristics with optic neuritis. Indeed this entity was formerly called "ischemic optic neuritis," a name that has been dropped because the pathogenesis is infarction, not inflammation. The affected blood supply belongs to the ciliary circulation within the laminar portion of the optic disc.[57] Both clinically and pathologically, ION resembles the lacunar infarction of the CNS.[27] Abrupt, fixed loss of function results from occlusion of vascular lumina by segmental fibrinoid necrosis and subendothelial hyalinization, a change encountered uniquely in hypertension. Hypertension has been recorded in 44% of patients with idiopathic ION in two retrospective series.[8,24] No other risk factors have been clearly identified.

The disc edema of ION has been described as "pallid swelling," often segmental, and accompanied by nerve fiber layer hemorrhages. However, the disc in optic neuritis has this appearance often enough so that the differential diagnosis must be made on nonophthalmoscopic grounds.

Treatment of ION is to no avail. As a completed stroke, recovery of established visual dysfunction does not occur, with or without therapy.[8] There is no rationale for prophylactic antiplatelet aggregants such as aspirin, dipyridamole (Persantin), or sulfinpyrazone (Anturane), because of lack of clinical or pathologic evidence for either thrombosis or embolism in the pathogenesis of ION. Instead, elimination of risk factors is the logical approach. Whether reduction of risk factors is effective in reducing the risk of later involvement of the fellow eye (25% to 40%) is not known, but studies clearly show that controlling hypertension prevents stroke.[85]

Ischemic infarction of the laminar disc also occurs in cranial arteritis,[45] as well as rarely in lupus and periarteritis nodosa. Connective tissue diseases should always be investigated, but cranial arteritis so rapidly threatens both optic nerves that the ophthalmologist's major consideration after making the diagnosis of ION is to rule out this disease. The initial key test is the erythrocyte sedimentation rate (ESR).

Cranial arteritis must be suspected in cases of ION in which visual function is devastated (finger counting or worse) or where there is evidence of bilateral simultaneous optic neuropathy. The presence of headache, jaw claudication, PMR syndrome (proximal muscle aches, stiffness), malaise, anorexia, fever, or scalp tenderness in patients (especially women) over age 60, or a markedly elevated ESR (>50 mm/per hour) implicate arteritis.[32]

Classic cases pose no diagnostic problems. But more often, the picture is incomplete, and the clinician is faced with some difficult options. The following facts may help.

Epidemiology.[32,50] There is conflicting information as to the prevalence of cranial arteritis; increased reports of this disease have been influenced by improved awareness. Prevalence increases with age and is estimated currently at about 3 cases per 100,000 over age 50 and approximately 55 per 100,000 in those over 80 with a predilection for northern latitudes and elderly white women (females:males = 2:1). The mean age of the affected population is 75, with a lower limit of 50, but a few well-documented cases below that age are reported. The mortality of patients with treated cranial arteritis is not greater than for age-matched controls. There is no significant familial association or linkage with other systemic diseases.

Nonophthalmic symptoms. The absence of headache, scalp and jaw pain, and PMR does not exclude the diagnosis but makes it extremely unlikely. Patients presenting with optic neuropathy as an isolated clinical sign have been reported (occult cranial arteritis).[21,78] They are considered rare but did constitute 24% in one series.[53] Since many of the symptoms of PMR are nonspecific and common in the elderly, one must be careful in history taking: headache should be recent, scalp tenderness should be exquisite, and jaw pain should be diffuse, related to chewing, and not localizable to the temporomandibular joint. These symptoms should respond dramatically to the institution of corticosteroids. In fact, if no relief has become evident within 48 hours, the diagnosis must be questioned.

The relationship between PMR and cranial arteritis is in dispute.[48] PMR is defined as morning stiffness and pain affecting especially the neck, shoulder, and pelvic girdle muscles, accompanied by an elevated ESR. Weight loss, fever, malaise, anorexia, and anemia may be present. Most authorities presently believe that PMR and cranial arteritis are part of a spectrum. This is based on the fact that 20% to 40% of PMR patients have positive temporal artery biopsies.[48]

Ophthalmic signs. Visual loss is reported in 12% to 50% of biopsy-proven cases, depending upon the source of the patient group.[32,50] A prodrome of transient monocular blindness is found in at least 10% of cases.[8,84] Fixed visual loss is caused chiefly by ION (90%) but may also be caused by central retinal artery occlusion (3%) or ischemic retinopathy (7%).[84] Occipital blindness is rare. This is because cranial arteritis tends to affect only arteries with an internal elastic lamina, a structure not present in the intradural portion of cerebral vessels.[86] Yet hemispheric and brain stem strokes are occasionally found, probably secondary to embolism from extradural portions of carotid and vertebral vessels involved with arteritis.[33]

If vision is to be affected, the infarction will involve the prelaminar disc substance or retinal circulation in at least 97% of cases,[84] so that in the acute phase, at least some signs should be visible ophthalmoscopically within 24 hours of the onset of visual loss. The ischemic nerve heads in the arteritic and nonarteritic forms of ION are ophthalmoscopically indistinguishable. The nerve fiber bundle field defects are also similar, except that the arteritic form typically produces more devastating visual loss and tends to involve both eyes within a shorter interval.

The untreated arteritic and nonarteritic forms of ION will both produce binocular involvement in approximately one third of cases.[32] But the interval before the second eye becomes involved in nonarteritic ION is typically months to years, while in the arteritic form, if fellow eyes become involved, one third will do so within 24 hours, another one third within a week, and most of the remainder within 4 weeks.[8,47,53,84] Visual loss has been reported as long as 22 years after initial diagnosis,[21] but very few fellow eyes become involved after 6 months.

Diplopia is reported in up to 10% of patients with cranial arteritis,[84] resulting from a ductional deficit. The only available pathology shows infarction of extraocular muscles.[4]

Sedimentation rate. Absence of a high ESR does not entirely rule out cranial arteritis. If the "normal" ESR is set at 40, there are instances of positive biopsies with normal ESRs.[33] However, the ESR should yield a value above 50 mm per hour in over 90% of the afflicted, and often over 90 mm per hour.[32] Values below 50 mm per hour begin to approach the upper limit seen in the elderly who are not ill.

Although the Westergren method of performing the sedimentation rate has been endorsed,[32] the popular Wintrobe method, if corrected for hematocrit, is adequate. A newer and less time-consuming method, the zeta sedimentation rate, has been found to be comparable to the Westergren and Wintrobe determinations.[10] Nonarteritic causes of an elevated ESR include arthritis and other collagenoses, occult infections, and neoplasms. Since laboratory error is not infrequent in this delicate test, it is worthwhile to repeat the test if it is not consonant with the clinical impression.

Biopsy. The temporal artery is the most accessible vessel with a high chance of pathologic involvement. Other branches of the external carotid would be the next choice. The selection of biopsy site should not be overly influenced by whether the vessel is tender, nodular, on the site of visual involvement, or angiographically abnormal. After some controversy[1,16,56] the issue of whether affected vessels may show intervals of normal histology (skip areas) is now settled. Skip areas do occur in as many as 28% of biopsies, and false-negatives can be minimized by removing at least a 2 cm length of artery and performing multiple serial sections.[56] Since at least 5% of cranial arteritis cases may involve only one temporal artery, a negative biopsy and high clinical suspicion warrant a biopsy on the other side.[56] Complications of biopsy are not reported. There have been several clinical reports of biopsy-negative cranial arteritis,[33] and one pathologic study in which 2 of 16 cases had widespread granulomatous arteritis without involving temporal vessels.[33] Still, we believe that bilateral negative biopsies of adequate length segments using appropriate pathologic criteria exclude the diagnosis except where clinical evidence is overwhelming.

The histopathology of cranial arteritis need not include giant cells.[21] It may show only intimal proliferation, fragmentation of the internal elastic lamina, and a mononuclear response involving the entire vessel wall (Plate 3, *B*). In the absence of giant cells it may be difficult to exclude polyarteritis nodosa, which should, however, demonstrate areas of focal vessel wall necrosis.[32]

How long will it take for steroid treatment to reverse pathologic changes? There is evidence that even after months of high-dose corticosteroid treatment, pathologic signs remain in the vessels,[42] indicating that treatment controls but does not cure the disease. Most authorities recommend biopsy within 1 week of starting corticosteroids.

Diagnosis (Chart 1-3). In consideration of the foregoing information, we recommend the following approach to the diagnosis of patients with ION:

1. An ESR should be drawn on all patients with ION, regardless of the patient's age or symptomatology. We consider the Westergren method most reliable.

2. If the Westergren ESR is ≥50 mm per hour and signs and symptoms of the PMR or giant cell arteritis (GCA) complexes are unequivocally present, the clinical diagnosis of GCA may be made presumptively; biopsy is optional. If such symptoms and signs are equivocally present or absent, a biopsy of at least 2 cm of temporal artery should be performed, preferably but not necessarily on the symptomatic side.

   Once a presumptive diagnosis of GCA is made, oral prednisone, 80 to 100 mg per day, should be started immediately—without waiting for the biposy to be performed. Biopsy should be performed within a few days of starting therapy, although it is doubtful if pathologic findings are reversed even within several weeks of initiating corticosteroids.

3. If temporal artery biopsy proves negative on adequate serial section, the other temporal artery must be biopsied because the combination of a high ESR and ION forces more defiinitive exclusion of GCA. A second negative biopsy is adequate evidence that the high ESR is caused by other disease.

4. If the ESR is <50 mm per hour, then the presence of PMR-GCA symptoms or signs must be scrupulously excluded. If this cannot be done with confidence, then the patient must be managed as if the ESR were >50 mm per hour (see 2 and 3 above). If there is no evidence of PMR-GCA complexes, the patient is diagnosed as having idiopathic ION.

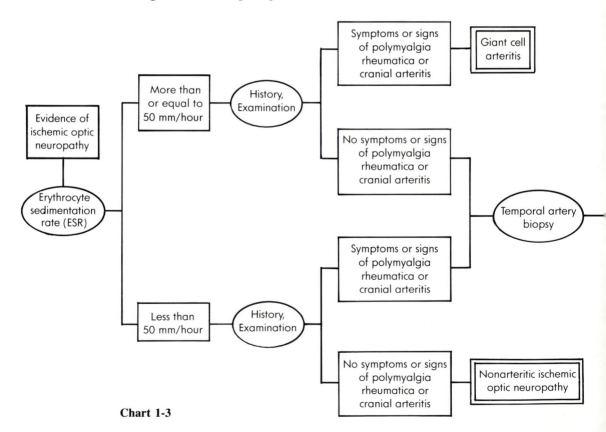

Chart 1-3

In effect, this approach places greatest reliance on the ESR because of the awareness that ION can be part of occult cranial arteritis,[21,78] where systemic signs and symptoms are absent. However, because of the few cases of GCA with normal ESRs,[33] the clinician must also place heavy reliance on history and physical examination.

Treatment and prognosis. Early treatment with at least the equivalent of prednisone 80 mg per day will largely prevent progression of the disease and produce rapid remission of nonvisual symptoms.[33] Treatment should be initiated promptly, before the biopsy is performed. Doses adequate to reverse PMR symptoms (prednisone 10 to 20 mg per day) will not prevent visual loss.[48] Involvement of the second eye in adequately treated patients is rare but may occur if inadequate steroid levels are used or tapering is premature.[33] Recovery of vision is extremely rare but apparently does occur, especially if visual loss is not severe at the time therapy is begun.[8]

After 2 to 4 weeks the majority of cases should have normalized their ESRs,[42] and gradual tapering may begin at 10% per week of the prevailing daily dose. If the ESR or PMR symptoms recrudesce, the dose must be raised. Most authorities suggest a maintenance dose of 5 to 15 mg per day for at least 1 year, although activation long after that is reported.[5] An alternate-day steroid regimen produces fewer side-effects and was as effective as daily administration in reducing inflammation in 18 of 27 (67%) patients in one series,[6] but in only 6 of 20 (30%) in another.[49] In the acute phase of treatment (first 4 months) we favor a daily steroid regimen; in the maintenance period an alternate-day regimen is acceptable, provided symptoms and ESR are controlled.

Some 20% of patients will maintain elevated ESRs despite clinical remission. If there are no symptoms of arteritis or PMR and no other explanation for the elevated ESR, we believe steroids should be cautiously tapered, using clinical signs as the principal

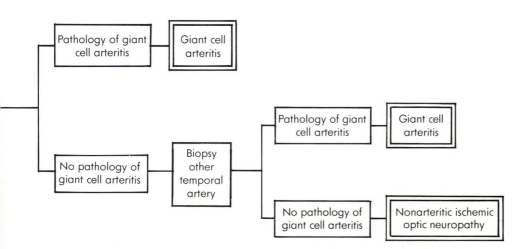

indicator, and being mindful of the fact that visual loss is rare after 4 months. Only if the ESR continues to inch upward should the clinician halt the steroid tapering. Since arteritis is responsible for only 3% of all cases of elevated ESRs,[33] more common causes should be sought.

The vicissitudes of long-term management of cranial arteritis revolve about the risks of chronic steroid therapy in the elderly population. These are exacerbation of diabetes, mood alteration, aseptic necrosis of bone, osteoporosis with vertebral fracture, exacerbation of tuberculosis and fungal disease, as well as an unattractive cushingoid appearance. For these reasons a diagnosis of cranial arteritis should always be supported by biopsy, except in absolutely classic clinical presentations. Every attempt must be made to reduce the steroid dosage. We suggest that after 6 months the ophthalmologist permit a somewhat "elevated" ESR, as long as it is not rising and the patient is symptom free. A persistently elevated ESR in the absence of symptoms of PMR or cranial arteritis should prompt investigation for other systemic inflammatory diseases. We do not recommend late rebiopsy[17] because pathologic signs are not necessarily indicative of clinical activity.

Treatment with other antiinflammatory agents has not been systematically evaluated, although PMR is known to respond to nonsteroidal antiprostaglandin agents.[32]

☐ Nutritional optic neuropathies

Alcoholic optic neuropathy. The optic neuropathy seen in chronic alcoholics is characterized by painless, progressive, bilateral, and symmetric involvement of papillomacular bundles to produce centrocecal scotomas and subnormal acuity at the level of 20/50 to 20/200.[62] Patients typically describe a fog or smudge in the center of their field of vision and note that colors look "washed out."

In advanced stages, diagnosis will be straightforward if the examiner is attune to the disease and reasonably adept at performing visual fields. Aside from the acuity and field changes, the only other ophthalmologic abnormality is temporal disc pallor. It is in the early cases that diagnosis is difficult to establish. At an acuity level of 20/50 or better, central or centrocecal scotomas are elusive, to be found only with small targets in very cooperative patients. The examiner will be tempted to conclude that the patient is malingering or to order radiologic studies in search of intracranial disease. The proper diagnosis can be improved by applying detailed central visual field techniques, including kinetic color (red) and static perimetry. The earliest field changes will be elevated thresholds in the area between fixation and the blind spot (Fig. 1-15). Patients often make many errors on conventional color vision tests. Neurologic examination may reveal findings indicative of peripheral neuropathy, superior vermis cerebellar degeneration, or Wernicke-Korsakoff syndrome.[83]

The optic neuropathy, the peripheral neuropathy, and the Wernicke-Korsakoff syndrome of alcohol abuse are precisely mimicked in patients with severe malnutrition. In both conditions, solid evidence supports the notion that the critical missing dietary substance is vitamin B_1 (thiamin).[83]

Carroll[12] found that the optic neuropathy of alcoholics could be reversed either by a well-balanced diet or by thiamin supplements (while subjects continued their drinking and poor diet). Many alcoholics do not avow a poor diet. However, even in the presence of adequate intake they absorb vitamins poorly, and because of liver disease they may not be able to convert them to bioactive forms.[83] Further the increased carbohydrate load

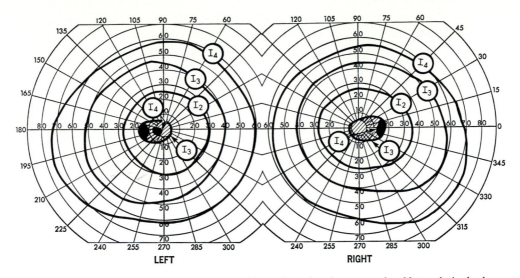

Fig. 1-15. Cecocentral scotomas in patient with nutritional optic neuropathy. Note relatively dense defect between fixation and physiologic blind spot in left eye, a typical finding. Similar defects are noted in patients with toxic optic neuropathy.

from alcohol ingestion consumes added amounts of thiamin, reducing the available stores.[83]

Pernicious anemia. Deficiency of vitamin B_{12} is rarely a factor in alcoholics and the severely malnourished because the ample reserves of B_{12} are repleted for a month with a single meal containing meat. Thus B_{12} deficiency is restricted to those patients who are unable to absorb it, either because of gastrointestinal disease or, more commonly, because of lack of a transport substance called gastric intrinsic factor. Intrinsic factor is secreted by stomach parietal cells; in pernicious anemia, autoantibodies against these cells impair their function. The lack of B_{12} interferes with red cell maturation, producing a megaloblastic anemia, and damages the posterior and lateral columns of the spinal cord to produce distal extremity paresthesias, loss of vibratory sense, weakness, and spasticity (subacute combined degeneration). Although not a prominent feature of pernicious anemia, optic neuropathy is reported with clinical characteristics similar to those of alcoholic optic neuropathy. Optic neuropathy may rarely be the presenting sign of pernicious anemia.[61] The diagnosis is made by having a high index of suspicion when confronted with bilateral subnormal acuity and central or centrocecal scotomas in nonalcoholic elderly (age >50 years) persons of northern European extraction with fair complexion and no family history of visual loss. Hematologic evaluation will reveal mild anemia with peripheral or bone marrow megaloblasts; neurologic examination may be normal or reveal the subtle findings described above. Serum B_{12} levels, now available by radioimmunoassay, will be below normal, and a Schilling test will reveal a significant increase in B_{12} absorption with the addition of intrinsic factor. Treatment is with monthly intramuscular B_{12} in 1,000 μg doses in perpetuity. Hematologic signs are reversible; neurologic signs will remit if not far advanced.

Tobacco amblyopia. The medical literature of the late nineteenth and early twentieth centuries is replete with admonitions as to the toxic effects of tobacco upon the optic nerves.[70] The neuro-ophthalmic syndrome described is exactly the same as seen in alcoholics and the severely malnourished and appears to occur primarily in pipe smokers, to a lesser degree in cigar smokers, snuff users, and tobacco chewers, and not at all in cigarette smokers. Later observations began to cast doubt on the toxic nature of this illness. The severity of optic neuropathy appeared to be independent of the amount of tobacco consumed; it tended to occur in patients who drank heavily but also ate poorly, and it could be reversed with either an adequate diet or thiamin.[70]

Several authors[11,28,44,87] have revivified the "toxic hypothesis" by showing that patients with tobacco amplyopia had significantly lower levels of thiocyanate in their plasma and urine than did comparable unaffected smokers. They postulated that the relatively few smokers who develop optic neuropathy have an inherent defect in detoxifying the cyanide of smoke and that the free cyanide damages the optic nerves. They cited experimental evidence showing that high doses of cyanide will produce axonal destruction in the optic nerves of animals.

They also showed that tobacco amblyopia patients have low or borderline levels of B_{12}, which is capable of binding cyanide ions. Four patients treated with cyanocobalamin did not improve, while four patients treated with hydroxycobalamin did manifest dramatic recovery of vision.[28] The authors postulated that the hydroxy form of B_{12} made available a binding site to absorb and sequester cyanide. Their work implies that the rare optic neuropathy in smokers is conditioned by relative B_{12} deficiency and that the pernicious anemia patients who develop optic neuropathy are smokers. Support for this hypothesis remains sparse.[62,70] However, making the etiology of the optic neuropathy in pernicious anemia and smokers multifactorial rescues it from confusing epidemiologic data.

Until more ample epidemiologic, experimental, and control clinical data are available, it is best to approach the diagnosis and management of symmetric, progressive, bilateral central or centrocecal scotomas with eclecticism. All such patients should be screened for pernicious anemia with serum B_{12} levels and checked for megaloblasts and myelopathy. If none of these are present (the usual case), then we suggest that patients wean themselves from alcohol and tobacco, eat a more balanced diet, and take multivitamins and thiamin, 25 mg three times a day. There is no objection to prescribing hydroxycobalamin 1000 µg intramuscularly each month, especially if the patient appears not to be an alcoholic. As an added precaution a careful drug history is important, and it may be necessary to screen for heavy metals in blood or urine, since lead and thallium are reported to cause similar changes.

☐ **Toxic optic neuropathies**

If cyanide has not been clearly established as an optic nerve toxin, there are several pharmacologic agents that have. The clinical picture produced by these drugs consists of insidious and painless bilateral loss of acuity and color vision, with central scotomas. In the early phases the optic disc may show mild swelling in some cases but is more commonly normal. In late phases, some temporal disc pallor may be evident. Among the many agents that have produced this syndrome, the most frequently implicated in current clinical practice is ethambutol, an antituberculosis drug.

Ethambutol optic atrophy. Since the initial description by Carr and Henkind in 1962,[11] further reports[34,60] have established ethambutol optic nerve toxicity as a dose-related retrobulbar neuropathy primarily but not exclusively involving papillomacular fibers.

Leibold[60] reported that in 59 patients treated at 35 mg/kg per day, optic neuropathy was seen in 11 (18%) patients. At 25 mg/kg per day the incidence of toxicity dropped to 2.25%. Others have confirmed this low risk, and present recommendations call for a dosage of 15 mg/kg per day.

The fundus is typically normal, although some hyperemia of the nerve head may rarely be seen. Visual acuity may be markedly reduced (hand movements) but is usually better than 20/100. Central and paracentral scotomas are the rule, although irregular constriction of central isopters and a case of bitemporal hemianopia are described.[59] Recovery occurs in the vast majority within 2 months of discontinuing the drug. No human pathologic material has been examined; in monkeys given 1300 to 1600 mg/kg/ per day, demyelination was found not only in optic nerves but in chiasm and tracts as well.[59]

What predisposes those rare individuals who develop ethambutol optic neuropathy at doses of 15 mg/kg/per day is unknown. Most authorities agree that the risk of irreversible toxicity at these dosage levels is too low to justify periodic ophthalmologic examination. Early manifestations of toxicity are exceedingly difficult to detect anyway. Thus the ophthalmologist's role is to be aware of the entity, to encourage safe dosage limits, and to recommend withdrawal of the agent at the first suggestion of stable or progressive unexplained visual loss.

One should be aware that isoniazid and streptomycin, other antituberculous drugs, are also optic nerve toxins.[34] Use of either of these agents with ethambutol may lower the toxic threshold.[54] While the toxicity of ethambutol is limited to the optic nerve, isoniazid is a general neurotoxin, causing peripheral neuropathy, seizures, and diffuse encephalopathy.[34] Alcoholics and those with hepatic or renal disease are at especial risk.[59] Recommended daily dosages are 300 mg/per day in adults. Optic neuropathy clinically similar to that of ethambutol toxicity has been reported at doses ranging from 200 to 900 mg/per day. The documentation of streptomycin optic nerve toxicity is too imprecise to offer helpful guidelines.[59]

Radiation optic neuropathy. Within the past decade, optic nerve toxicity from a nonpharmacologic source has been well documented: megavoltage x-irradiation. In patients with malignancies of the ethmoid and sphenoid sinuses, especially when the orbit has been invaded, neither the eyes nor the optic nerves can be shielded if the proper therapeutic radiation levels are to reach the tumor. In nasopharyngeal tumors that have extended to the cranial base the eyes are not included in the treatment field, but the optic nerves are. At standard total dosage schedules of 6,000 to 7,000 rad a majority of patients whose eyes are not shielded will develop ischemic retinopathy; those whose eyes are shielded but whose optic nerves are exposed will develop ischemic retrobulbar optic neuropathy. After a latency that varies from 1 to 5 years,[77] vision may be lost abruptly or in a gradual stepwise progression. Final visual outcome is frequently legal blindness in both eyes, because lateral fields include both optic nerves. There appear to be two distinct manifestations, depending upon whether the optic disc and retina or the retrobulbar optic nerve and chiasm are the principal sites of damage.

If radiation doses of more than 4,000 rad reach the retina and optic nerve, the fundus may show microaneurysms, hemorrhages, exudates, and neovascularization—a picture similar to that seen in diabetes. However, one may also see telangiectatic vessels, venous stasis, cotton-wool spots, pallid disc swelling, arteriolar narrowing, and focal retinal pigment epithelial loss, indicating compromise of retinal, ciliary, and choroidal vessels[14,68] (Plate 3, *C*). In fact, the fundus appearance resembles that seen in carotid and ophthalmic artery occlusive disease, giving rise to "ischemic oculopathy." The clinical course may be static but tends to be slowly progressive, leading to severe, if not total, visual loss and to intractable neovascular glaucoma.

If the eyes escape the brunt of the radiation, but the optic nerves do not, then optic neuropathy without retinopathy will typically occur at total tumor doses above 6,000 rad and daily dose fractions above 180 rad. The patient presents with acute loss of sight, and the only abnormal findings are a relative afferent pupillary defect and visual fields that show either a prechiasmal (nerve fiber bundle) defect limited to the symptomatic eye, or a junctional or bitemporal pattern indicating a lesion at the chiasm. The patient is usually misdiagnosed as having "optic neuritis," or worked up for a compressive lesion. Radiography is uniformly unrevealing.

Radiation retinopathy and optic neuropathy are acknowledged risks of potentially life-saving x-irradiation of ocular, orbital, sinus, and nasopharyngeal neoplasms. They are not expected but have also occurred, albeit rarely, after irradiation of tumors of the sellar area.[3,43] Harris and Levene[43] reported 18% radiation-induced visual loss in 55 patients treated for pituitary adenomas and craniopharyngiomas. All cases occurred in patients treated with dose fractions of 250 rad per day; none occurred at lower fractions. Arishzabal et al.[3] noted a 4% incidence of visual loss in 122 patients treated for pituitary adenomas. They believed that a total dose greater than 4500 rad was most responsible for this complication. Schatz et al.[75] have described three cases of visual loss after treatment for middle fossa masses at 5,000 rad in 200-rad daily fractions. The clinical syndrome was stereotypic: visual loss occurred suddenly in one eye between 6 months and 2 years after completion of treatment. There were no fundus abnormalities at first. Visual fields disclosed either prechiasmal (nerve fiber bundle) or chiasmal (hemianopic) defects. Later, visual acuity and field continued to deteriorate, often in a stepwise fashion, and optic pallor appeared. Steroids and hyperbaric oxygen have been used unsuccessfully. Although data are not conclusive, the risk of radiation toxicity seems to be especially high where the optic nerve has already been compromised by previous compression by tumor. Patients with diabetes and hypertension are also particularly vulnerable, probably because of underlying vascular disease.[13]

Pathologic studies of optic nerve and chiasm in all autopsied cases of radiation toxicity to the anterior visual pathway show changes similar to those encountered in delayed radiation effects on the spinal cord and brain: vascular endothelial proliferation and fibrinoid necrosis, necrosis of white and gray matter, and reactive astrocytosis.[20,30,72]

☐ Hereditary optic neuropathies

So rarely are cases of hereditary optic neuropathy seen in clinical practice that they are usually misdiagnosed. Though the afflicted cannot be treated, they deserve to be given a sage prognosis and to be spared unnecessary studies. This entity, whose ophthalmologic manifestations are similar to those of nutritional and toxic optic neuropathies, occurs both as an isolated condition and as part of a degenerative CNS disease.

Isolated hereditary optic neuropathy. Glaser[31] has clarified the classification of these conditions by dividing them into the rare, recessively inherited type and the relatively more common, dominantly inherited type.

The recessive ("simple") optic atrophy is probably congenital, produces severe and stable central visual loss (20/200, hand movements) with nystagmus, achromatopsia, and optic disc pallor. The normal caliber of the retinal arterioles and a normal ERG distinguish it from Leber's amaurosis.

The dominant optic atrophy becomes symptomatic between the ages of 4 and 8 years, produces moderate visual impairment (20/40 to 20/200), slow progression, no nystagmus, moderate disc pallor (Plate 4, *A* and *B*), centrocecal scotomas, and a tritanopic color defect.

Complicated hereditary optic atrophy. Optic atrophy with central or centrocecal scotomas is a manifestation of a wide variety of neurodegenerative states. The familial eponymic spinocerebellar degenerations such as Friedreich's, Marie's, and Behr's, as well as the polyneuropathy of Charcot-Marie-Tooth, may include optic atrophy.[35] Optic atrophy may also be seen in the neurologic diseases of inborn metabolic errors that manifest retinal pigmentary degeneration, maculopathy, and cherry red spots. In most of these conditions, visual loss and optic neuropathy occur either concomitantly or follow other neurologic signs. There is no treatment.

Leber's optic atrophy. In 1871, Leber[58] described a hereditary optic neuropathy affecting first one eye and then the other, after an interval of days to weeks. Most of the cases afflict males in their second and third decade, producing rapid visual loss to a variable level (usually 20/200 to finger counting), which is usually unremitting. Fundoscopy is often normal in the acute phase, although some observers report hyperemia and telangiectasia of peripapillary retinal capillaries and swelling of the nerve fiber layer adjacent to the disc[31] (Plate 4, *C* and *D*). Ultimately the patient develops optic atrophy and centrocecal scotomas.

Leber's optic atrophy has defied classification as a purely hereditary disease because (1) it violates mendelian X-linked inheritance by absence of transmission through males and (2) the visual acuity may improve months to years after onset. At present the best explanation appears to be a genetically conditioned viral illness. In treatment of Leber's, corticosteroids, hydroxycobalamin, and craniotomy for lysis of opticochiasmatic adhesions all have their adherents[31]; no treatment has achieved widespread acceptance.

DIAGNOSIS OF OPTIC ATROPHY WITHOUT BENEFIT OF HISTORY OR VISUAL FIELD

Many patients are unable to give a precise history as to the duration and course of their visual loss. In such patients the examiner may have to rely upon the appearance of the fundus, especially if the visual fields are not trustworthy.

A retrospective study of stereofundus photographs of 163 cases of optic atrophy reviewed as unknowns by several examiners[80] revealed that (1) ipsilateral attenuation of retinal arterioles is a specific sign of old central retinal artery occlusion (Plate 3, *D*), (2) healed papillitis (inflammatory or ischemic) causes narrowing of the retinal arterioles only in their papillary segment, after which they actually enlarge slightly in caliber as they traverse the fundus (Plate 3, *E*), and (3) substantial disc excavation is likely to indicate glaucoma except if there is pallor of the temporal neuroretinal rim (Plate 4, *E* and *F*), in which case a nonglaucomatous process such as intracranial neoplasia or old retrobulbar neuritis is responsible. Otherwise, fundus signs are not specific for any particular etiology, and diagnosis must be obtained from nonophthalmoscopic findings.

In summary, optic atrophy, together with marked attenuation of the retinal arterioles, generally means retinal disease and should restrain the urge to perform intracranial studies.[80,81] On the other hand, if substantial arteriolar narrowing is not present and the clinical course is unclear, a CT scan should be performed in any patient with optic atrophy.

CENTRAL RETINAL ARTERY OCCLUSION

The diagnosis of acute central retinal artery occlusion (CRAO) or branch retinal arterial occlusion (BRAO) is usually straightforward (Fig. 1-16). Management is the problem.

Patients present with sudden painless loss of vision. Although monocular transient visual loss often precedes the fixed deficit in vision, it generally has been present less than 48 hours. The extent of visual loss depends upon the segment of retina that has been

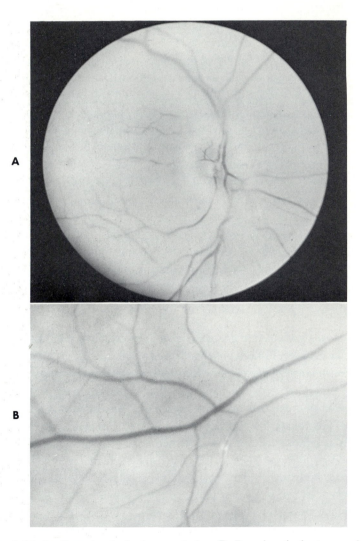

Fig. 1-16. A, Central retinal artery occlusion. **B,** Branch retinal artery occlusion.

COLOR PLATES 2, 3, and 4

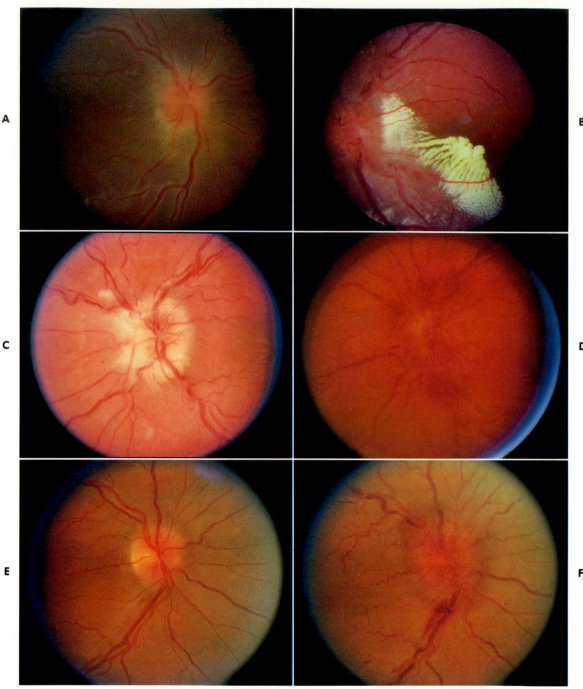

Plate 2. A, Papillitis with periphlebitis. **B,** Papillitis with retinal exudates, cotton-wool spots indicative of "neuroretinitis." **C,** Segmental papillitis with cotton-wool spots. **D,** Leukemic infiltration of optic nerve head. **E,** Moderate disc swelling in dysthyroid orbitopathy. **F,** Marked disc swelling in same eye, **E,** as disease worsens.

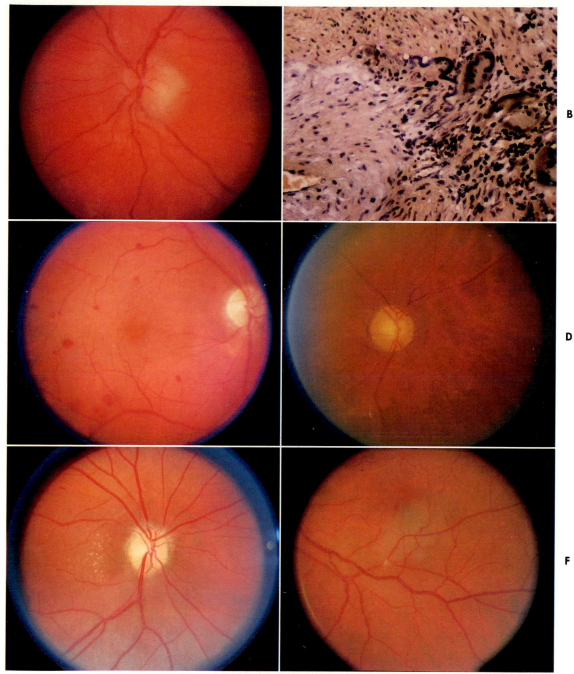

Plate 3. A, Cranial arteritis. Note segmental infarction of optic disc. **B,** Cranial arteritis. Note giant cells and disrupted elastic lamina in temporal artery biopsy (Verhoeff elastic stain). **C,** Radiation-induced ischemic retinopathy and papillopathy. Note perivenous hemorrhages, sheathed and attenuated retinal arterioles, and disc pallor. **D,** Old central retinal artery occlusion. Note markedly attenuated and sheathed arterioles and disc pallor. **E,** Old papillitis. Note residual retinal exudates and that arterioles are narrowed at disc but of normal caliber elsewhere (reverse taper sign of healed papillitis). **F,** Branch retinal arterial occlusion. Note intraluminal plaque.

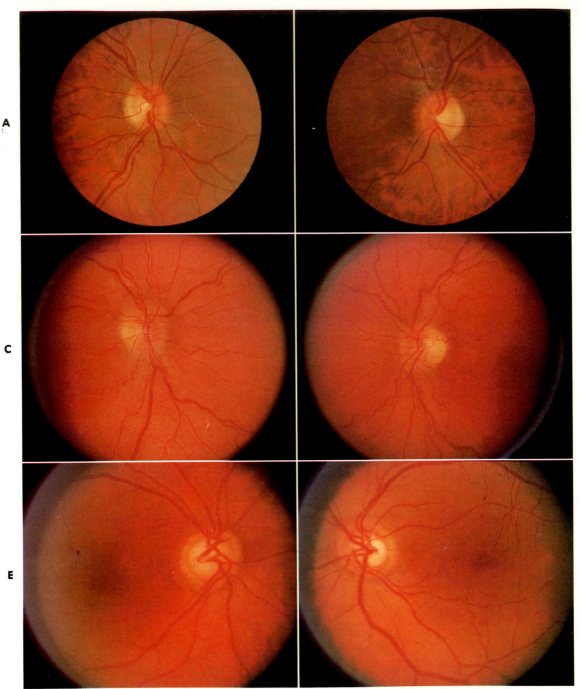

Plate 4. A and **B,** Dominant optic atrophy. Note wedge-shaped, symmetric temporal disc pallor. Similar findings may be seen in nutritional and toxic optic neuropathies. **C** and **D,** Leber's optic neuropathy. Right eye, **C,** in acute phase shows opacification of nerve fiber layer at upper and lower poles of optic nerve head, together with telangiectasia. Left eye, **D,** in chronic phase shows nerve fiber layer obscuration but no telangiectasia. Note disc pallor. **E** and **F,** Nonglaucomatous optic disc excavation. Patient had compression of right optic nerve by subfrontal meningioma. Note temporal rim pallor in right eye, a clue that excavation is unlikely to be caused by glaucoma.

infarcted. The event is termed a CRAO if most of the retina has been affected, and a BRAO if only a small portion is involved. BRAO infarctions often do not extend to the optic disc, originating instead at the point of termination of an embolus (Plate 3, *F*) or the crossing of the affected arteriole and a vein. The infarcted retina has lost its transparency and appears milky white, especially in its thickest region around the macula. The transmission of the normal orange-red choroidal color in the macular area contrasts with the surrounding milky retinal pallor and gives the appearance of a cherry red spot. The retinal turbidity is gradually lost after an interval of 10 to 14 days, and for the next 40 days the diagnosis may be difficult to make on ophthalmoscopic grounds. The retinal arterioles will gradually become attenuated and often sheathed, the nerve fiber layer atrophic, and the disc pale. Visual field defects are nerve fiber bundle in configuration and typically involve the fixation area unless a cilioretinal artery has been spared.

Treatment of the acute event is based on the principle of reducing external pressure and dilating the retinal vasculature. Pressure is lowered by means of digital massage of the globe, anterior chamber paracentesis, and agents that block aqueous secretion. Ocular massage is advised especially if an embolus is visible, in hopes of dislodging it and promoting distal migration. Dilatation of retinal vessels is fostered by paper bag rebreathing to build up carbon dioxide and by injecting vasodilator agents retrobulbarly.

Only anecdotal evidence points to the efficacy of these maneuvers,[79] and most authors consider them hopeless if more than 6 hours have elapsed from the onset of the fixed deficit. In spite of the absence of better data, we would support the traditional heroic measures, even if 24 hours have elapsed, acknowledging that reversal of visual loss is rare. There would appear to be little rationale for using systemic vasodilators since these only tend to shunt blood to healthier, more responsive vessels.

The workup of patients with CRAO or BRAO after the acute treatment period is very problematic. The considerations are similar to those involved in evaluating patients with transient visual loss and are best dealt with in Chapter 2.

REFERENCES

1. Albert, DM, Ruchman, MC, and Keltner, JL: Skip areas in temporal arteritis, Arch Ophthalmol 94:2072, 1976.
2. Altrocchi, PA, Remhardt, PM, and Eckman, PB: Blindness and meningeal carcinomatosis, Arch Ophthalmol 88:508, 1972.
3. Arishzabal, S, Caldwell, WL, and Avila, J: The relationship of time-dose fractionation factors to complications in the treatment of pituitary tumors by irradiation, Radiat Oncol Biol Phys 2:667, 1977.
4. Barricks, ME, Traviesa, DB, and Glaser, JS: Ophthalmoplegia in cranial arteritis, Brain 100:209, 1977.
5. Beevers, DG, Harper, JE, and Turk, KAD: Giant cell arteritis—the need for prolonged treatment, J Chron Dis 26:571, 1973.
6. Bengtsson, B, and Malmvall, B: An alternate-day corticosteroid regimen in maintenance therapy of giant cell arteritis, Acta Med Scand 209:347, 1981.
7. Bird, AC: Is there a place for corticosteroids in the treatment of optic neuritis? In Brockhurst, RM, Boruchoff, SA, Hutchinson, BT, and Lessell, S, editors: Controversy in ophthalmology, Philadelphia, 1977, WB Saunders Co, p 882.
8. Boghen, DR, and Glaser, JS: Ischaemic optic neuropathy, Brain 98:689, 1975.
9. Bradley, WG, and Whitty, WM: Acute optic neuritis: its clinical features and their relation to prognosis for recovery of vision, J Neurol Neurosurg Psychiatry 30:531, 1967.
10. Bull, BS, and Brecher, G: An evaluation of the relative merits of the Wintrobe and Westergren sedimentation methods, including hematocrit correction, Am J Clin Pathol 62:502, 1974.
11. Carr, RE, and Henkind, P: Ocular manifestations of ethambutol: toxic amblyopia after administration of an experimental antituberculous drug, Arch Ophthalmol 67:566, 1962.
12. Carroll, F: Etiology and treatment of tobacco-alcohol amblyopia, Am J Ophthalmol 47:713, 1944.

13. Chacko, DC: Considerations in the diagnoses of radiation injury, JAMA 245:1255, 1981.
14. Chee, PHY: Radiation retinopathy, Am J Ophthalmol 66:860, 1969.
15. Chiappa, KH, Harrison, JL, Brooks EB, and Young, RR: Brainstem auditory evoked responses in 200 patients with multiple sclerosis, Ann Neurol (in press).
16. Cohen, D, and Smith, T: Skip areas in temporal arteritis: myth versus fact, Trans Am Acad Ophthalmol Otolaryngol 78:772, 1974.
17. Cohen, DA: Temporal arteritis: improvement in visual prognosis and management with repeat biopsies, Trans Am Acad Ophthalmol Otolaryngol 177:74, 1973.
18. Cohen, MM, Lessell, S, and Wolf, PA: A prospective study of the risk of developing multiple sclerosis in uncomplicated optic neuritis, Neurology (Minneap) 29:208, 1979.
19. Compston, DAS, Batchelor, JR, Earl, CJ, and McDonald, WI: Factors influencing the risk of multiple sclerosis developing in patients with optic neuritis, Brain 101:495, 1978.
20. Crompton, MR, and Layton, DD: Delayed radionecrosis of the brain following therapeutic irradiation of the pituitary, Brain 84:85, 1961.
21. Cullen, JF, and Coleiro, JA: Ophthalmic complications of giant cell arteritis, Surv Ophthalmol 20:247, 1976.
22. Dutton, JJ, Burde, RM, and Klingele, TG: Autoimmune optic neuritis, Am J Ophthalmol 94:11, 1982.
23. Earl, CJ, and Martin, B: Prognosis of optic neuritis related to age, Lancet 1:74, 1967.
24. Ellenberger, C: Ischemic optic neuropathy as a possible early complication of vascular hypertension, Am J Ophthalmol 88:1045, 1979.
25. Ellis, W, and Little, HC: Leukemic infiltration of the optic nerve head, Am J Ophthalmol 75:867, 1973.
26. Ellison, GW, and Myers, L: A review of systemic non-specific immunosuppressive treatment of multiple sclerosis, Neurology (Minneap) 28(2):132, 1978.
27. Fisher, CM: Lacunes: small, deep cerebral infarcts, Neurology (Minneap) 15:774, 1965.
28. Foulds, WS: Surv Reply, Ophthalmol 17:334, 1973.
29. Frey, T: Optic neuritis in children: infectious mononucleosis as an etiology, Doc Ophthalmol 34:183, 1973.
30. Ghatak, NR, and White, BE: Delayed radiation necrosis of the hypothalamus, Arch Neurol 21:425, 1969.
31. Glaser, JS: Heredofamilial disorders of the optic nerve. In Goldberg, MF, editor: Genetic and metabolic eye disease, Boston, 1974, Little Brown & Co, p 463.
32. Goodman, BW: Temporal arteritis, Am J Med 67:839, 1979.
33. Goodwin, JA: Temporal arteritis. In Vinken, PJ, and Bruyn, GW, editors: The handbook of clinical neurology, vol 39, Amsterdam, 1980, Elsevier-North Holland, p 313.
34. Grant, WM: Toxicology of the eye, Springfield, Ill, 1974, Charles C Thomas, Publisher, p 459.
35. Greenfield, JG: The spinocerebellar degenerations, Oxford, 1954, Blackwell Scientific Publications.
36. Gudas, PP: Optic nerve myeloma, Am J Ophthalmol 71:1085, 1971.
37. Hackett, ER, Martinez, RD, Larson, PF, et al: Optic neuritis in systemic lupus erythematosus, Arch Ophthalmol 31:9, 1974.
38. Halliday, AM, Halliday, E, Kriss, A, McDonald, WI, and Mushin, J: The pattern-evoked potential in compression of the anterior visual pathway, Brain 99:357, 1976.
39. Halliday, AM, McDonald, WI, and Mushin J: Delayed visual evoked response in optic neuritis, Lancet 1:982, 1972.
40. Halliday, AM, and Mushin, J: The visual evoked potential in neuro-ophthalmology. In Sokol, S, editor: Electrophysiology and psychophysics: their use in ophthalmic diagnosis, Int Ophthalmol Clin 20(1):155, 1980.
41. Halliday, AM, McDonald, WI, and Mushin, J: Visual evoked response in diagnosis of multiple sclerosis, Br Med J 4:661, 1973.
42. Hamilton, CR, Shelley, WM, and Tumulty, PA: Giant cell arteritis: including temporal arteritis and polymyalgia rheumatica, Medicine 50:1, 1971.
43. Harris, JR, and Levene, MB: Visual complications following irradiation for pituitary adenomas and craniopharyngiomas, Radiology 120:167, 1976.
44. Heaton, JM, McCormick, AJA, and Freeman, AG: Tobacco amblyopia: a clinical manifestation of vitamin B_{12} deficiency, Lancet 2:286, 1958.
45. Henkind, P, Charles, NC, and Pearson, J: Histopathology of ischemic neuropathy, Am J Ophthalmol 69:78, 1970.
46. Hershey, LA, and Trotter, JC: The use and abuse of the cerebrospinal fluid IgG profile in the adult: a practical evaluation, Ann Neurol 8:426, 1980.
47. Hollenhorst, RW, Brown, JR, Wagener, HP, and Schick, RM: Neurologic aspects of temporal arteritis, Neurology (Minneap) 10:490, 1960.
48. Hunder, GG, Disney, TF, and Ward, LE: Polymyalgia rheumatica, Mayo Clin Proc 44:849, 1969.

49. Hunder, GG, Sheps, SG, Allen, GL, and Joyce, J: Daily and alternate-day corticosteroid regimens in treatment of giant cell arteritis. Comparison in a prospective study, Ann Intern Med 82:613, 1975.

50. Huston, KA, Hunder, GG, Lie, JT, Kennedy, RH, and Elvebach, LR: Temporal arteritis. A 25 year epidemiologic, clinical and pathologic study, Ann Intern Med 88:162, 1978.

51. Jampol, LM, Woodfin, W, and McLean, EB: Optic nerve sarcoidosis: report of a case, Arch Ophthalmol 87:355, 1972.

52. Johnson, KP, and Nelson, BJ: Multiple sclerosis: diagnostic usefulness of cerebrospinal fluid, Ann Neurol 2:425, 1977.

53. Jonasson, F, Cullen, JF, and Elton, RA: Temporal arteritis. A 14 year epidemiological, clinical and prognostic study, Scott Med J 24:111, 1979.

54. Karmon, G, Savir, H, Zevin, D, and Levi, V: Bilateral optic neuropathy due to combined ethambutol and isoniazid treatment, Ann Ophthalmol 11:1013, 1979.

55. Kennedy, C, and Carroll, FD: Optic neuritis in children, Arch Ophthalmol 63:747, 1960.

56. Klein, RG, Campbell, RJ, Hunder, GG, and Carney, JA: Skip lesions in temporal arteritis, Mayo Clin Proc 51:504, 1976.

57. Knox, DL, and Duke, JR: Slowly progressive ischemic optic neuropathy, Trans Am Acad Ophthalmol Otolaryngol 75:1065, 1971.

58. Leber, T: Ueber hereditare und congenitalangelegte Sehnervenleiden, Albrecht Von Graefes Arch Klin Exp Ophthalmol 17:249, 1871.

59. Leibold, JE: Drugs having a toxic effect on the optic nerve. In Ellis, PP, editor: Side effects of drugs in ophthalmology, Int Ophthalmol Clin 11(2):137, 1971.

60. Leibold, JE: The ocular toxicity of ethambutol and its relation to dose, Ann NY Acad Sci 135:904, 1966.

61. Lerman, S, and Feldman, AC: Centrocecal scotomata as the presenting sign in pernicious anemia, Arch Ophthalmol 65:381, 1961.

62. Lessell, S: Toxic and deficiency optic neuropathies. In Smith, JL, and glaser, JS, editors: Neuro-ophthalmology Symposium of the University of Miami and the Bascom Palmer Eye Institute, vol 7, St Louis, 1973, The CV Mosby Co.

63. Link, H, Norrby, E, and Olsson, JE: Immunoglobulins and measles antibodies in optic neuritis, N Engl J Med 289:1103, 1973.

64. McAlpine, D: The benign form of multiple sclerosis, Brain 84:186, 1961.

65. Nikoskelainen, E: Later course and prognosis of optic neuritis, Acta Ophthalmol 53:273, 1975.

66. Nikoskelainen, E: Symptoms, signs, and early course of optic neuritis, Acta Ophthalmol 53:254, 1975.

67. Nikoskelainen, E, Frey, H, and Salmi, A: Prognosis of optic neuritis with special reference to cerebrospinal fluid immunoglobulins and measles virus antibodies, Ann Neurol 9:545, 1981.

68. Perrers Taylor, M, Brinkley, D, and Reynolds, T: Choroidoretinal damage as a complication of radiotherapy, Acta Radiol 3:431, 1965.

69. Poser, CM: Diagnostic techniques in multiple sclerosis, Surv Ophthalmol 25:91, 1980.

70. Potts, AM: Tobacco amblyopia, Surv Ophthalmol 17:313, 1973.

71. Regan, D, Milver, BA, and Heron, JR: Delayed visual perception and delayed visual evoked potentials in the spinal form of multiple sclerosis and in retrobulbar neuritis, Brain 99:43, 1976.

72. Ross, HS, Rosenberg, S, and Friedman, AH: Delayed radiation necrosis of the optic nerve, Am J Ophthalmol 76:683, 1978.

73. Sandberg-Wollheim, M: Optic neuritis: studies on the cerebrospinal fluid in relation to clinical course in 61 patients, Acta Neurol Scand 52:167, 1975.

74. Sandberg-Wollheim, M: Optic neuritis studies on the cerebrospinal fluid in relation to clinical course in 61 patients, Acta Neurol Scand 52:167, 1975.

75. Schatz, NJ, Lichtenstein, S, and Corbett, JJ: Delayed radiation necrosis of the optic nerves and chiasm. In Glaser, JS, and Smith, JL, editors: Neuro-ophthalmology Symposium of the University of Miami and the Bascom Palmer Eye Institute, vol 8, St. Louis, 1975, The CV Mosby Co, p 131.

76. Shahrokhi, F, Chiappa, KH, and Young, RR: Pattern shift visual evoked responses. Two hundred patients with optic neuritis and/or multiple sclerosis, Arch Neurol 35:65, 1978.

77. Shukovsky, LJ, and Fletcher, GH: Retinal and optic nerve implications in a high dose irradiation technique of ethmoid sinus and nasal cavity, Radiology 104:629, 1972.

78. Simmons, RJ, and Cogan, DG: Occult temporal arteritis, Arch Ophthalmol 68:8, 1962.

79. Stone, R, Zink, H, Klingele, T, and Burde, RM: Visual recovery after central retinal artery occlusion: two cases, Ann Ophthalmol 9:445, 1977.

80. Trobe, JD, Glaser, JS, and Cassady, JC: Optic atrophy. Differential diagnosis by fundus observation alone, Arch Ophthalmol 98:1040, 1980.

81. Trobe, JD, Glaser, JS, Cassady, JC, Herschler, J, and Anderson, DR: Non-glaucomatous excavation of the optic disc, Arch Ophthalmol 98:1046-1050, 1980.
82. Trobe, JD, Glaser, JS, and LaFlamme, P: Dysthyroid optic neuropathy. The clinical course and rationale for management, Arch Ophthalmol 96:1199, 1978.
83. Victor, M: Tobacco alcohol amblyopia. A critique of current concepts of this disorder, with special reference to the role of nutritional deficiency in its causation, Arch Ophthalmol 70:313, 1963.
84. Wagener, HP, and Hollenhorst, RW: The ocular lesions of temporal arteritis, Am J Ophthalmol 45:617, 1958.
85. Whisnant, JP: Epidemiology of stroke: emphasis on transient cerebral ischemia attachs and hypertension, Stroke 5:68, 1974.
86. Wilkinson, IMS, and Russell, RWR: Arteries of the head and neck in giant cell arteritis. A pathological study to show the pattern of arterial involvement, Arch Neurol 27:378, 1972.
87. Wokes, F: Tobacco amblyopia, Lancet 2:526, 1958.
88. Younge, BR: Fluorescein angiography and retinal venous sheathing in multiple sclerosis, Can J Ophthalmol 11:31, 1976.

PART III

Chiasmal visual loss

It has been estimated that 25% of all brain tumors occur in the chiasmal area, and of these almost one half will produce the initial complaint of visual loss.[37] Of the lesions causing chiasmal compression, pituitary tumors are the most common (50% to 55%), followed by craniopharyngiomas (20% to 25%), meningiomas (10%), and gliomas (7%). The other causes of chiasmal compression, including aneurysm, are relatively rare.

The major, and sometimes only, symptoms produced by these gradually enlarging benign masses is progressive visual loss. Because of this the ophthalmologist is likely the first physician consulted and by virtue of his training the best suited to establish the diagnosis.

The role of the ophthalmologist in the patient with visual field evidence of chiasmal compromise is as follows:

1. To establish the diagnosis clinically and to effect an appropriate referral for specific neuroradiologic investigations based on the clinical information.
2. To document asymptomatic visual loss in a patient with a known chiasmal or parachiasmal lesion.
3. To evaluate patients after they have been treated for a chiasmal or parachiasmal mass to chart the course of visual function.

DIAGNOSIS OF CHIASMAL SYNDROME
Symptoms of chiasmal syndrome

Visual loss. Decreased vision is the primary symptom of chiasmal compression. Slow-growing neoplasms produce a gradual, insidious, painless visual loss that may progress for months or years before being discovered by the patient. Decreased acuity and not the realization of a peripheral field constriction usually prompts the patient with chiasmal compression to seek medical care. The pattern of visual loss will depend on the anatomic relationship of the causative mass lesion to the optic chiasm (see Signs of Chiasmal Syndrome, p. 59).

Rarely visual loss may be rapidly progressive or even apoplectic in onset. An apoplectic loss of vision is highly suggestive of rapid expansion of a pituitary tumor because of infarction or hemorrhage (see Pituitary Apoplexy, below).

Diplopia. Double vision may be caused by lateral extension of the tumor into the cavernous sinus (Fig. 1-17), resulting in dysfunction of the third, fourth, or sixth cranial nerve. Another form of diplopia occurs without obvious muscle paresis (nonparetic dip-

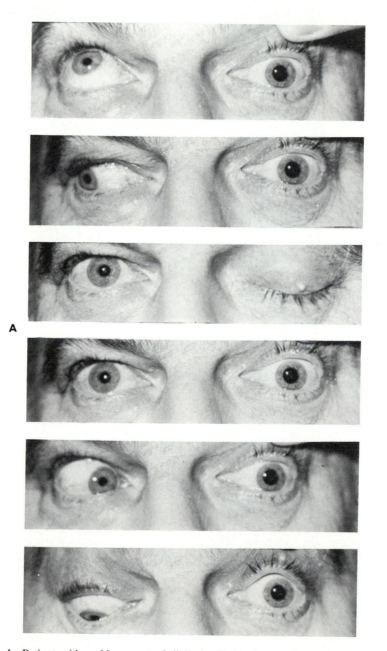

A

Fig. 1-17. A, Patient with sudden onset of diplopia. Patient has total ophthalmoplegia with the pupil involved.

Continued.

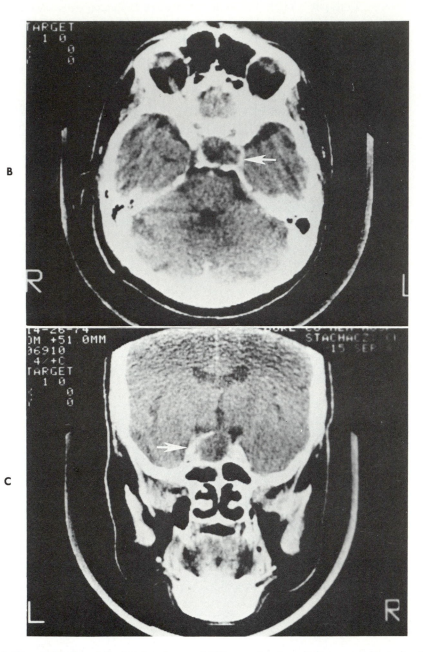

Fig. 1-17, cont'd. B and **C,** Axial and coronal CT scan showing pituitary mass (arrow) extending toward left cavernous sinus. No visual field defect was present.

lopia). The patient's complaint of vertical (or horizontal) diplopia is explained by the absence of a temporal field in either eye to act as a physiologic linkage. As a result of this inability to maintain the two nasal fields in juxtaposition, exo-, eso-, or hyperdeviations occur. This has been dubbed the *hemifield slide phenomenon*.[48,70] Elkington[25] described 98 of 260 patients with pituitary adenoma who complained of double vision. However, only 14 patients had a demonstrable ocular motor palsy. Of 1,000 patients with pituitary tumors seen at the Mayo Clinic, 62 had extraocular muscle palsies, but no description of diplopia from the hemifield slide phenomenon was recorded.[37] Thus the prevalence of nonparetic diplopia in patients with chiasmal lesions is unknown.

Nystagmus. A peculiar type of dissociated nystagmus termed see-saw nystagmus occasionally accompanies mass lesions in the chiasmal area. When see-saw nystagmus is present, a bitemporal hemianopia must be sought.[23] (See Chapter 6.)

Headache. Headache is a significant complaint in all series of pituitary tumor patients. Hollenhorst and Younge[37] report that 13% of 1000 patients with pituitary tumors had headache as a presenting complaint. Elkington[25] recorded severe headache in one third of his 260 patients (11 had pituitary apoplexy), while another one third complained of slight headache. The headache is usually frontal in location and attributed to stretching of the diaphragma sella.

Endocrine dysfunction. The endocrine abnormalities associated with chiasmal mass lesions are discussed under each individual entity.

Signs of chiasmal syndrome

Perimetry is the cornerstone upon which rests the clinical diagnosis of chiasmal disorders. To understand the localizing value and clinical implications of chiasmal visual field defects, certain aspects of gross and microscopic fiber anatomy of the chiasm must be kept in mind.

The optic chiasm is formed by the confluence of the optic nerves. An average vertical distance of 10 mm separates the chiasm from the dorsum sellae and the pituitary fossa. Pituitary lesions must have a substantial suprasellar extension before visual field defects are produced, since chiasmal visual loss is observed only when the chiasm and its vascular supply are greatly compressed and distorted (Fig. 1-18). Small intrasellar lesions never produce visual field defects.

The chiasm does not bear a constant relationship to the pituitary gland. The body of the chiasm is situated over the pituitary in 80% of patients, over the tuberculum sellae (prefixed) in 9%, and over the dorsum sellae (postfixed) in 11%. Pituitary tumors are likely to produce optic tract visual field defects in prefixed chiasms and unilateral optic nerve involvement in postfixed chiasms.[8] In a study of 1,000 pituitary tumors, bitemporal defects were the most common (67%), while junction scotoma (29%), homonymous hemianopia (7%), and prechiasmal visual field loss (2%) occurred with less regularity.[37]

The chiasm is bordered laterally by the supraclinoid portion of the carotid arteries, superiorly by the anterior cerebral and anterior communicating arteries, and below by the posterior cerebral, basilar, and posterior communicating arteries.[8] Although these arteries (especially the carotid artery) can produce grooving of the chiasm, the production of visual field defects corresponding to these grooves are difficult to document.

The inferior nasal (crossed) fibers are the first to decussate in the chiasm. A few fibers actually course forward to occupy a portion of the contralateral optic nerve (Wil-

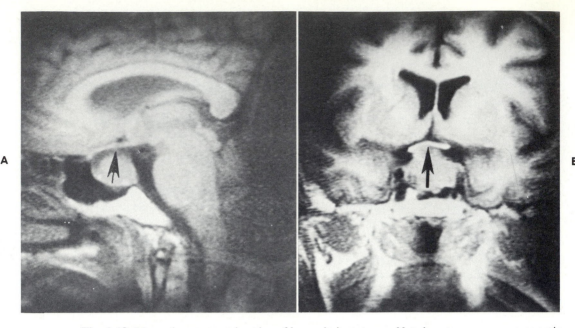

Fig. 1-18. Magnetic resonance imaging of large pituitary tumor. Note how tumor compresses optic chiasm (arrow) in both the sagittal, **A,** and coronal sections, **B.**

brand's knee). The superior nasal fibers cross mainly in the superoposterior portion of the chiasm. Almost the entire median portion of the chiasm is occupied by macular crossing fibers. There is no discrete macular bundle within the chiasm, although these fibers are mostly concentrated centrally and dorsally.[40]

Utilizing the knowledge of chiasmal fiber anatomy, we can understand that there are essentially four visual field defects possible with parachiasmal mass lesions. The visual field defects shown (Fig. 1-19) all localize lesions to the optic chiasm, and when any of these defects is encountered, neuroradiologic studies are mandatory to establish the precise localization of the mass lesion.

Central scotoma (prechiasmal compression) (Fig. 1-19, *A*). Visual loss is usually slowly progressive and manifests optic nerve characteristics; but the visual field in the contralateral eye is full. This implies compression of the intracranial prechiasmal portion of the optic nerve. The causes, however, are identical to the causes of a chiasmal syndrome, but the visual field differs either because the chiasm is postfixed or because the lesion is located anteriorly. The central scotoma is the most consistent perimetric finding in prechiasmal compressive lesions. While central scotomas are most frequently caused by inflammatory optic neuropathies, this form of visual field defect may be absent in approximately 25% of patients with optic neuritis.[86] Therefore the time course of the development of the optic neuropathy is as critical to diagnosis as the pattern of the visual field loss. In any patient with a slowly progressive optic neuropathy a compressive etiology must be sought.

Junction scotoma (Fig. 1-19, *B*). Lesions that involve the intracranial optic nerve frequently will extend backward toward the chiasm. Since the nasal crossing fibers from the fellow eye course anteriorly into the opposite optic nerve, the ipsilateral central

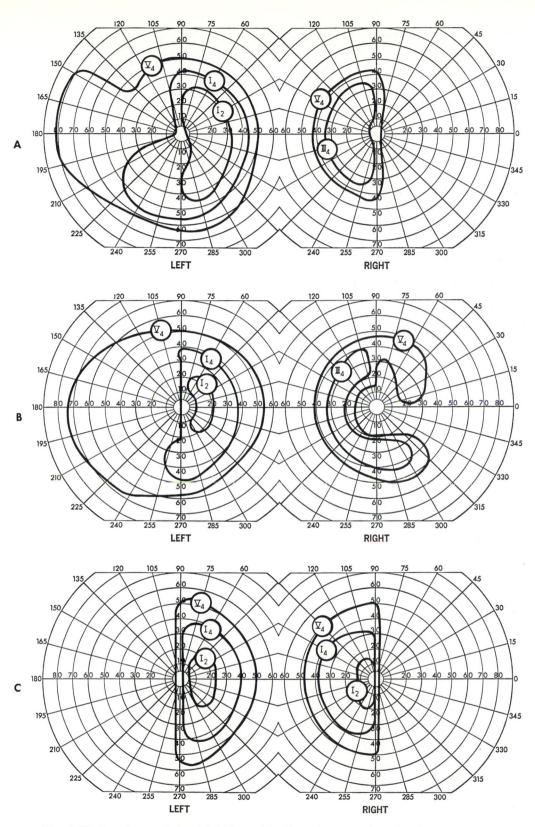

Fig. 1-19. Four forms of visual field loss with chiasmal compression. **A,** Right central scotoma: from prechiasmal compression that evolved into a junctional defect as the mass enlarged. **B,** Junctional defect: right central scotoma with left temporal hemianopia due to lesion at junction of right optic nerve and chiasm. **C,** Bitemporal hemianopia: complete defect to largest isopters.

Continued.

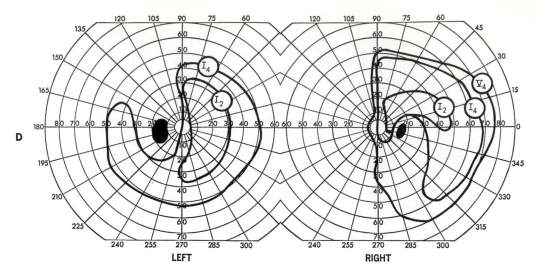

Fig. 1-19, cont'd. D, Incongruous homonymous hemianopia: from involvement of right optic tract.

scotoma may be accompanied by a contralateral, supratemporal visual field depression (junction syndrome). The detection of such a combination of visual field defects exquisitely localizes the lesion to the junction of the involved optic nerve and chiasm and should prompt investigation identical to that for a bitemporal hemianopia.

Bitemporal hemianopia (Fig. 1-19, *C*). The hallmark of chiasmal involvement is the bitemporal hemianopia. In practice, however, it is unusual to see an isolated bitemporal defect with no loss of central acuity in at least one eye. Visual loss occurs because the causative mass lesions are large and tend to distort the entire chiasm and compromise the optic nerves as well. Thus central acuity depression in one or both eyes is the rule; a pure bitemporal hemianopia with intact acuity is the exception.

Bitemporal hemianopias may be complete or incomplete and symmetric or asymmetric. At times the hemianopia may be exclusively paracentral and will be overlooked unless the central field is explored carefully, utilizing small white or large red test objects. It is unwise to predict the site of the mass lesion from the character of the hemianopia. Inferior visual field defects do not invariably imply compression by a suprachiasmal lesion.

Incongruous homonymous hemianopia (Fig. 1-19, *D*). Posteriorly the optic chiasm forms the optic tracts. Optic tract lesions usually produce incongruous homonymous hemianopias, often with decreased acuity in one eye. The most frequent cause of the optic tract syndrome is craniopharyngioma or other large parachiasmal mass lesion.[81]

Once the ophthalmologist has determined that the lesion is parachiasmal, further investigation falls to the neuro-ophthalmologist, neuroradiologist, and endocrinologist. Treatment of these lesions may include surgery, radiation, or medical therapy, alone or in combination.

POSTTHERAPY FOLLOW-UP EVALUATION

The ophthalmologist should determine the amount of change in visual function that has occurred as a result of treatment. Return of vision following surgical decompression

Table 1-2. A proposed schedule for follow-up visual field testing

Treatment	Visual field follow-up
Surgery alone	Immediately postoperatively
	4 to 6 weeks postoperatively
	At 4-month intervals for 1 year
	Yearly for 5 years
	Then every 2 years
Radiation alone	At the midpoint and end of radiotherapy
	At 3-month intervals for 1 year
	At 6-month intervals for 1 year
	Then yearly
Surgery and radiation	Immediately postoperatively
	At completion of radiotherapy
	At 3-month intervals for 1 year
	Yearly for 5 years
	Then every 2 years
Medical (bromocriptine)	Monthly for large tumors or during pregnancy for tumors of any size
	At 6-month intervals in microadenomas for 1 year, then yearly

is rapid. In a small series, Kayan and Earl[45] document return of acuity and visual field within 48 hours of decompression. However, the bulk of vision probably returns even earlier. Therefore, if possible, vision should be evaluated in the recovery room as soon as the patient can respond. If vision is poorer than the preoperative level, CT scan should be obtained to rule out hematoma, air, or a migrated pituitary fossa muscle pack that may be compressing the chiasm. The first postoperative visual field may be done within days of surgery. If postoperative radiation is administered, perimetry should be repeated at the end of radiation. It is unusual for vision to deteriorate during postsurgical radiation therapy.

If, however, the original treatment is radiation alone, the visual field should be monitored at the midpoint and at the completion of radiation therapy. This is because of the unlikely but real possibility of a radiation-induced tumor swelling, producing further visual loss or on rare occasions pituitary apoplexy.[91] Should apoplexy occur, immediate surgical evacuation of the tumor is required.

The utilization of bromocriptine in the treatment of prolactin-secreting pituitary tumors has had promising initial results. It is not possible at present to say at what intervals visual field examination in these patients should be performed. Our recommendations are listed in Table 1-2. Larger tumors should be followed more frequently than microadenomas.

Following the apparently successful treatment of a parachiasmal mass lesion with initial return of visual function, the patient may experience a deterioration of vision or a worsening of the visual field defects. In this circumstance the following causes should be considered.

Tumor recurrence

Recurrence or continued growth of treated pituitary adenoma must be considered as a cause of progressive visual loss. Hollenhorst and Younge[37] reported 213 recurrences in 781 patients following treatment for pituitary tumors. However, they did not differentiate between patients who received radiation following surgery and those who did not. Ray and Patterson[76] reported that the recurrence rate following surgery combined with radiation was 8%, while the recurrence rate following surgery alone was 22%.

In the pre-CT era, diagnosis of tumor recurrence was dependent largely upon the reappearance or progression of visual signs or symptoms. Muhr et al.[68] examined the CT scans of 25 asymptomatic patients 10 to 15 years after surgical treatment of pituitary tumors. Recurrence with suprasellar extension was found in six patients (25%). Interestingly only three of the six patients had progressive visual field defects. This suggests that reliance on perimetry alone may result in drastic underestimation of tumor recurrence rates. Conversely, the tissue seen on CT may represent residual tumor and not regrowth, since the patients reported had no immediate postoperative CT scans. In a second communication, Muhr et al. report recurrence or regrowth of pituitary adenomas up to 9 years following treatment.[67] Therefore it appears that patients treated for pituitary tumors should have repeat perimetry and sequential CT scanning in perpetuity.

Craniopharyngioma also may recur or regrow following surgery, even after so-called total excision.[1] Sequential perimetry therefore is mandatory following treatment of craniopharyngioma, although CT has the distinct advantage of detecting recurrence before it becomes visually symptomatic. Rapid deterioration of visual function in the postoperative period may reflect reformation of a cyst within a craniopharyngioma or the shifting of residual tumor into the chiasmal area. This sudden loss of vision requires immediate CT scan and further surgical decompression if indicated.

Empty sella syndrome with chiasmal prolapse

Successful treatment of pituitary tumors leaves the sella enlarged but now devoid of tumor and therefore "empty." It is stated that the chiasm may prolapse into the enlarged empty sella with the resultant traction producing chiasmal visual field loss. Olson et al.[72] reported three patients with visual loss secondary to chiasmal prolapse. The first patient experienced sudden worsening of vision following surgery. Intracranial exploration revealed downward displacement of the chiasm into the empty sella. Correction of the prolapse resulted in slight improvement of vision but not of the bitemporal hemianopia. The second patient was an acromegalic who received radiation therapy. Vision in one eye was said to improve following surgery, but no acuities or visual fields were documented. The third patient had a suprasellar cyst, and vision was said to be improved following drainage. Decker and Carras[21] reported an isolated instance of chiasmal prolapse with preoperative and postoperative visual field documentation, showing dramatic visual improvement following elevation of the chiasm from within the sella.

Mortara and Norrell[66] state that visual loss with a deficient sellar diaphragm may be produced by the pushing down or kinking of an optic nerve or chiasm. Five of their ten patients were said to have experienced visual loss. However, two patients had "tubular" fields, which were likely to have been functional; one patient had acute visual loss, headache, and a bitemporal hemianopia, probably representing pituitary apoplexy with destruction of the tumor. Of the two remaining patients with bitemporal hemianopias, one had previous radiation therapy, and at surgery dense arachnoidal adhesions were noted. In this case the hemianopia may have been secondary to radiation effect. The last patient had an incomplete bitemporal hemianopia (fields not shown), but at surgery it only "appeared" as if the chiasm dipped into the sella.

Given the number of transsphenoidal procedures performed for pituitary tumors that then result in a secondary empty sella, the infrequency of chiasmal prolapse speaks to the rarity of this syndrome. If chiasmal prolapse is suspected, CT scan with metrizamide injection should reveal the empty sella with the prolapsed chiasm. Without this documentation, we advocate that ''chiasmopexy'' with packing of the sella and elevation of the chiasm is to be avoided.

Radiation injury to anterior visual pathways

The onset of radiation injury syndrome typically occurs 12 to 24 months after radiation therapy has been completed (see Part II of this chapter) and may be signaled by a rather sudden and dramatic loss of visual function following months of sustained improvement.

Chiasmal radiation doses of over 200 rads per day have been implicated as the cause of this syndrome, even if the total dose remains within accepted limits (4,500 to 5,000 rads).[34,59] The mechanism by which the visual defect is produced remains speculative. Direct radiation effect with necrosis of the chiasm or necrosis secondary to vasculitis are the two theories most frequently advanced. However, an allergic reaction has been suggested as the reason for the typical delay from time of radiation to the onset of visual loss.[17] Acromegalic patients may be more susceptible to developing decreased vision as a result of the radiotherapy than are patients radiated for other parachiasmal mass lesions.[2]

The patient who has the reappearance of chiasmal or prechiasmal visual loss months after radiation therapy must have a CT scan. If there is no evidence of tumor recurrence or cyst formation in the suprasellar cistern, the diagnosis of optic nerve or chiasmal radiation necrosis should be entertained. We believe that these patients should not be subjected to surgical exploration to rule out the remote possibility of arachnoiditis (see below).

Systemic corticosteroid therapy can improve the edema associated wtih radiation necrosis of the brain parenchyma but not the necrosis itself. In these patients corticosteroids should be instituted but should not be continued beyond 2 weeks if no clinical improvement is evident.[59]

Chiasmal arachnoiditis

Chiasmal arachnoiditis is characterized by inflammatory changes in the arachnoid of the chiasm producing chiasmal visual field defects. This entity enjoyed wide acceptance in the early part of this century, but with more sophisticated neuroradiologic techniques and a better understanding of optic nerve dysfunction the significance of this disorder as a frequent cause of visual loss is questionable. There is little doubt, however, that rarely chiasmal adhesions can follow meningitis, trauma, irradiation, or surgery in the parachiasmal area.

Several reports have proposed that this disorder occurs frequently but is often overlooked. However, there is reason to question the authenticity of the diagnosis of chiasmal arachnoiditis in many of the cases. Two brothers were reported as having chiasmal arachnoiditis (case 1/A); however, one patient probably had demyelinating disease. His brother's bilateral central scotomas also failed to improve following surgery. A second sibling pair experienced bilateral acute optic neuropathy with pallor in the papillomacular bundle (''temporal half of the discs''). The third set of young brothers had bilateral acute optic neuropathies, the first (case 3/A) having bilateral "papilledema." In addition there was a history of visual loss in a maternal uncle. These last two sibling pairs are clinically indistinguishable from patients with Leber's hereditary optic neuropathy.[42]

Iraci et al.[43] reported their experience in 82 patients with chiasmal arachnoiditis. Patients with previous neurosurgery, irradiation, or trauma were excluded from consideration. It is stated that neuroradiologic studies were not always reliable in making the diagnosis, nor were the visual field defects (none are shown in the report) recognizable as typically chiasmal defects. Given these two factors, it is difficult to be sure that the localization for the visual loss is truly chiasmal. These authors urge, on the basis of their review, that surgery be performed on all suspected cases of optochiasmatic arachnoiditis. They state that the risks of craniotomy do not seem to outweigh the potential benefits of surgery. However, close inspection of their data shows a mortality rate of 6.1% (5/82), while only 9 of 82 patients regained useful vision. Their data do not appear to support their conclusions regarding the existence or proposed treatment of optochiasmatic arachnoiditis. Because of the probable varied causes of the visual deficits in these 82 patients, we would discourage surgical exploration of the chiasm in the absence of a recognizable chiasmal visual field defect or abnormal neuroradiologic studies including metrizamide cisternography.

SPECIFIC CAUSES OF THE CHIASMAL SYNDROME
Pituitary tumors

Pituitary adenomas are the lesions that most frequently cause chiasmal visual field defects in adults. In a series from the Mayo Clinic[37] 42% of patients with pituitary adenomas had visual loss as the presenting complaint. Chamlin et al. report bitemporal hemianopias in 96% of their 109 patients with chromophobe adenomas.[14]

Visual loss is typically slowly progressive so that the patient is usually unaware of peripheral field loss. Frequently there are only vague complaints of visual difficulty, whose true nature goes undetected until perimetry is performed. Although the progression of visual field defects is usually slow, there is a rather dramatic form of chiasmal syndrome associated with apoplectic visual loss/pituitary apoplexy.

Pituitary apoplexy. Pituitary apoplexy is precipitated by the rapid expansion of a pituitary tumor due to either infarction of or hemorrhage into the tumor. The exact mechanism for this event remains unknown. Rapid tumor growth outstripping its blood supply or compression of the tumor's vascular supply by the mass itself may cause ischemic necrosis of the tumor.[9,78]

In one series of 560 consecutive cases of pituitary adenoma 51 (9.1%) patients had symptoms of pituitary apoplexy, with 38 of the events being classified as major (disturbances of consciousness, hemiparesis, loss of vision, or ocular motor palsy). Forty-two patients (7.5%) had hemorrhaged into their tumors but had manifested no clinical symptoms of pituitary apoplexy.[89] Apoplexy probably occurs more frequently than is clinically apparent.

Symptoms of pituitary apoplexy. *Headache* is usually of sudden onset and severe enough to be frequently mistaken for a ruptured aneurysm. It may be generalized or retrobulbar in location. *Double vision* may be due to unilateral or bilateral ophthalmoplegia. The third, fourth, and sixth cranial nerves are usually compromised in the cavernous sinus. *Subarachnoid hemorrhage* is not present in all patients with pituitary apoplexy. While a grossly bloody CSF is the rule, xanthochromia, pleocytosis, or a normal CSF may be encountered. Headache, double vision, and subarachnoid hemorrhage have been called the classic triad of pituitary apoplexy.[20]

Visual loss does not occur in every patient with pituitary apoplexy. However, when vision is compromised, the patient may be blind bilaterally or manifest any of the patterns of chiasmal visual loss (Fig. 1-19).

Coma was an almost constant finding in the earlier publications dealing with pituitary apoplexy. It is now recognized that some patients may have a relative paucity of symptoms and still have undergone apoplexy.

Diagnosis. Any patient with a preexisting pituitary tumor who develops these rapidly evolving symptoms must be considered to have pituitary apoplexy. Patients who present with headache, ophthalmoplegia, and signs of meningeal irritation are usually diagnosed as having a ruptured intracranial aneurysm. A skull roentgenogram that reveals changes in the sella turcica should alert the clinician to the possibility of apoplexy. While CT scanning is frequently helpful diagnostically, even with high-resolution scanning there are no recognized pathognomonic signs of pituitary apoplexy.[75]

Contributing factors. Several factors have been clearly implicated in precipitating pituitary apoplexy: radiation therapy[91] and trauma and pregnancy.[20,88] Maygar and Marshall[58] found that with the use of clomiphene citrate to induce pregnancy, 39% of women with pituitary tumors developed headache and visual disturbance (type unspecified) during gestation and 30% (22 patients) required surgery or radiation therapy or both for an enlarging pituitary tumor during the pregnancy or in the puerperium. Another study described 31 induced pregnancies in 28 women following the treatment of hyperprolactinemia with bromocriptine.[7] Although the sella was enlarged radiographically in four postpartum women, the pregnancies came to term and were clinically uneventful. Bromocriptine was discontinued when pregnancy was achieved.

It appears that women with hyperprolactinemia may carry a pregnancy to term without developing pituitary apoplexy. These women, however, should be observed closely for evidence of visual fluctuation that could signal enlargement of the preexisting prolactin-secreting pituitary tumor.

Treatment. Corticosteroid replacement therapy is the first therapeutic maneuver in pituitary apoplexy. This is especially important if the patient is to be subjected to a variety of stressful neurodiagnostic procedures. Neurosurgical decompression of the anterior visual pathways is mandatory if decreased vision is present. The transsphenoidal approach has become the procedure of choice in most centers.[16,49]

Endocrinologic signs and symptoms of pituitary tumors. While visual symptoms are more common with endocrinologically inactive pituitary tumors, visual loss may be an initial complaint in all adenomas.[14,37] The endocrine changes of Cushing's disease usually prompt investigation long before the tumor achieves significant suprasellar extension, but about 37% of acromegalics in one series had visual field defects.[37] About 70% of tumors in children and adolescents are endocrinologically active and are therefore usually detected prior to the onset of visual loss.[77]

The traditional cellular classification of pituitary tumors was based on light microscopy characteristics of the tumor's chief cellular component. Recently, newer classifications of these cell types and tumors have been constructed utilizing clinical hormonal criteria as well as immunocytochemical and electromicroscopic techniques. It must be cautioned that inconsistencies exist between these newer methods of classification.[60] An adenoma may be hormonally active or inactive regardless of its cell type.

Endocrinologic abnormalities will depend on the predominant secreting (or non-secreting) cell of the tumor. A more frequent clinical problem is the female patient with amenorrhea-galactorrhea or the male patient with impotence, decreased libido, or infertility. Prolactin levels must be obtained in these patients since many will harbor prolactinomas. Prolactin levels may be elevated without clinical signs of increased prolactin secretion. Therefore serum prolactin determination is an essential portion of the pituitary tumor workup.[3] Current interest in these prolactin-secreting tumors is responsible for their early detection before suprasellar extension and visual loss occurs. Nevertheless the possibility of tumor growth with subsequent suprasellar extension supports the advisability of sequential perimetry in these patients.

Special forms of pituitary tumors

Nelson's syndrome. Nelson's syndrome is characterized by acquired cutaneous hyperpigmentation, increased concentration of ACTH, and pituitary tumor growth following total adrenalectomy for Cushing's disease.[71] The frequency with which these ACTH-producing tumors develop following adrenalectomy varies from approximately 10%[65] to 38% or higher[15] in adults and 25% in children.[38]

Any patient with Cushing's disease should have high-resolution CT scans of the sella turcica prior to adrenalectomy. Changes in the configuration of the sella may develop from months to years after adrenalectomy.[15,65] Sequential visual field testing and CT scans are recommended in these patients.

Multiple endocrine neoplasia (MEN). On occasion pituitary tumors are associated with other endocrine tumors:

MEN type I: Pituitary, parathyroid, and pancreatic tumors.
MEN type II: Pheochromocytoma plus medullary thyroid carcinoma.
MEN type III: Type II plus multiple mucosal neuromas. Prominent corneal nerves
               are visible on biomicroscopy.

"Malignant" pituitary adenomas. There is some controversy as to the existence of a truly malignant pituitary adenoma. The presence of mitosis or abnormal appearing cells does not necessarily imply malignancy. Invasive pituitary adenoma is said to be a more appropriate term.[57] These tumors produce bone destruction, escape from their capsule, invade cavernous sinus and brain (producing cranial nerve palsies and seizures), and frequently produce elevated serum prolactin levels. True carcinomas of the pituitary, on the other hand, which are characterized by blood-borne metastases, are rare.

Neuroradiologic diagnosis of pituitary adenoma

1. Skull roentgenograms show abnormalities of the sella turcica. The sella is usually enlarged, but bone destruction is seen with more invasive adenomas.
2. Hypocycloidal polytomography is an excellent modality to detect subtle thinning of sella bony structures or slanting of the floor of the pituitary fossa. This is a particularly helpful technique in women with amenorrhea-galactorrhea who frequently harbor microadenomas and in whom standard skull x-ray studies would be "normal." However, a cautionary note was sounded by Burrow et al.[12] when they found frequent false-negative as well as false-positive evidence of sellar abnormalities in 120 autopsy specimens of sphenoid bone and pituitary glands. The predictive value of a positive

tomograph was 22% and of a negative tomograph 72%, with an overall accuracy of 61%.

3. Computerized tomography (CT) has greatly simplified the radiologic diagnosis of pituitary tumors. With axial and coronal techniques the extent of the tumor can readily be appreciated so that pneumoencephalography has all but been replaced. The introduction of water-soluble contrast material (metrizamide) into the CSF during CT scanning will outline suprasellar extension. This contrast material is most helpful in visualizing isodense suprasellar cystic lesions such as craniopharyngiomas.

4. Cerebral arteriography: Transsphenoidal removal of a pituitary tumor may be accomplished safely without prior angiography. Those who prefer to perform arteriography preoperatively do so for these reasons:

   a. To be absolutely certain that the lesion is a pituitary tumor and not an aneurysm. As the resolution of CT scanning improves, this distinction becomes less difficult.

   b. To ascertain the position of the carotid arteries in relation to the planned operative field. CT scanning with contrast enhancement can frequently localize these arteries sufficiently.

   c. To detect the presence of any intracavernous vascular channel in the floor of the sella.

5. Pneumoencephalography has largely disappeared from the neuroradiologic evaluation of chiasmal syndrome in most centers.

Treatment of pituitary tumors

Surgery. Transsphenoidal microsurgical removal of pituitary tumors has become the surgical procedure of choice. It has significantly decreased the mortality and morbidity rates in patients with pituitary tumors.[52,92]

The relative and absolute indications and contraindications for transfrontal craniotomy or transsphenoidal surgery vary from surgeon to surgeon and need not be enumerated here. Large pituitary tumors as well as smaller ones may be removed via the transsphenoidal route with excellent results.[73]

Tumors with extensive extrasellar extension are difficult (or impossible) to excise totally. The goal of surgery in this situation should be to decompress the anterior visual pathways. Residual tumor may then be treated with other modalities (e.g., radiotherapy). If the surgeon does attain "total" tumor removal, radiotherapy is, or course, not indicated. Sequential CT scanning to detect possible recurrence is recommended for the long-term follow-up of both irradiated and nonirradiated patients.[67]

Radiation therapy. The role of radiation in the treatment of pituitary tumors remains controversial. CT scanning now permits sequential visualization of the original tumor bed to detect recurrence or regrowth of tumor. Many clinicians routinely utilize radiotherapy following transsphenoidal decompression since the recurrence rate of nonradiated tumors may be as high as 100%.[83] Ray and Patterson[76] found a 22% recurrence rate following surgery alone, but with radiation following surgery the rate fell to 8%.

The use of radiation as the primary treatment modality for pituitary tumors has certain disadvantages:

1. Surgery results in immediate decompression of the anterior visual pathways, whereas the beneficial effects of radiation are delayed.

2. The tissue type of the tumor and thus its radiosensitivity can only be ascertained with certainty by histologic examination. Epidermoid tumors or craniopharyn-

giomas can, at times, be indistinguishable radiographically from pituitary adenomas.

3. Even radiosensitive tumors may have cystic components that are relatively radioresistant.

It is difficult to compare meaningfully the efficacy of surgery and radiation. Many patients treated with radiation alone are in poorer medical condition, and frequently their tumors have little to no suprasellar extension. There is no doubt that the mortality and morbidity rate with radiation is lower than that of surgery. However, when visual loss is present, rapid decompression (surgical) of the optic nerves and chiasm seems more reasonable, although no data exist to prove this unequivocally. Moreover, radiation therapy is not without complications. Radiation may produce delayed vasculitis of the optic nerves or chiasm with subsequent visual loss and has been implicated as a contributing factor to pituitary apoplexy. There is also some evidence that acromegalic patients treated with radiation are at risk to develop radiation vasculitis.[2] Given the technical advancements in microneurosurgery, the transsphenoidal excision of these usually small pituitary adenomas is recommended.[87]

Medical treatment. Bromocriptine is a welcome alternative to the risks of surgery and radiation in the therapy of pituitary tumors. Most clinically inactive pituitary tumors actually have a high prolactin-secreting portion. These tumors are thus susceptible to shrinkage with bromocriptine, an ergot derivative and dopamine agonist. The exact mechanism(s) by which bromocriptine lowers prolactin levels and reduces tumor size remains unknown. Dopamine receptors are present on pituitary lactotrophs, and their stimulation (by ergot derivatives) probably causes decreased synthesis and release of prolactin. There is, in addition, likely a direct (but yet unknown) effect on the hypothalamus. In animals, dopamine agents reduce mitotic activity of pituitary cells that are stimulated by estrogen.[85] Recent reports have documented dramatic reduction in tumor size and the reversal of visual loss with bromocriptine.[29,62,63,85]

It is not yet clear if these prolactin-secreting tumors will reappear with the cessation of bromocriptine therapy. It has been shown that patients with large tumors will experience sustained suppression of prolactin secretion following bromocriptine withdrawal. This sustained effect was not appreciated in patients with microadenomas or macroadenomas with only moderately elevated serum prolactin levels.[26]

Craniopharyngioma

These tumors arise from nests of squamous epithelial cells that are the remnants of Rathke's pouch and that lie between the anterior and posterior lobes of the pituitary gland. They are found in children (13% of all intracranial tumors) more frequently than in adults (3% of all tumors). Craniopharyngiomas may be solid, cystic, or a combination of the two. The cysts are frequently filled with a thick viscous fluid and glistening cholesterol-like material.

The clinical manifestations of craniopharyngioma vary according to the time of life in which the tumor presents (Table 1-3). In children under 15, visual difficulty and headache are the most frequent findings.[5,6,47,61] Growth retardation or other endocrinologic disturbances and papilledema occur in at least one half of the patients in this age group. In older patients visual loss is still of paramount importance, but papilledema is uncommon. Endocrinologic abnormalities occur as well, and about one third of patients in the older age group are demented or have some other problem with mentation.

Table 1-3. Clinical signs and symptoms in craniopharyngioma

	Banna et al.[5]	Matson and Crigler[61]	Kennedy and Smith[47]	Bartlett[6]
Children under age 15	N = 57	N = 57	N = 19	N = 30
Visual defects	64%	64%	60% (VF 50%)	76%
Papilledema	31%	31%	45%	73%
Endocrine abnormalities	94%	47%	43%	46%
Headache	66%	80%	100%	—
Vomiting	50%	34%	65%	—
Adults	N = 85		N = 26	N = 55
Visual defects	80%	—	64% (VF 64%)	74%
Endocrine abnormalities	57%	—	75%	32%
Dementia	10%	—	35%	32%
Papilledema	15%	—	15%	5%
Headache	39%	—	60%	—

VF = visual fields.

Visual field abnormalities are found in the majority of patients with craniopharyngioma. This slowly expanding, at times cystic, tumor results in compression and distortion of the chiasm and surrounding structures. The bitemporal hemianopia is the single most frequently detected abnormality; however, incongruous homonymous hemianopia of optic tract origin is plotted as well.[81]

The diagnosis of craniopharyngioma is made on the basis of the clinical findings, which vary according to the patients age and in particular with the plotting of chiasmal or optic tract visual field defects. Skull roentgenograms may be abnormal in over 90% of childhood craniopharyngiomas, with calcification being the rule in this age group.[4] Computerized tomography reveals the extent of the lesion and whether it is solid or cystic. Certain craniopharyngiomas may escape initial CT detection since their radiodensity may be similar to that of surrounding normal brain or have a large cystic component. Metrizamide studies will on occasion be necessary in order to outline these tumors (Fig. 1-20).

The preferred therapy of craniopharyngioma is controversial and varies from total resection[36,61] to radiotherapy following biopsy[50] to a combination of surgery and radiation.[82] Recent technologic developments have repopularized the transsphenoidal approach to these tumors.[51]

Meningioma

Meningioma of the suprasellar area (tuberculum sellae and planum sphenoidale) are slow-growing tumors that frequently are undiagnosed before significant visual loss is sustained.[27] The visual loss initially may be monocular. Pregnancy may stimulate the rapid growth of these tumors and accelerate the tempo of visual loss.[24]

The pattern of visual field deficit is dependent on the site of the tumor and the position of the chiasm (see earlier discussion at the beginning of this chapter). One or both optic discs are usually pale. Rarely, however, one disc may be edematous while its fellow is atrophic, a combination of findings that constitutes part of the Foster-Kennedy syndrome (which also includes anosmia and dementia).[46] The Foster-Kennedy syndrome is seen with large subfrontal masses of any type that compress one optic nerve (ipsilateral

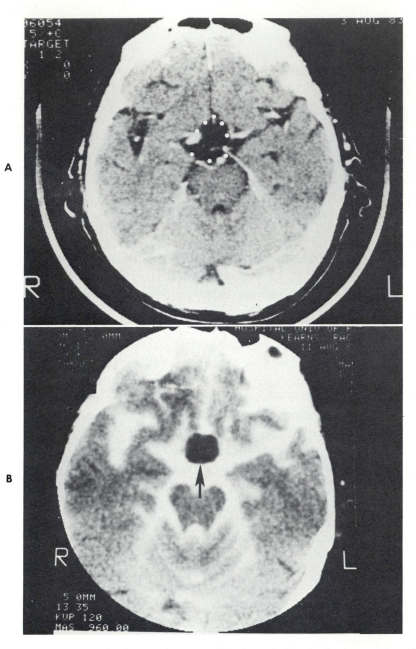

Fig. 1-20. Suprasellar arachnoid cyst. **A,** Suprasellar cistern (white dots) appears enlarged, but no mass is seen. **B,** After metrizamide is injected in subarachnoid space a prominent mass (arrow) is seen on axial as well as coronal, **C,** images.

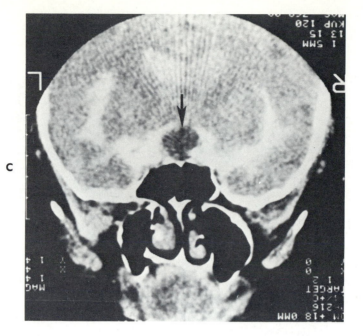

Fig. 1-20, cont'd. For legend see opposite page.

disc pallor) and the foramen of Monro, causing hydrocephalus and therefore contralateral papilledema.

Neuroradiologic investigations may reveal alteration in surrounding bone (blistering) even on plain x-ray films or polytomography. Although not pathognomonic,[54] this hyperostosis is a rather sensitive indicator of meningioma. CT scanning will reveal a mass lesion with various degrees of contrast enhancement depending on the vascularity of the tumor. Since meningiomas are frequently vascular, arteriography is a prudent step prior to attempted neurosurgical extirpation.

The preferred treatment of meningioma is surgical removal. However, total removal may not always be possible or advisable if critical structures are densely encased by tumor. There is, as yet, no convincing evidence that meningiomas are radiosensitive.

Glioma

Optic glioma is a term that has been applied to gliomatous infiltration of one or both optic nerves and to its extension into the optic chiasm, hypothalamus, optic tract, and third ventricle. Since the natural history of the disorder is far from clear, the role or efficacy of treatment remains debatable.

Gliomas usually occur in children below age 10. Miller et al.[64] have suggested a topographic distinction into three groups: (1) glioma of only one optic nerve, (2) glioma of the optic chiasm, and (3) glioma with involvement of the hypothalamus and third ventricle structures. The first two groups (anterior tumors) are associated with a favorable prognosis, while the latter group (posterior tumors) has a poorer but not invariably fatal outcome. In essence it is the location rather than the cytologic characteristics that affects prognosis.[35,74] These are histologically benign tumors that become functionally "malignant" when vital structures are involved.

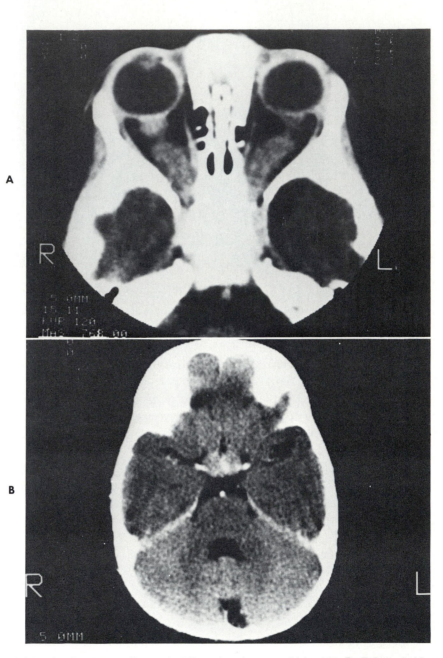

Fig. 1-21. Visual pathway glioma. **A,** Bilateral optic nerve thickening. **B,** Enlarged chiasm with calcification. **C,** Extension of glioma into both optic tracts.

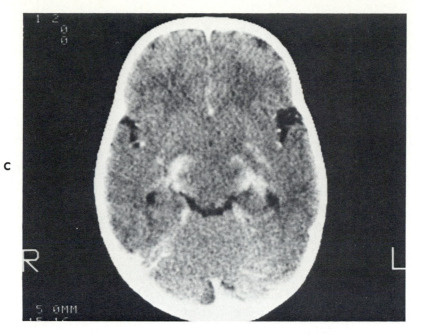

Fig. 1-21, cont'd. For legend see opposite page.

The typical patient with a chiasmal glioma presents with headache and visual loss and has a 20% to 30% incidence of neurofibromatosis. Proptosis usually indicates optic nerve involvement. The visual field deficits are not overwhelmingly chiasmal in nature despite the localization of the tumor.[30] In posterior tumors, diabetes insipidus, the diencephalic syndrome, or other hypothalamic signs or symptoms are evident.

The diagnosis of optic glioma may be suggested neuroradiologically, especially with high-resolution CT scanning[19] (Fig. 1-21). Surgical exploration and biopsy has its advocates,[56,64,69] as does nonintervention.[30,39] Others favor excision of optic nerve lesions and radiation of chiasmal gliomas should progression be documented neuroradiologically or neuro-ophthalmologically.[74]

A more aggressive form of optic glioma is found in adults. The syndrome occurs in middle-aged patients with a possible male predominance and is characterized by rapid visual loss mimicking optic neuritis. The visual loss progresses within 5 to 6 weeks to total blindness and is invariably fatal within months. Funduscopic examination shows disc edema, which may progress to complete arterial and venous occlusion.

Histopathologically the tumor involves the entire anterior optic pathway and appears to spread via the subpial and dural routes. No effective treatment is known; in fact the diagnosis is rarely entertained before death.[33,41]

Many unusual mass lesions in the chiasmal area will produce one of the four visual field abnormalities of chiasmal disease. It is not the specific etiology of the chiasmal syndrome that should be of concern initially, but the localization as indicated by the visual fields.

Aneurysm

Aneurysmal dilatation of the vessels of the circle of Willis is an infrequent cause of chiasmal syndrome.[90] The combination of CT scanning and cerebral arteriography serves to establish the origin of the aneurysm as well as the extent of its mass effect.

Infection

Infective processes of the sphenoid sinus or intrasellar abscess formation may masquerade as pituitary tumors.

Mucoceles in the posterior ethmoid and sphenoid sinuses may produce slowly progressive visual loss or more infrequently sudden visual loss similar to pituitary apoplexy. Chiasmal syndromes from sphenoid mucoceles, while they do exist, are rare. Mucoceles more often produce unilateral or bilateral optic nerve involvement.[31]

Pituitary abscess is uncommon but of importance because of its curability if promptly diagnosed. Patients may present with signs of a chiasmal syndrome or meningitis. In almost all instances the sellar area is abnormal radiologically. Interestingly, abscess formation may occur in a preexisting tumor in the area.[22]

The source of the infection is not always easily identified. Cultures are said to be "sterile" in more than half the patients.[55] It has been proposed, however, that this may be due to the abscesses' being caused largely by anaerobic organisms.[22]

Transsphenoidal drainage of the abscess combined with the appropriate antibiotic coverage is the treatment of choice. The prognosis is guarded since the overall mortality is 28%, increasing to 45% if meningitis develops.[22]

Nontumorous causes of chiasmal syndromes

When a chiasmal visual field abnormality is noted, the physician should go to all reasonable lengths to exclude a mass lesion. Rarely, however, a mass is not present, and the visual defect is due to one of the following noncompressive lesions.

Inflammation. Inflammatory optic neuropathies rarely may be associated with a superior temporal visual depression in the fellow eye (junction scotoma). Bitemporal hemianopias have been reported with demyelinating disease[79,84] and sarcoidosis.[32] CT scanning may reveal an enlarged chiasm, but tumors are readily excluded.

Ischemia. Ischemic chiasmal syndrome may be produced by a variety of causes.[53] Again, the duty of the physician is to diagnose the site of the lesion (by perimetry) and to rule out a compressive lesion.

Trauma. Traumatic chiasmal syndrome is usually, but not invariably, accompanied by skull fracture, severe frontal trauma, and associated neurologic signs and symptoms. Diabetes insipidus is a frequent finding.[80]

Traction. Prolapse of the chiasm into a primary empty sella has been implicated as a cause of chiasmal visual loss, but we are not convinced of a cause-and-effect relationship. The empty sella syndrome (ESS) probably results from extension of the subarachnoid space into the sella through a congenitally incompetent diaphragma sellae.

Jordon et al.[44] described 12 patients with primary ESS, two of whom had "generalized peripheral field constrictions." No chiasmal field defects were found. Cupps and Woolf[18] reported a 58-year-old woman with ESS with vision remaining only in the left inferior homonymous quadrant. At surgery, however, neither optic nerve was under tension, nor had the chiasm prolapsed into the sella.

An association does exist between the ESS and pseudotumor cerebri. In one report, four of eight patients with both entities had visual field loss. However, all patients with visual field defects had papilledema. One patient was said to have "bitemporal hemianopia," but no fields were shown. The other field defects could all be attributed to the disc edema and not the ESS with chiasmal prolapse. No patient with ESS without papilledema had a visual field defect.[28]

Buckman et al.[10] presented a thoroughly evaluated (neuro-ophthalmologically and neuroradiologically) alcoholic patient with a subtle bitemporal hemianopia. Since an empty sella was found, this was said to be the cause of the hemianopia. Craniotomy was not performed; therefore positive proof of chiasmal prolapse is lacking.

The prevalence of ESS as determined at autopsy is approximately 5%.[13] If ESS is a significant cause of visual loss, we would expect to see visual loss more frequently. Thus diagnosis of an empty sella as the cause of chiasmal visual field loss should be made cautiously. In most instances the true etiology will be an undetected mass lesion.

REFERENCES

1. Amacher, AL: Craniopharyngioma. The controversy regarding radiotherapy, Childs Brain 6:57, 1980.
2. Atkinson, AB, Allen, IV, Gordon, DS, et al: Progressive visual failure in acromegaly following external pituitary irradiation, Clin Endocrinol 10:469, 1979.
3. Balagura, S, Frantz, AG, Housepian, EM, et al: The specificity of serum prolactin as a diagnostic indicator of pituitary adenoma, J Neurosurg 51:42, 1979.
4. Banna, M. Craniopharyngioma: based on 160 cases, Br J Radiol 49:206, 1976.
5. Banna, M, Hoare, RD, Stanley, P, et al: Craniopharyngioma in children, J Pediatr 83:781, 1973.
6. Bartlett, JR: Craniopharyngiomas: a summary of 85 cases, J Neurol Neurosurg Psychiatry 34:37, 1971.
7. Bergh, T, Nillius, SJ, Larsson, SG, et al: Effects of bromocriptine-induced pregnancy on prolactin-secreting pituitary tumours, Acta Endrocrinol 98:333, 1981.
8. Bergland, RM, Ray, BS, and Torack, RM: Anatomical variations in the pituitary gland and adjacent structures in 225 human autopsy cases, J Neurosurg 28:93, 1968.
9. Brougham, P, Heusner, AP, and Adams, RD: Acute degenerative changes in adenomas of the pituitary body with special reference to pituitary apoplexy, J Neurosurg 7:421, 1950.
10. Buckman, MT, Husain, M, Carlow, TJ, et al: Primary empty sella syndrome with visual field defects, Am J Med 61:124, 1976.
11. Burde, RM: Pituitary tumors reassessed, Am J Ophthalmol 89:874, 1980.
12. Burrow, GN, Wortzman, G, Rewcastle, NB, et al: Microadenomas of the pituitary and abnormal sellar tomograms in an unselected autopsy series, N Engl J Med 304:156, 1981.
13. Busch, W: Die Morphologie der Sella Turcica und ihre Beziehungen zur Hypophyse, Arch Pathol Anat 320:437, 1951.
14. Chamlin, M, Davidoff, LM, and Feiring, EH: Ophthalmologic changes produced by pituitary tumors, Am J Ophthalmol 40:353, 1955.
15. Cohen, KL, Noth, RH, and Pechinski, T: Incidence of pituitary tumors following adrenalectomy, Arch Intern Med 138:575, 1978.
16. Conomy, JP, Ferguson, JH, Brodkey, JS, et al: Spontaneous infarction in pituitary tumors: neurologic and therapeutic aspects, Neurology (Minneap) 25:580, 1975.
17. Crompton, MR, and Layton, DD: Delayed radionecrosis of the brain following therapeutic x-radiation of the pituitary, Brain 84:85, 1961.
18. Cupps, TR, and Woolf, PD: Primary empty sella syndrome with panhypopituitarism, diabetes insipidus, and visual field defects, Acta Endocrinol 89:445, 1978.
19. Daniels, DL, Haughton, VM, Williams, AL, et al: Computed tomography of the optic chiasm, Radiology 137:123, 1980.
20. David, NJ, Gargano, FP, and Glaser, JS: Pituitary apoplexy in clinical perspective. In Glaser, JS, and Smith, JL, editors: Neuroophthalmology symposium of the University of Miami and the Bascom Palmer Eye Institute, vol 8, St Louis, 1975, The CV Mosby Co, p 140.
21. Decker, RE, and Carras, R: Transsphenoidal chiasmapexy for correction of posthypophysectomy traction syndrome of the optic chiasm, J Neurosurg 46:527, 1977.
22. Dominque, JN, and Wilson, CB: Pituitary abscesses, J Neurosurg 46:601, 1977.
23. Druckman, R, Ellis, P, Kleinfeld, J, et al: See-saw nystagmus, Arch Ophthalmol 76:668, 1966.

24. Ehlers, N, and Malmros, R: The suprasellar meningioma. A review of the literature and presentation of a series of 31 cases, Acta Ophthalmol [Suppl] 121:1, 1973.

25. Elkington, SG: Pituitary adenoma. Preoperative symptomatology in a series of 260 patients, Br J Ophthalmol 52:322, 1968.

26. Eversmann, T, Fahlbusch, R, Rjosk, HK, et al: Persisting suppression of prolactin secretion after long-term treatment with bromocriptine in patients with prolactinomas, Acta Endocrinol 92:413, 1979.

27. Finn, JE, and Mount, LA: Meningiomas of the tuberculum sellae and planum sphenoidale. A review of 83 cases, Arch Ophthalmol 92:23, 1974.

28. Foley, KM, and Posner, JB: Does pseudotumor cerebri cause the empty sella syndrome? Neurology (Minneap) 25:565, 1975.

29. George, SR, Burrow, GN, Zinman, B, et al: Regression of pituitary tumors, a possible effect of brom-ergocryptine, Am J Med 66:697, 1979.

30. Glaser, JS, Hoyt, WF, and Corbett, J: Visual morbidity with chiasmal glioma, Arch Ophthalmol 85:3, 1971.

31. Goodwin, JA, and Glaser, JS: Chiasmal syndrome in sphenoid sinus mucocele, Ann Neurol 4:440, 1978.

32. Gudeman, SK, Selhorst, JB, Susac, JO, and Waybright, EA: Sarcoid optic neuropathy, Neurology (Minneap) 32:597, 1982.

33. Harper, CG, and Stewart-Wynne, EG: Malignant optic gliomas in adults, Arch Neurol 35:731, 1978.

34. Harris, JR, and Levene, MB: Visual complications following irradiation for pituitary adenomas and craniopharyngiomas, Radiology 120:167, 1976.

35. Heiskanen, O, Raitta, C, and Torsti, R: The management and prognosis of gliomas of the optic pathways in children, Acta Neurochir 43:193, 1978.

36. Hoffman, HJ, Hendrick, EB, Humphreys, RP, et al: Management of craniopharyngioma in children, J Neurosurg 47:218, 1977.

37. Hollenhorst, RW, and Younge, BR: Ocular manifestations produced by adenomas of the pituitary gland: analysis of 1000 cases. In Kohler, PO, and Ross, GT, editors: Diagnosis and treatment of pituitary tumors, New York, 1973, American Elsevier Publishing Co, p 53.

38. Hopwood, NJ, and Kenny, FM: Incidence of Nelson's syndrome after adrenalectomy for Cushing's disease in children, Am J Dis Child 131:1353, 1977.

39. Hoyt, WF, and Baghdassarian, SB: Optic glioma of childhood. Natural history and rationale for conservative management, Br J Ophthalmol 53:793, 1969.

40. Hoyt, WF, and Luis, O: The primate chiasm, Arch Ophthalmol 70:69, 1963.

41. Hoyt, WF, Meshel, LG, Lessell, S, et al: Malignant optic glioma of adulthood, Brain 96:121, 1973.

42. Iraci, G, Gerosa, LT, Gerosa, M, et al: Opto-chiasmatic arachnoiditis in brothers, Ann Ophthalmol 11:479, 1979.

43. Iraci, G, Secchi, AG, Gerosa, M, et al: Opto-chiasmatic ''flogosis.'' Doc Ophthalmol Proc Series 17:261, 1979.

44. Jordon, RM, Kendall, JW, and Kerber, CW: The primary empty sella syndrome, Am J Med 62:569, 1977.

45. Kayan, A, and Earl, CJ: Compressive lesions of the optic nerves and chiasm. Pattern of recovery of vision following surgical treatment, Brain 98:13, 1975.

46. Kennedy, F: Retrobulbar neuritis as an exact diagnostic sign of certain tumors and abscesses in the frontal lobe, Am J Med Sci 142:355, 1911.

47. Kennedy, HB, and Smith, RJS: Eye signs in craniopharyngioma, Br J Ophthalmol 59:689, 1975.

48. Kirkham, TH: The ocular symptomology of pituitary tumors, Proc R Soc Med 65:517, 1972.

49. Kosary, IZ, Braham, J, Tadmor, R, et al: Transsphenoidal surgical approach in pituitary apoplexy, Neurochirurgia 19:55, 1976.

50. Kramer, S, Southard, M, and Mansfield, CM: Radiotherapy in the management of craniopharyngiomas: further experiences and late results, Am J Roentgenol Radium Ther Nucl Med 103:44, 1968.

51. Laws, ER, Jr: Transsphenoidal microsurgery in the management of craniopharyngiomas, J Neurosurg 52:661, 1980.

52. Laws, ER, Jr, and Kern, EB: Complications of transsphenoidal surgery. In Tindal, GT, and Collins, WF, editors: Clinical management of pituitary disorders, New York, 1979, Raven Press, p 435.

53. Lee, KF, Schatz, NJ, and Savino, PJ: Ischemic chiasmal syndrome. In Glaser, JS, and Smith, JL, editors: Neuroophthalmology, Symposium of the University of Miami and the Bascom Palmer Eye Institute, vol 8, St Louis, 1975, The CV Mosby Co, p 115.

54. Lee, KF, Whiteley, WH, III, Schatz, NJ, et al: Juxtasellar hyperostosis of non-meningiomatous origin, J Neurosurg 44:571, 1976.

55. Lindholm, J, Rasmussen, P, and Korsgaard, O: Intrasellar or pituitary abscess, J Neurosurg 38:616, 1973.

56. Lowes, M, Bojsen-Moller, M, Vorre, P, et al: An evaluation of gliomas of the anterior visual pathways. A 10-year survey, Acta Neurochir 43:201, 1978.

57. Lundberg, PO, Drettner, B, Hemmingsson, A, et al: The invasive pituitary adenoma, Arch Neurol 34:742, 1977.

58. Magyar, DM, and Marshall, JR: Pituitary tumors and pregnancy, Am J Obstet Gynecol 132:739, 1978.

59. Martin, AN, Johnston, JS, Henry, JM, et al: Delayed radiation necrosis of the brain, J Neurosurg 47:336, 1977.

60. Martinez, AJ, Lee, A, Moossy, J, et al: Pituitary adenomas: clinicopathological and immunohistochemical study, Ann Neurol 7:24, 1980.

61. Matson, DD, and Crigler, JF, Jr: Management of craniopharyngioma in childhood, J Neurosurg 30:377, 1969.

62. McGregor, AM, Scanlon, MF, Hall, K, et al: Reduction of size of a pituitary tumor by bromocriptine therapy, N Engl J Med 300:291, 1979.

63. McGregor, AM, Scanlon, MF, Hall, R, et al: Effects of bromocriptine in pituitary tumor size, Br Med J 2:700, 1979.

64. Miller, NR, Iliff, WJ, and Green, WR: Evaluation and management of gliomas of the anterior visual pathways, Brain 97:743, 1974.

65. Moore, TJ, Dluhy, RG, Williams, GH, et al: Nelson's syndrome: frequency, prognosis and effect of prior pituitary irradiation, Ann Intern Med 85:731, 1976.

66. Mortara, R, and Norrell, H: Consequences of a deficient sellar diaphragm, J Neurosurg 32:565, 1970.

67. Muhr, C, Bergström, K, Enoksson, P, et al: Follow-up study with computerized tomography and clinical evaluation 5 to 10 years after surgery for pituitary adenoma, J Neurosurg 53:144, 1980.

68. Muhr, C, Bergström, K, Hugosson, R, and Lundberg, PO: Pituitary adenomas: computed tomography and clinical evaluation in a follow-up after surgical treatment, Eur Neurol 19:171, 1980.

69. Myles, ST, and Murphy, SB: Gliomas of the optic nerve and chiasm, Can J Ophthalmol 8:508, 1973.

70. Nachtigaller, H, and Hoyt, WF: Storungen des Seheindruckes bei bitemporaler Hemianopsie und Verschiebung der Sehachsen, Klin Monatsbl Augenheilkd 156:821, 1970.

71. Nelson, DH, Meakin, JW, Dealy, JB, et al: ACTH-producing tumor of the pituitary gland, N Engl J Med 259:161, 1958.

72. Olson, DR, Guiot, G, and Derome, P: The symptomatic empty sella. Prevention and correction via the transsphenoidal approach, J Neurosurg 37:533, 1972.

73. Orr, LS, Schatz, NJ, Savino, PJ, et al: Transsphenoidal surgery for large pituitary tumors. In Glaser, JS, editor: Neuro-ophthalmology Symposium of the University of Miami and the Bascom Palmer Eye Institute, vol 9, St Louis, 1977, The CV Mosby Co, p 128.

74. Oxenhandler, DC, and Sayers, MP: The dilemma of childhood optic gliomas, J Neurosurg 48:34, 1978.

75. Post, MJD, David, NJ, and Glaser, JS, et al: Pituitary apoplexy: diagnosis by computed tomography, Radiology 134:665, 1980.

76. Ray, BS, and Patterson, RH, Jr: Surgical experience with chromophobe adenomas of the pituitary gland, J Neurosurg 34:726, 1971.

77. Richmond, IL, and Wilson, CB: Pituitary adenomas in childhood and adolescence, J Neurosurg 49:163, 1978.

78. Rovit, RL, and Fein, FM: Pituitary apoplexy: a review and reappraisal, J Neurosurg 37:280, 1972.

79. Sacks, JG, and Melen, O: Bitemporal visual field defects in presumed multiple sclerosis, JAMA 234:69, 1975.

80. Savino, PJ, Glaser, JS, and Schatz, NJ: Traumatic chiasmal syndrome, Neurology 30:963, 1980.

81. Savino, PJ, Paris, M, Schatz, et al: Optic tract syndrome: a review of 21 patients, Arch Ophthalmol 96:656, 1978.

82. Sharma, A, Tandon, PN, Saxena, KK, et al: Craniopharyngiomas treated by a combination of surgery and radiotherapy, Clin Radiol 25:13, 1974.

83. Sheline, GE: Treatment of chromophobe adenomas of the pituitary gland and acromegaly. In Kohler, PO, and Ross, GT, editors: Diagnosis and treatment of pituitary tumors, New York, 1973, American Elsevier Publishing Co, p 201.

84. Spector, RH, Glaser, JS, and Schatz, NJ: Demyelinative chiasmal lesions, Arch Neurol 37:757, 1980.

85. Thorner, MO, Martin, WH, Rogol, AD, et al: Rapid regression of pituitary prolactinomas during bromocriptine treatment, J Clin Endocrinol Metab 51:438, 1980.

86. Trobe, JD, and Glaser, JS: Quantitative perimetry in compressive optic neuropathy and optic neuritis, Arch Ophthalmol 96:1210, 1978.

87. Tucker, HSG, Grubb, SR, Wigand, JP, et al: The treatment of acromegaly by transsphenoidal surgery, Arch Intern Med 140:795, 1980.
88. Van Wagenen, A: Hemorrhage into a pituitary tumor following trauma, Ann Surg 95:626, 1932.
89. Wakai, S, Fukushima, T, Teramoto, A, et al: Pituitary apoplexy: its incidence and clinical significance, J Neurosurg 55:187, 1981.
90. Walsh, FB: Visual field defects due to aneurysms at the circle of Willis, Arch Ophthalmol 71:15, 1964.
91. Weisberg, LA: Pituitary apoplexy, Am J Med 63:109, 1977.
92. Wilson, CB, and Dempsey, LC: Transsphenoidal microsurgical removal of 250 pituitary adenomas, J Neurosurg 48:13, 1978.

PART IV

Postchiasmal visual loss

Lesions posterior to the optic chiasm produce homonymous hemianopias. Patients with homonymous hemianopia may present with a variety of visual signs or symptoms.

CLINICAL PRESENTATIONS

Reduced visual acuity. Decreased visual acuity in a patient with homonymous hemianopia may be seen in two circumstances. The first is the patient with a lesion that involves the area of the optic tract. The optic tract is formed by visual fibers that extend from the posterior portion of the optic chiasm to synapse at the lateral geniculate nucleus (LGN). The tracts diverge, one from the other, to sweep around the cerebral peduncles.

Lesions of the optic tract are seldom small or discrete but may involve the optic nerve or chiasm as well; therefore it is more appropriate to speak of an optic tract syndrome than an optic tract lesion. This syndrome is characterized by an incongruous homonymous hemianopia, a relative afferent pupillary defect in the eye with reduced central acuity or greater visual field loss, or both, and "hemioptic" optic atrophy (see Chapter 3). Associated neurologic signs and symptoms are not essential to the diagnosis. The lesions most frequently causing this syndrome are craniopharyngiomas, aneurysms, and pituitary tumors. A mass lesion must be excluded when an optic tract syndrome is encountered.[23]

Lesions of the LGN occur infrequently. They may result from tumors,[13] demyelination,[30] or infarction.[10]

The second circumstance in which patients may have reduced central acuity is when bilateral occipital lobe lesions occur. Sometimes the dysfunction in one occipital lobe is only temporary and is attributed to "diaschisis." This phenomenon is thought to be due to a primary decrease in metabolic rate and blood flow in the fellow occipital lobe that is, in some unknown manner, a result of the contralateral infarction.[17]

Homonymous hemianopia: reduced visual perception on one side of visual space. Patients themselves may notice difficulty with peripheral vision, such as in parking their cars. The presence of a hemianopia may be brought dramatically to their attention when a large object suddenly appears out of a previously unrecognized hemianopic field. More frequently, however, patients will have vague complaints, which they will localize to one eye, not realizing that the true difficulty is a homonymous visual field deficit. Some will complain of difficulty reading. The patient with a right homonymous hemianopia has difficulty finding the next word and continually loses his place reading across the page; the patient with a left homonymous defect cannot accurately locate the next line of print. If the homonymous hemianopia is paracentral and not complete, a tangent screen examination may be needed to plot the small defect. When a patient has difficulty reading and has normal acuity, visual field examination may reveal hemianopic defects.

Hallucinations in a homonymous field. The most frequent cause of a homonymous visual field defect is migraine. Migraineurs will also experience visual hallucinatory phenomena in a homonymous distribution. The visual abnormality is usually a small scotoma surrounded by sharp-edged lines (fortification scotoma). This small paracentral defect gradually expands to involve the entire homonymous field over a period of approximately 20 to 30 minutes and then disappears.

If a headache occurs upon resolution of the scotoma, the term *classic migraine* is applied. The scotoma is not followed by headache in *acephalgic migraine*. *Common migraine*, which is the most frequent form, does not have a visual aura preceding the headache.

Occipital tumors or arteriovenous malformations (AVM) may cause migrainelike visual symptoms. These symptoms are usually brief and not associated with the fortification spectra of classic migraine.[28] Rarely hallucinatory phenomena indistinguishable from migraine may be caused by occipital AVMs. The monotonous unilaterality of the hallucinatory phenomenon or the headache phase preceding the visual phase mandates CT scanning to search for a structural lesion[27] (Fig. 1-22).

The visual hemianopia of migraine is usually fleeting, but in rare instances a fixed neurologic deficit may be produced.[2] In these instances CT scanning demonstrates the area(s) of infarction.[3] There is some indication that the migraineur is more likely to experience complications with arteriography.[21] Oral contraceptives may precipitate or

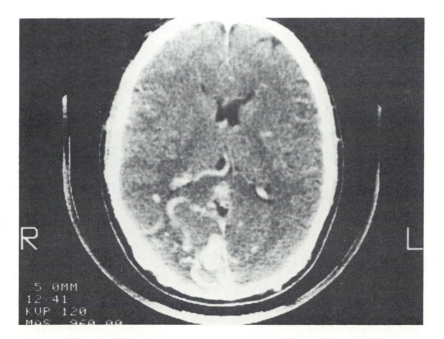

Fig. 1-22. Patient with symptoms of fortification scotoma lasting 20 minutes followed by headache always in same location. CT shows extensive AVM involving right occipital lobe.

aggravate preexisting migraine.[8] Women with migraine should avoid these drugs.

Homonymous hemianopia: associated with neurologic signs or symptoms. Lesions of the temporal and parietal lobes produce homonymous hemianopias. However, it would be distinctly unusual for these patients to present with a chief complaint of a visual disturbance since their neurologic deficits tend to outweigh any visual abnormality.

Homonymous hemianopia detected on routine examination. Patients with homonymous hemianopias may be asymptomatic, with their hemianopia being discovered on routine examination. If the patient is otherwise asymptomatic, this almost assuredly represents a silent occipital lobe infarction.[26] However, it is prudent to obtain a CT scan in all patients with homonymous hemianopias since tumors may present in an identical fashion.

DIAGNOSIS

The patient with a predominantly visual symptom who proves to have a homonymous hemianopia will usually have a lesion of the optic tract or occipital lobe. It is unlikely for patients with involvement of the temporal or parietal lobe to present initially to the ophthalmologist, since the wealth of neurologic signs and symptoms that accompany lesions in these regions usually prompt neurologic evaluation before the visual symptomatology becomes noticed by or bothersome to the patient.

The location of a lesion may be inferred by the character of the visual field loss (see below). The visual fibers in the anterior portion of the optic radiations are less highly segregated than they are posteriorly. Therefore the field defect from an anterior lesion will be less congruous than will a defect from a posterior lesion. It should be stressed, however, that complete unilateral destruction of the visual pathway at any point posterior to the chiasm will produce a total homonymous hemianopia. A total hemianopia is not localizing. Once a homonymous hemianopia is detected, CT scanning is mandatory. While sudden onset implies a vascular etiology and while a progressive course suggests a mass lesion, there is enough variability in the presentation of any lesion to make CT scanning obligatory.

SPECIFIC LESIONS OF OPTIC TRACT AND RADIATIONS
Optic tract

Isolated lesions of the optic tract or lateral geniculate body are rare. Clinically, large mass lesions that also involve the optic chiasm will produce the optic tract syndrome.[23]

Lateral geniculate nucleus

The fibers that originate in the retina synapse in the LGN, which is a triangular structure composed of six layers. Visual fibers enter the LGN anteriorly on the convex surface. Fibers from the ipsilateral eye terminate in layers 2, 3, and 5, while the contralateral fibers synapse in layers 1, 4, and 6. The superoposterior aspect of the LGN gives rise to the optic radiations.

The hallmark of LGN disease is the wedge-shaped homonymous visual field defect. The LGN obtains its vascular supply from the distal anterior choroidal and the lateral choroidal arteries. Frisén has suggested that two different syndromes result from vascular occlusion of one or the other artery. Likewise the syndrome of the distal anterior choroidal artery is characterized by loss of upper and lower homonymous sectors in the visual field with corresponding sectoral optic disc pallor.[9] The second syndrome—of the lateral choroidal artery—consists of homonymous, horizontal sectoranopia and sectoral optic atrophy.[10]

Temporal lobe

As visual fibers leave the LGN, the inferior fibers (subserving superior visual field) course anteriorly around the temporal horn to form Meyer's loop. These inferior fibers are also in close approximation to the internal capsule and the temporal isthmus. Blood supply to the temporal isthmus is provided by the anterior choroidal artery. Vascular episodes (or tumors) in this region will produce the syndrome of the temporal isthmus. If the dominant temporal lobe is affected, the patient will be aphasic, hemianopic, and will experience contralateral motor difficulties especially in the leg. A nondominant lesion produces contralateral hemianopia, hemianesthesia, and loss of body recognition.[5]

The typical temporal lobe visual field defect is a homonymous superior quadrantanopia (Fig. 1-23). There is some disagreement concerning the congruity of the visual field loss with temporal lobe lesions. Perhaps the best evidence is to be found in the patients who have undergone temporal lobectomy for epilepsy. Van Buren and Baldwin[29] encountered incongruous field defects in 23 of 33 patients subjected to temporal lobectomy for relief of epilepsy. Walker and Walsh[31] also studied field defects in patients who had undergone lobectomy. They concluded that characteristic temporal lobe visual field defects were pie-shaped sectors that extended from the vertical meridian with a sharp, congruous, straight vertical border and an irregular, ill-defined, sloping horizontal margin. They emphasized that the criteria for congruity of each examiner, as well as the results obtained with various perimetric techniques, may be different. Scrutiny of the visual field defects in both of these series shows incongruity, but the magnitude of incongruity is usually minimal. In the examination of the visual fields of 69 patients following temporal lo-

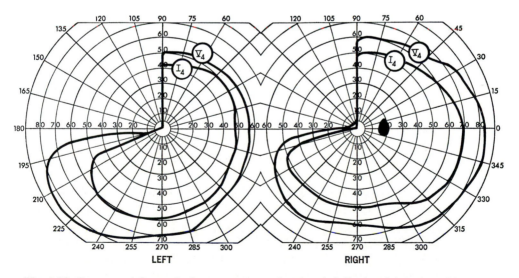

Fig. 1-23. Congruous left superior homonymous quadrantanopia following right temporal lobectomy for epilepsy.

bectomy, Jensen and Seedorff detected visual field incongruity in 20 of 51 patients who had field defects.[14] It should be noted that these authors considered 5° as the maximum allowable difference between "congruous" fields. Furthermore, temporal lobectomy may compromise the blood supply to the ipsilateral optic tract.[16] The postoperative field defect in such a case would be incongruous, but on the basis of optic tract rather than temporal lobe involvement.

Temporal lobe dysfunction may produce a variety of neurologic disturbances. Seizures may be generalized or localized. They are often preceded by an aura of an unpleasant odor or taste (uncinate fit). Dreamlike states with a feeling of déjà-vu and visual hallucinations that are usually vivid and formed are important signs of temporal lobe disease.

Parietal lobe

As the visual fibers course toward the calcarine area, their topographic organization becomes more highly segregated. However, patients with extensive parietal lobe lesions routinely have neurologic signs and symptoms that overshadow their homonymous hemianopia or inferior quadrantanopia. Lesions of the nondominant parietal lobe produce neglect of the contralateral part of the patient's visual and nonvisual environment. Formal visual fields are frequently unrewarding ventures, which are frustrating for both the patient and perimetrist. Dominant parietal lobe lesions may produce Gerstmann's syndrome, which is characterized by finger agnosia, agraphia, acalculia, right-left confusion, and a right homonymous hemianopia. Two neuro-ophthalmic signs have been described in patients with parietal lesions.

Spasticity of conjugate gaze. Cogan[6] suggests that tonic deviation of the eyes to the side opposite parietal lesions during an attempt at producing a Bell's phenomenon is a useful sign of parietal lobe localization.

Optokinetic asymmetry. Optokinetic asymmetry with the evoked nystagmus being dampened when the stimuli are moved in the direction of the damaged parietal lobe appears to be a deficit of the ipsilateral slow component,[1] although proponents of an abnormality of the saccadic component exist.[11]

Occipital lobe

Optic radiation fibers become totally segregated when the visual cortex is reached. Therefore the hallmark of occipital lobe disease is exquisite congruity whether the visual field defects be quadrantic in nature or involve a lesser area of field (homonymous scotoma) (Fig. 1-24). Total hemianopias occur, but these cannot be considered congruous. Two perimetric peculiarities are observed with occipital lobe disease.

Preservation of the temporal crescent. An area of visual cortex lying anteriorly in the interhemispheric fissure corresponds to the broader nasal retina.[24] At times the portion of cortex subserving this area of retina will be spared in occipital strokes (Fig. 1-25). This temporal crescent preservation may appear as an incongruous hemianopia on first glance. However, when this portion of the field is eliminated from consideration, the extreme congruity of the defect can be appreciated. Less frequently the area of the temporal crescent may be the only portion of the visual cortex that is abnormal, resulting in loss of the temporal portion of only one field.

Macula sparing. Some occipital hemianopias appear to preserve or retain a small area around fixation (macula sparing) in contrast to the more typical respecting of the

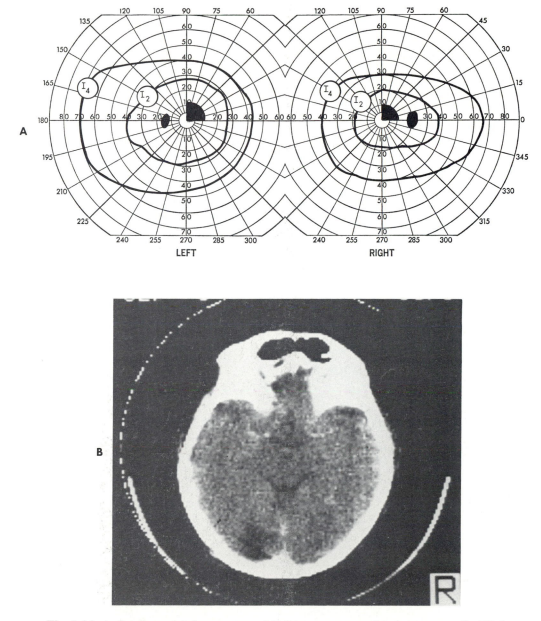

Fig. 1-24. A, Small exquisitely congruous right homonymous quadrantic scotomas. **B,** CT shows hypodense area of infarction at left occipital pole.

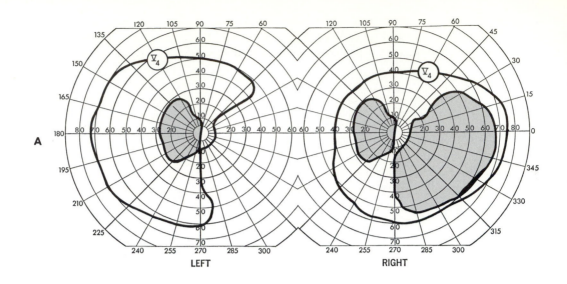

A

LEFT   RIGHT

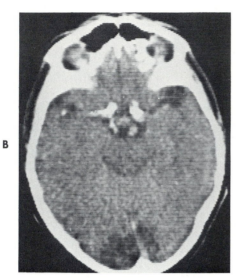

B

Fig. 1-25. Temporal crescent sparing with bilateral occipital infarction. **A,** There is a highly congruous left homonymous scotoma. Right homonymous defect appears incongruous until it is realized that the persistent peripheral rim of vision in right temporal field is a preserved crescent. **B,** CT scan showing bilateral occipital infarcts.

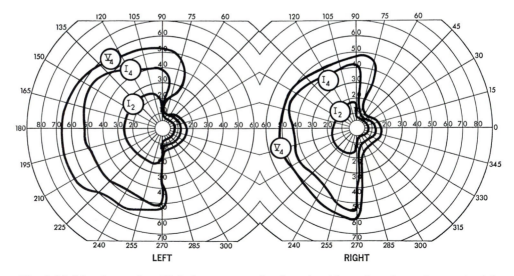

LEFT   RIGHT

Fig. 1-26. Macular sparing. Right homonymous hemianopia with sparing of macular area in right homonymous field.

vertical meridian through fixation (macula splitting) (Fig. 1-26). Sparing may be due to the dual vascular supply of the occipital pole by branches of either the posterior cerebral or middle cerebral artery. However, by injecting horseradish peroxidase into one lateral geniculate nucleus of monkeys, it has been shown that retinal ganglion cells projecting ipsilaterally and contralaterally are intermixed.[4] This appears to reestablish bilateral macular representation as an explanation of some instances of macular sparing. It now appears that either mechanism may be involved in producing this phenomenon.[19]

Special manifestations of occipital lobe disease. Several occipital lobe syndromes should be recognized.

Cortical blindness. This syndrome consists of total blindness due to bilateral occipital lobe lesions. The pupillary reactions are intact, and the funduscopic examination is normal. These two findings frequently lead to the misdiagnosis of functional blindness. This impression may be fortified since these patients may deny their blindness and fabricate an imaginary visual environment (Anton's syndrome).

The most frequent cause of cortical blindness is bilateral infarction of the occipital lobes. The infarcts may occur simultaneously during severe blood loss or hypotensive shock[20] or following arteriography,[25] but the same syndrome may result from sequential occipital infarctions.

Riddoch phenomenon. The perception of movement without the perception of form (statokinetic dissociation) was originally thought to be a specific indicator of occipital lobe disease. It is now apparent that this phenomenon may be detected in lesions at any point along the visual system and is not a pathognomonic sign of occipital lobe disease.[22]

Cerebral dyschromatopsia. Although acquired alteration of color vision is predominantly a sign of anterior visual pathway disease, there is an unusual form of dyschromatopsia associated with occipital lobe disease. These patients have bilateral occipital lesions but may not have extensive visual field defects. When they have defects, they are usually superior, indicating a lesion inferiorly in the occipital area. Prosopagnosia (inability to recognize faces) is a frequent associated finding.[12]

Disconnection syndromes. A variety of other higher cortical dysfunctions are associated with primary and associational visual cortex.[15]

Alexia without agraphia. This patient is unable to read but can write and speak intelligently. The lesions producing this syndrome are in the left occipital zone and the splenium of the corpus callosum. The occipital lesion produces a right homonymous defect, depriving the left hemisphere of visual information. The information from the right hemisphere cannot be transmitted to the left side because of the splenium lesion.

Palinopsia. The persistence or recurrence of visual images after the stimulus has been removed is referred to as palinopsia. The patient usually, but not invariably, experiences these false images in an area of homonymous hemianopic defect. The causative lesion is occipital in location.[18]

Hallucinations. Although unformed visual hallucinations are classically ascribed to occipital lobe disease, formed images may also be experienced with occipital lesions. Unformed hallucinations rarely may indicate temporal lobe malfunction, although in this area formed images are the rule.[7,32]

The lesions that produce occipital lobe dysfunction may be vascular (infarction), neoplastic (meningioma, metastatic disease, glioma), congenital (porencephaly, arterio-

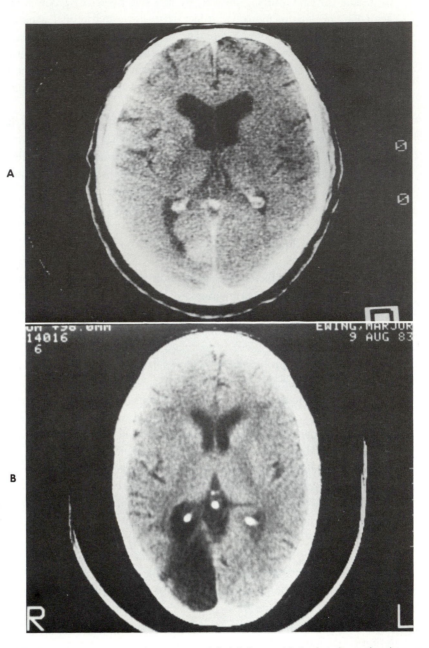

Fig. 1-27. Occipital infarction. **A,** Acute occipital infarct with brain edema that is contrast enhancing. Surrounding structures are not displaced as they would be with a mass lesion. **B,** Long-standing occipital infarct with area of lucency in territory of posterior cerebral artery. **C,** Partial occipital infarct involving only a portion of right occipital lobe.

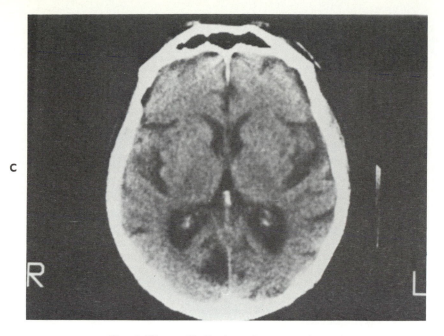

C

R L

Fig. 1-27, cont'd. For legend see opposite page.

venous malformations), traumatic, or toxic. The single most important test in differentiating among these various etiologies is the CT scan (Fig. 1-27). Any patient with a fixed homonymous hemianopia must have a CT scan.

REFERENCES

1. Baloh, RW, Yee, RD, and Honrubia, V: Optokinetic nystagmus and parietal lobe lesions, Ann Neurol 7:269, 1979.
2. Boisen, E: Strokes in migraine: report of seven strokes associated with severe migraine attacks, Dan Med Bull 22:100, 1975.
3. Bousser, MG, Baron, JC, Iba-Zizen, MT, et al: Migranous cerebral infarction: a tomographic study of cerebral blood flow and oxygen extraction fraction with the oxygen—15 inhalation techniques, Stroke 11:145, 1980.
4. Bunt, AH, and Minckler, DS: Foveal sparing. New anatomical evidence for bilateral representation of the cerebral retina, Arch Ophthalmol 95:1445, 1977.
5. Cogan, DG: Neurology of the visual system, Springfield, Ill, 1966, Charles C Thomas, Publisher, p 254.
6. Cogan, DG: Neurology of the visual system, Springfield, Ill, 1966, Charles C Thomas, Publisher, p 267.
7. Cogan, DG: Visual hallucinations as release phenomena, Albrecht Von Graefes Arch Klin Exp Ophthalmol 188:139, 1973.
8. Dalton, K: Migraine and oral contraceptives, Headache 15:247, 1976.
9. Frisén, L: Quadruple sectoranopia and sectorial optic atrophy—a syndrome of the distal anterior choroidal artery, J Neurol Neurosurg Psychiatry 42:590, 1979.
10. Frisén, L, Holmegaard, L, and Rosencrantz, M: Sectorial optic atrophy and homonymous, horizontal sectoranopia: a lateral choroidal artery syndrome? J Neurol Neurosurg Psychiatry 41:374, 1978.
11. Gay, AJ, Newman, Keltner, JL, and Stroud, MH: Eye movement disorders, St Louis, 1974, The CV Mosby Co, p 50.
12. Green, GJ, and Lessell, S: Acquired cerebral dyschromatopsia, Arch Ophthalmol 95:121, 1977.
13. Gunderson, CH, and Hoyt, WF: Geniculate hemianopia: incongruous homonymous field defects in two patients with partial lesions of the lateral geniculate nucleus, J Neurol Neurosurg Psychiatry 34:1, 1971.
14. Jensen, I, and Seedorff, HH: Temporal lobe epilepsy and neuro-ophthalmology. Ophthalmological findings in 74 temporal lobe resected patients, Acta Ophthalmol 54:827, 1976.

15. Lessell, S: Higher disorders of visual function: negative phenomena. In Glaser, JS, and Smith, JL, editors: Symposium of the University of Miami and the Bascom Palmer Eye Institute, vol 8, St Louis, 1975, The CV Mosby Co, p 1.

16. Lindenberg, R, Walsh, FB, and Sachs, JG: Neuro-pathology of vision—an atlas. Philadelphia, 1973, Lea & Febiger, p 332.

17. Meyer, JS, Shinohara, Y, Kanda, T, et al: Diaschisis resulting from acute unilateral cerebral infarction, Arch Neurol 23:241, 1970.

18. Michel, EM, and Troost, BT: Palinopsia—cerebral localization with computed tomography, Neurology 30:887, 1980.

19. Miller, NR, editor: Walsh and Hoyt's clinical neuro-ophthalmology, Baltimore, 1982, The Williams & Wilkins Co, p 147.

20. Nepple, EW, Appen, RE, and Sackett, JF: Bilateral homonymous hemianopia, Am J Ophthalmol 86:536, 1978.

21. Patterson, RH, Goodoll, H, and Dunning, HS: Complications of carotid arteriography, Arch Neurol 10:513, 1964.

22. Safran, AB, and Glaser, JS: Statokinetic dissociation in lesions of the anterior visual pathways, Arch Ophthalmol 98:291, 1980.

23. Savino, PJ, Paris, M, Schatz, NJ, et al: Optic tract syndrome, Arch Ophthalmol 96:656, 1978.

24. Stensaas, SS, Eddington, KD, and Dobelle, WH: The topography and variability of the primary visual cortex in man, J Neurosurg 40:747, 1974.

25. Studdard, WE, Davis, DO, and Young, SW: Cortical blindness after cerebral angiography, J Neurosurg 54:240, 1981.

26. Trobe, JD, Lorber, ML, and Schlezinger, NS: Isolated homonymous hemianopias: a review of 104 cases, Arch Ophthalmol 89:377, 1973.

27. Troost, BT, Mark, LE, and Maroon, JC: Resolution of classic migraine after removal of an occipital lobe AVM, Ann Neurol 5:199, 1979.

28. Troost, BT, and Newton, TH: Occipital lobe arteriovenous malformation. Clinical and radiologic features in 26 cases with comments on the differentiation from migraine, Arch Ophthalmol 93:250, 1975.

29. Van Buren, JM, and Baldwin, M: The architecture of the optic radiation in the temporal lobe of man, Brain 31:2, 1958.

30. Vedel-Jensen, N: Optic tract neuritis in multiple sclerosis, Acta Ophthalmol 37:537, 1959.

31. Walker, AE, and Walsh, FB: The visual disturbances in temporal lobectomized patients. In Smith, JL, editor: Neuro-ophthalmology Symposium of the University of Miami and the Bascom Palmer Eye Institute, vol 4, St Louis, 1968, The CV Mosby Co, p 230.

32. Weinberger, LM, and Grant, FC: Visual hallucinations and their neuro-optical correlates, Arch Ophthalmol 23:166, 1940.

CHAPTER 2

Transient visual loss

Transient visual loss (TVL), or "amaurosis fugax," is a reversible deficit in visual function that lasts less than 30 minutes. The term should be reserved for discrete events in which patients describe an abrupt loss of all or a portion of their field of vision in one or both eyes. Sometimes it is difficult to distinguish TVL from the fluctuations in visual clarity without abrupt onset that occur in other conditions such as diabetes, corneal edema, and multiple sclerosis (MS). MS patients typically describe blurred vision after increases in body temperature from a hot bath or exercise (Uhthoff's phenomenon).

MECHANISMS OF TVL

The above definition makes TVL a subtype of transient ischemic attack (TIA), a reversible focal neurologic deficit of 24 hours' duration or less. In fact the principal mechanism for TVL is ischemic. The other accepted mechanism, believed to be less common, is epileptic discharge.[56] Seizures within the visual cortex are caused by neoplasms, arteriovenous malformations, meningoencephalitis, ischemia, or trauma and typically have an excitatory component as well. That is, the patient experiences hallucinations, usually of unformed images, at some time during the abnormal discharge. The hallucinations usually consist of flickering lights that do not move across the visual field as they do in migraine.[81]

Ischemia produces TVL by (1) vascular occlusion or (2) reduced blood flow through nonoccluded vessels.

Occlusion

TVL results from vascular occlusion in three circumstances: thromboembolism, vasospasm, and compression (Fig. 2-1).

Thromboembolism. The circulation to the eye or visual cortex may be temporarily blocked by an embolus originating from a diseased arterial wall, or heart valve or wall, and turbulent or sluggish blood flow. The commonest source of embolism is atheromatous ulceration of large arteries, but inflammation, dysplasia, tumor, trauma, and exogenous injection of particles must also be considered. Atheromas collect fibrin and platelets, forming a thrombus that may or may not totally occlude the vessel lumen. Parts of the thrombus break off and drift downstream to plug distal vessels. Whether transient arterial thrombosis or embolism is the cause of most TIAs in patients with atheromatous extracranial disease is unsettled. However, embolism is the presumed mechanism in patients with cardiac valve or wall abnormalities.

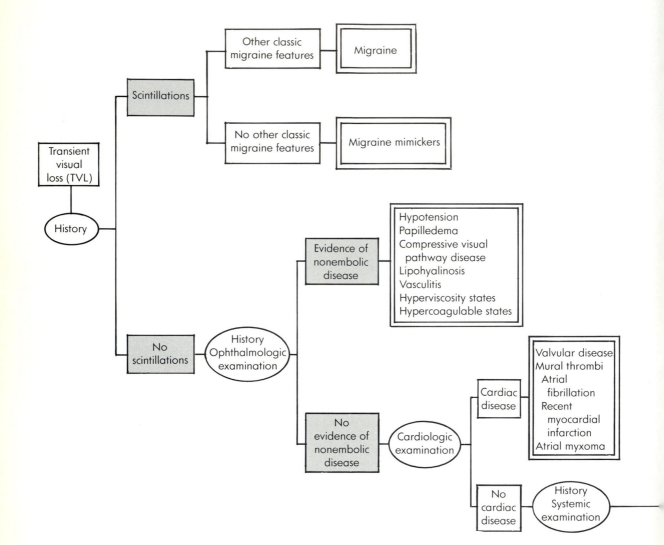

Chart 2-1

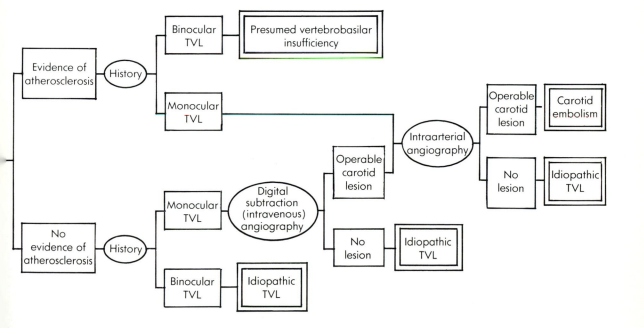

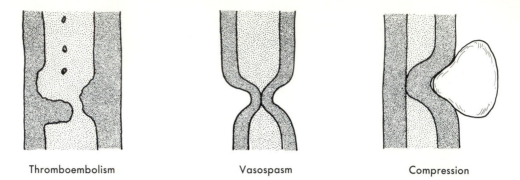

Thromboembolism   Vasospasm   Compression

Fig. 2-1. The three mechanisms of vaso-occlusion associated with transient visual loss.

TVL may also occur from thrombosis of a feeder vessel close to the eye or visual cortex. In addition to atherosclerosis, other processes affect these smaller vessels, especially lipohyalinosis, vasculitis, and hypercoagulable states. Lipohyalinosis, the hyperplastic process associated with systemic hypertension that obliterates the lumen of small arterioles, is believed responsible for the nonarteritic form of ischemic optic neuropathy (ION).[10,25,40] TVL is associated with vasculitis most commonly in giant cell arteritis, less commonly in Takayasu's (pulseless) disease, lupus erythematosus, rheumatoid arthritis, and polyarteritis nodosa. Hypercoagulable states causing TVL include sickle cell anemia, macroglobulinemia, and multiple myeloma.

The TVL associated with thromboembolism usually lasts 5 minutes or less.[20] It will be monocular if it affects the eye, and binocular if it affects the visual cortex. In either case the TVL is frequently an isolated symptom. The TVL associated with lipohyalinosis or vasculitis is comparably brief but has the distinction of being typically limited to a 48-hour period before infarction occurs.[10,25]

Vasospasm. A temporary narrowing of muscular arteries may occur without any evidence of structural vessel wall abnormality, thromboembolism, or external compression, Contraction is mediated by local vasoactive substances, including histamine, serotonin, bradykinin, and prostaglandins. Vasospasm is the mechanism believed to mediate cerebral ischemia in migraine, subarachnoid hemorrhage, and hypertensive crisis. In migraine, when the target organ is the visual cortex, TVL is typically binocular, homonymous, and preceded by a sensation of flashing lights or lines called a scintillation (classic or occipital migraine). Monocular TVL without scintillations may arise if ocular vessels become spastic (ocular migraine).

Markedly elevated blood pressure (greater than 120 diastolic) may give rise to encephalopathy and monocular or binocular TVL. Retinal arterioles are extremely attenuated, but visual loss may result from ischemia in the visual cortex[50] as well as in the retina and optic nerve.[48] Lowering of blood pressure is curative but must be accomplished slowly; otherwise optic disc infarction may occur.[48]

Vasospasm may also account for the frequently idiopathic monocular and binocular TVL described by otherwise healthy young adults.

Compression. A relatively rare cause of TVL is external compression of blood vessels that nourish the visual pathway. This mechanism is involved in papilledema, in

---

PRINCIPAL MECHANISMS OF TVL

I. Ischemia
   A. Vascular occlusion
      1. Thromboembolism
         a. Atheromatous
         b. Nonatheromatous
            (1) Cardiac
            (2) Other
      2. Vasospasm
         a. Migraine
         b. Malignant hypertension
         c. Subarachnoid hemorrhage
         d. Idiopathic
      3. External compression
         a. Papilledema
         b. Tumors
   B. Reduced flow through nonoccluded vessels
      1. Hypotension
         a. Cardiac
         b. Orthostatic
      2. Hyperviscosity
II. Seizures
      1. Occipital lobe
      2. General cerebral

---

which pressure on vessels in the swollen nerve head causes blackout of vision over the entire field of one or both eyes, lasting a second or two (transient obscurations). The episodes, which are so brief that the patient is apt to ignore them at first, may be precipitated by standing up or by Valsalva maneuvers. Fundus examination shows markedly swollen discs, and the intracranial pressure is generally above 200 mm of water. Normalization of the pressure eliminates the symptom.

Compression of a part of the visual pathway by an adjacent or intrinsic tumor generally causes slowly progressive visual loss but rarely will produce TVL.[13] For example, an intraorbital tumor may intermittently compress the optic nerve as the eye is rotated into eccentric gaze positions.

Reduced flow through nonoccluded vessels

The visual pathway may become ischemic even if blood vessels are patent, but cerebral perfusion is reduced as a result of subnormal cardiac output or hyperviscosity. Patients most often experience binocular TVL accompanied by dizziness, light-headedness, confusion, nausea, headache, and occasionally photopsias. Clinical and experimental evidence[7] suggests that cardiogenic hypoperfusion rarely produces TVL as an isolated symptom.

Hyperviscosity states may produce ischemia not only by sluggish blood flow but also by an increased propensity to thrombosis. In patients with such disorders TVL may be a prominent symptom. A study of 511 polycythemia patients (457 with polycythemia vera) found that 11% complained of TVL that was relieved by phlebotomy.[77]

The symptoms and signs of TVL are not specific enough to attribute them to a given mechanism in a great many cases. Largely on the basis of circumstantial evidence, atheromatous thromboembolism is considered responsible for the vast majority of TVL episodes in those over 40 years of age. Among patients 40 years old or younger most cases of TVL remain unexplained, although migraine and atheromatous thromboembolism are often invoked as mechanisms. In both age groups, cardiac emboli, nonatheromatous vasculopathies, and papilledema must always be excluded.

DIAGNOSIS AND MANAGEMENT OF TVL

In the workup of patients with TVL we suggest the examiner proceed as follows:
1. Determine if the scintillations of migraine are present.
2. If scintillations are not present, use history and ophthalmologic examination to differentiate embolic from nonembolic causes of TVL and to distinguish monocular from binocular TVL. If a nonembolic cause is found, which will be unusual, refer to the appropriate specialist or treat.
3. If an embolic cause is suggested or cannot be excluded, refer for cardiac evaluation. This step is necessary both to rule out a cardiac source for emboli and to establish that there is adequate cardiac reserve in case carotid endarterectomy is contemplated.
4. If cardiac evaluation is negative for an embolic source, patients suitable for carotid endarterectomy who have signs of arteriosclerosis and monocular TVL should have transarterial cerebral angiography to rule out an operable extracranial carotid lesion.

Patients without arteriosclerosis, who are usually under 50 years of age, should have digital subtraction angiography (DSA), the most reliable noninvasive study of the extracranial carotid, because of its reduced risk and a relatively lower expectation of vasculopathy. If a lesion is found with DSA, transarterial cerebral angiography should be performed. Patients with no lesions should be placed on aspirin (one every other day).

Patients with binocular TVL and no cardiac source for emboli need no further studies and may also be treated with aspirin, especially if other arteriosclerotic signs or symptoms suggest vertebrobasilar insufficiency (VBI).

☐ **Ruling out migraine** (Chart 2-1, *A*)

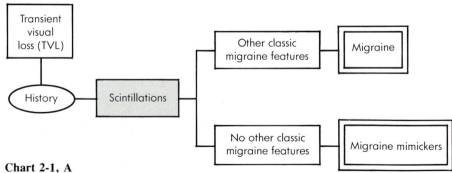

Chart 2-1, A

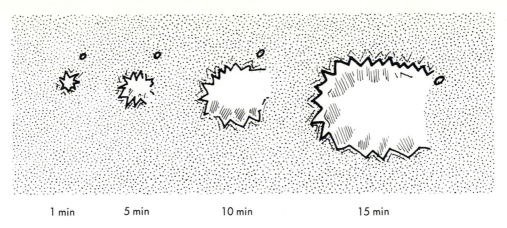

| 1 min | 5 min | 10 min | 15 min |

Fig. 2-2. Scintillating scotoma of migraine. Small area of visual disturbance initially just eccentric to fixation, slowly expanding over a 15- to 20-minute period (left to right) to fade away at onset of headache in classic migraine. Similar events can occur in patients without the headache phase. The center of the scotoma may appear black or gray or may just contain blurred imagery.

The first step in history taking is to determine if the patient is experiencing scintillations. If these are present, especially with fortification, the diagnosis is likely to be migraine. If the symptom complex consists of a stereotyped hallucination followed by a scotoma lasting approximately 15 to 20 minutes, then the diagnosis is assured.

Pathogenesis. Migraine is a disease of vascular hyperreactivity, affecting 20% of the general population.[83] Its manifestations are probably caused by local vasoactive agents that produce an initial intracranial vasoconstriction (aura), followed by extracranial vasodilatation (headache). Although substantiated by cerebral blood flow studies, these vascular changes have never been verified angiographically. There is some evidence that the aura-headache cycle is related to platelet aggregation.[34]

Symptoms. In the classic form of migraine, patients experience sensory or motor prodromes (auras), the most common of which are visual. These auras are typically followed by headaches of mounting intensity and variable duration, often confined to one side of the head. The aura and headaches typically shift sides from episode to episode, but there are many patients in whom the same side is always involved. Patients often report the headaches as throbbing and associated with nausea and disequilibrium and say that they feel compelled to lie down and sleep.

The visual aura in its classic form consists of a flickering zigzag line (fortification scotoma) (Fig. 2-2), which appears in an eccentric position of field and spreads across it. Some patients merely report stationary flickering lights and colors that often have elementary forms such as stars, pinwheels, rings, and triangles. Others describe foggy vision or "heat waves." The hallucination lasts 15 to 20 minutes and during this period frequently traverses the visual field from center to periphery or vice versa. It is this stereotyped "march" or "buildup" that is so characteristic of migraine. These hallucinations differ from those associated with mechanical deformation of retinal receptors from vitreous tug (phosphenes), which typically last only seconds and are precipitated by eye movement. Fisher[29] points out that VBI manifests hallucinations that may have the form of fortifications, but they are typically stationary. The hallucinations of occipital epilepsy also tend to lack a buildup and vary in duration from episode to episode.[81]

The visual auras of migraine may terminate with scotomas, which in rare cases remain as permanent homonymous defects. The entire symptom complex often occurs without headache. If so, and if the flickering lights last 15 to 20 minutes, the symptom is considered a migraine equivalent, or acephalgic migraine. This relatively stereotyped hallucinatory symptom complex is believed to represent ischemia of the visual cortex caused by temporary vasospasm. The gradual movement of the scintillations across the visual field, followed by scotoma, probably represents a traveling excitatory wave in cortical cells, which are then rendered exhausted. Electroencephalography during this phase has not shown the signs of a seizure disorder.[34]

The vast majority of visual auras of this type occur in patients who have a personal or family history of ''sick headaches'' beginning before age 20. However, a substantial number will give no such history, their first attack occurring after age 40. Such patients probably still qualify for the diagnosis of primary migraine, even those who do not report the typical buildup of scintillations. Fisher[29] states that as many as 25% of migraine patients will describe a ''visual display that becomes maximum almost immediately.'' As the atypical features mount, however, we believe that the examiner must begin to consider the possibility that the migraine complex is a manifestation of an underlying disease, such as VBI, occipital epilepsy, lupus erythematosus, head injury, or viral meningoencephalitis (migraine mimickers or secondary migraine).[9]

Patients with migraine histories may also experience transient monocular visual loss (ocular migraine). However, the symptoms are so nonspecific that diagnosis is always presumptive and is only made after excluding all other causes. Visual loss rarely lasts longer than a few minutes, and there are no hallucinations and no headache. In those cases where the fundus has been observed during an attack, retinal arteriolar and venous narrowing, retinal edema, venous dilatation, and delayed flourescein filling of retinal vessels have been noted.[53,86] If retinal ischemia is severe, infarction results. Migraine patients may rarely suffer ischemic papillopathy and central serous retinopathy. The underlying abnormality is considered to be vasospasm of opthalmic, retinal, or choroidociliary circulations.

☐ **Differentiating embolic from nonembolic causes of TVL** (Chart 2-1, *B*)

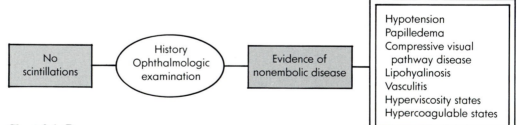

Chart 2-1, B

Having excluded migraine as a cause of TVL, the examiner must direct the history toward discovering if the TVL has an embolic or nonembolic cause. Clues are provided from history and ophthalmologic examination.

○ **History**

Other concurrent cerebral ischemic symptoms. If dizziness, confusion, seizures, or syncope accompanied the TVL, the diagnosis of global cerebral ischemia is suggested, possibly caused by cardiogenic hypotension. If the episode was precipitated by assuming an upright posture, then orthostatic hypotension must be considered. If diplopia, dysarthria, vertigo, or disequilibrium accompanied TVL, the diagnosis is probably brain stem ischemia from cardiac or vertebrobasilar atheromatous thromboembolism. If ipsilateral hemispheric ischemic symptoms coincided with monocular TVL, then cardiac or carotid emboli are likely.

Arteriosclerotic risk factors. Hypertension, diabetes, familial arteriosclerotic disease, and a personal history of heavy smoking are risk factors associated not only with extracranial atheromatous thromboembolism but also with cardiac disease.

Heart disease. The finding of prosthetic valves or abnormal cardiac rhythm (especially atrial fibrillation) establishes a special risk for cardiac emboli.

Constitutional symptoms. Fever, chills, headache, malaise, and lethargy establish a possibility of endocarditis, cardiac myxoma, giant cell arteritis, or hyperviscous states. Transient blurred vision is a complaint in patients with increased serum viscosity, as in polycythemia vera, thrombocytosis, multiple myeloma, macroglobulinemia, cryoglobulinemia, and sickle cell anemia.

Rheumatologic disease. The finding of serositis, arthritis, and dermatitis suggests a possibility of vasculitis.

Migraine. Even if there are no scintillations and TVL is monocular, a strong history of migraine fortifies a suspicion of ocular migraine, especially in young people.

Birth control pill ingestion, pregnancy, and postpartum or dehydrated states. These conditions may produce a hypercoagulable state. Although strokes often occur in these settings, they are rarely preceded by TIAs. It is not yet possible to predict which of these patients is at risk of stroke.

Head or neck trauma. If head or neck trauma has occurred, it suggests the possibility of bony compression or a dissecting aneurysm of neck vessels.

○ **Ophthalmologic examination**

Anterior segment and adnexal signs. Conjunctivitis, uveitis, and scleritis may be part of a picture of vasculitis or of anterior segment ischemia. Although often associated with proximal (carotid artery) atherosclerosis, anterior segment ischemia reflects, in our view, atheromatous compromise of distal (ophthalmic artery) circulation to the eye.

Fundus signs

Papilledema. The presence of swollen discs suggests increased intracranial pressure as a possible cause of TVL and directs the investigation away from the more common extracranial sources.

Plaques in the retinal vessels (Plate 5, *A* and *B*). Although intraluminal plaques implicate an extracranial embolic source, the appearance of the plaques is not often distinctive enough to indicate their precise origin (vessel or heart).

Venous tortuosity, peripheral perivenous hemorrhages, and microaneurysms. These signs suggest reduced flow (Plate 5, *C*). Cotton-wool and Roth spots (Plate 5, *D* and *E*) suggest arteritis, hypertension, or embolism. Attenuated arterioles suggest hypertension; peripheral sea fans and sunbursts suggest sickle cell anemia (Plate 5, *F*), and pallid disc swelling implies ischemic optic neuropathy (vasculitis or lipohyalinosis).

Visual field defects. Patients with TVL caused by compressive visual pathway disease will generally also have a fixed deficit apparent in the visual field examination. The history and opthalmologic examination together should provide evidence of the relatively rare nonembolic causes of TVL, including hypotension, papilledema, compressive visual pathway disease, lipohyalinosis, vasculitis, hyperviscosity, and hypercoagulable states (see Mechanisms of Transient Visual Loss, above).

☐ **Ruling out cardiac source of emboli** (Chart 2-1, *C*)

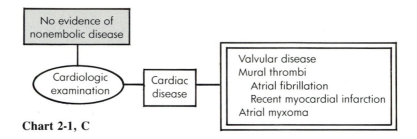

Chart 2-1, C

If nonembolic causes of TVL have been excluded, one must turn to the consideration of emboli, and the heart should first be excluded as a source.

The central nervous system (CNS) is a target of an estimated 75% of cardiac emboli.[64] Although such emboli are an established cause of retinal and occipital infarction,[65] there are no adequate data on how frequently they cause TVL. In a series of 54 patients with rheumatic heart disease, 33% of patients had TVL, but none mentioned the symptoms spontaneously, none had coincident TIAs, and none had retinal strokes.[80] The frequency of TVL episodes was unrelated to anticoagulation. Therefore it is unclear whether the TVL episodes were of embolic origin.

Cardiac emboli may originate from heart valves, from endocardial thrombi, and from tumor. The diagnosis of a cardiac source for TVL is made difficult by the fact that patients often have coexisting hypertensive or atheromatous arterial disease and by the fact that visual system symptoms and signs of cardiac emboli are indistinguishable from those caused by artery-to-artery emboli. The orange-yellow reflective cholesterol (Hollenhorst) plaque is said to come from a carotid atheromatous source, while the large white retinal arteriolar calcific plaque derives from a cardiac valve or wall lesion, and the platelet-fibrin plaque may derive from either source.[43,47] We often consider it difficult to differentiate ophthalmoscopically between these three types of retinal emboli. The only firm criterion for suspecting a cardiac source of embolus is a history or clinical findings of cardiac disease together with evidence of recent infarction in multiple parts of the brain and body. The absence of risk factors for or signs of cervical atheromatous disease adds further support to the diagnosis of a cardiac source. Cardiac emboli occur with the following disorders.

☐ **Valvular disease.** The most common valvular causes of emboli are rheumatic heart disease and prosthetic valves.[49,64,65] Rheumatic heart disease is a source of cerebral emboli both from platelet-fibrin vegetations on mitral (and aortic) valve leaflets and from associated atrial fibrillation, which causes stagnation of blood flow and secondary mural thrombus formation. If patients are in congestive failure because of valvular disease, the

COLOR PLATE 5

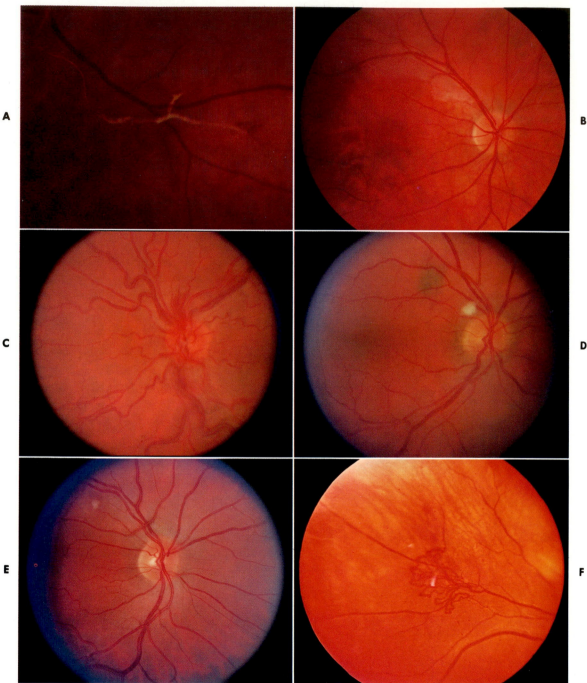

Plate 5. A, Retinal vascular plaque. **B,** Retinal vascular plaque (at emergence of vessel from disc substance) with infarction. **C,** Retinal venous congestion in polycythemia vera. **D,** Cotton-wool spot. **E,** Roth spot. **F,** Sea fan in sickle cell anemia.

correct management is valvuloplasty or replacement. Otherwise, patients should be anticoagulated indefinitely.

Embolization remains one of the principal long-term risks of prosthetic valves. In a study of the Starr-Edwards 2400 aortic valve, Dale[18] found a 7% per year incidence of stroke in spite of anticoagulation. This risk diminishes markedly after the third postoperative year. Procine (homograft) valves have a lower incidence of emboli, 1% per year in one series.[16] One report[57] emphasizes that long-term warfarin anticoagulation reduces the likelihood of embolization tenfold in the presence of prosthetic heart valves.

Infective endocarditis causes cerebral emboli in an estimated 10% to 50% of cases.[3] It should be suspected whenever the patient has either fever, chills, night sweats, or retinal nerve fiber layer hemorrhages with white centers (Roth spots, nonspecific indicators of retinal infarction) (Plate 5, *E*). Acute endocarditis usually occurs in individuals with normal hearts whose valves are infected with *Staphylococcus aureus*. Subacute endocarditis usually affects patients with rheumatic or congenital valvular disease or prosthetic valves; *Streptococcus viridans* is the major causative organism. Physical findings include cardiac murmurs, skin petechiae, nailbed splinter hemorrhages, and splenomegaly. Early intensive antibiotic therapy is often effective in preventing serious complications.

Nonbacterial thrombotic (marantic) endocarditis occurs in cancer patients, particularly those with mucinous adenocarcinomas, and in other chronic debilitating conditions. These patients may develop vegetations of the mitral (60%) or aortic (40%) valves.[3] Noninfective vegetations may also occur in lupus erythematosus (Libman-Sacks endocarditis).[33] The incidence of clinical embolism in these conditions is considered rare.

Fibromyxomatous degeneration of the mitral valve (prolapsing mitral valve, Barlow's syndrome) may give rise to cerebral emboli and TVL, with an incidence of stroke estimated at 1:100,000 per year.[74] In 1963, Barlow[5] associated a typical midsystolic cardiac clicking sound with evidence of a prolapsing motion of the mitral valve leaflets (Fig. 2-3). Since then the pathology has been defined as fibromyxomatous degeneration of these leaflets and of the chordae tendineae with uncommonly short papillary muscles. This disorder occurs in up to 6% of otherwise healthy young adults but has also been linked to angina, endocarditis, and sudden death. Barnett[6] reported 12 patients without any stroke risk factors who had TIA or stroke and prolapsing mitral valves. The presence of prolapse was much more common in these patients than in age-matched controls, leading the authors to postulate that emboli originated from valvular vegetations that have been noted on autopsy.[70] Because of the high incidence of mitral valve prolapse, it has been considered the cause of as many as one quarter of strokes in young adults without other known contributory disease.[31] Diagnosis of the valvular abnormality is often but not always straightforward: the click may be difficult to hear, and the echocardiogram may not be diagnostic. There is no evidence that treatment helps, but symptomatic patients are managed on platelet antiaggregation agents.

☐ **Mural thrombi.** Atrial fibrillation (AF) appears to constitute an important risk factor for cerebral emboli, whether the AF is associated with rheumatic, ischemic, or myopathic heart disease. In one autopsy study,[42] symptomatic systemic emboli had occurred in 41% of patients with AF and rheumatic mitral valve disease, 35% with AF and ischemic heart disease, and 17% with AF and other heart disease. Emboli were found in only 7% of control patients with ischemic heart disease but without AF. The emboli are believed to originate from endocardial clots that accumulate in stagnant atrial flow. Patients

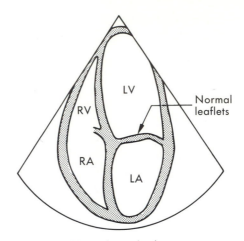

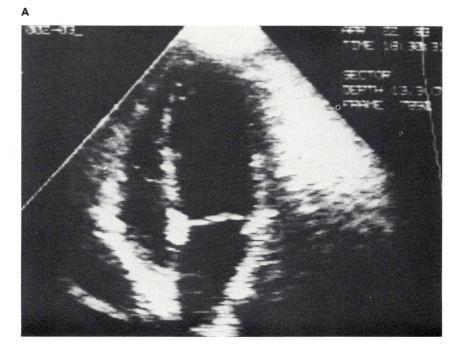

Fig. 2-3. A, Two-dimensional echocardiogram in a normal heart.

should be treated with anticoagulants for at least 6 months and perhaps indefinitely, especially if AF is intermittent. Cardioversion should be attempted after several weeks of anticoagulation in recent-onset AF.

Cerebral emboli may arise from the mural thrombi associated with myocardial infarction. It is generally believed that if mural thrombi are to form after myocardial infarction, they will usually do so within the first 8 weeks.[65] However, ventricular wall segments rendered akinetic by infarction may allow thrombi to form many months after the acute event. Diagnosis is made by two-dimensional echocardiography.

☐ **Atrial myxoma.** Atrial myxoma rarely may give rise to TVL and stroke.[14,42] Cardiac myxomas are rare tumors (1 in 4000 autopsies) and an even rarer cause of stroke. Most

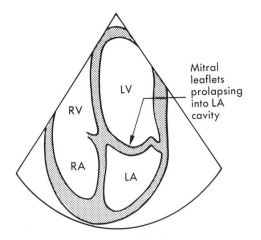

Prolapsed mitral valve

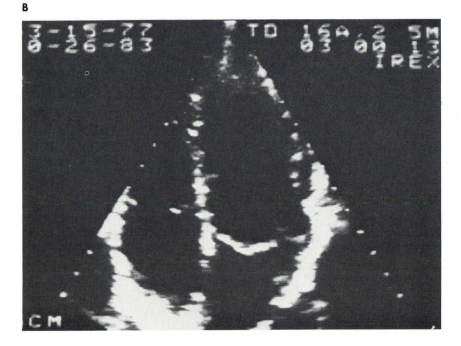

Fig. 2-3, cont'd. B, Two-dimensional echocardiogram in a heart with mitral valve prolapse.

myxomas occur in the left atrium, appearing in individuals between the ages of 30 and 60 years.[14] About 50% of patients with these tumors will develop emboli, chiefly to the brain. Patients will often have unexplained malaise, weight loss, fever, petechiae, and abdominal pain. The myxoma generally has little effect on cardiac function but may give rise to subtle, changing murmurs and rarely to signs of mitral insufficiency. Whenever the diagnosis of endocarditis is entertained, atrial myxoma should be on the list. The diagnosis is made by echocardiography and cardiac catheterization. Treatment is surgical removal.

In the evaluation of patients suspected of having a cardiac source of emboli, if clinical examination and electrocardiographic studies are normal, recent reports[54,60] indicate that echocardiography (2-dimensional, M mode) is unlikely to discover a cardiac source of emboli.

If the cardiologic examination has ruled out cardiac sources of cerebral emboli, then the examiner must turn to the consideration of cervical atheromatous thromboembolism as a cause of TVL.

☐ **Ruling out operable extracranial carotid atheromatous disease** (Chart 2-1, *D*)

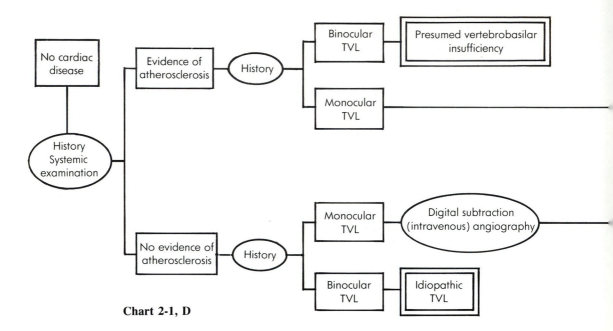

Chart 2-1, D

Atherosclerosis of the internal carotid system is found primarily at the origin of the internal carotid and to a lesser extent in its intracavernous (siphon) portion and proximal middle and anterior cerebral branches. The vertebrobasilar system is occluded by atheroma at the takeoff of the vertebral arteries, at the junction of the vertebral and basilar arteries, and at the junction of the basilar and superior cerebellar arteries. Atheromatous involvement of these vessels is believed to produce cerebral ischemia either by generating emboli or by temporarily occluding them and reducing perfusion to vulnerable distal territories.[52]

Symptoms. The TVL associated with carotid atheromatous disease consists of brief monocular attacks lasting 1 to 15 minutes, but usually less than 5 minutes.[20] Patients may describe a shade or veil descending or ascending over a portion of their field, a wedge defect or central scotoma, peripheral loss with central sparing, or a Swiss cheese pattern of irregularly spared areas. Some will describe a blackout, others a brownout or grayout, but many patients will simply report that vision was diffusely blurred. Rarely, patients will describe momentary flashes or spots of light (photopsias). There are usually no coincident nonvisual symptoms.

Visual cortical ischemia caused by vertebrobasilar atheroma produces binocular visual loss. Attacks are typically briefer than with carotid disease, lasting a minute or two.[20] Visual loss may be an isolated symptom but is often accompanied by brain stem ischemic symptoms, which include disequilibrium, diplopia, dysarthria, dysphagia, sudden weakness of the legs (drop attack), and perioral and extremity numbness. Flashing lights may rarely be perceived during an attack, but a progression of fortifications (zigzag lines) across the visual field is not reported. Loss of vision may be total. If partial, it will be homonymous, but the patient is frequently unaware of its binocularity, localizing it to the eye with the temporal field loss.

TVL may be a frequent and often isolated symptom of carotid and vertebrobasilar atheroma because (1) TVL is a symptom readily noticed by the patient, (2) metabolic demands of the eye and visual cortex are relatively high, (3) laminar flow somehow

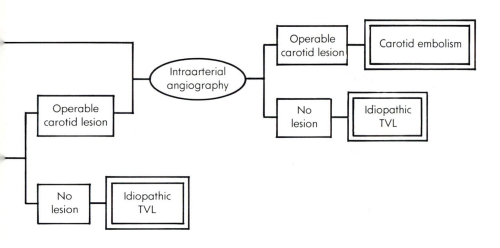

favors these areas, so that emboli are carried here, (4) these tissues are served by a poorly collateralized circulatory bed (retina), or constitute watershed areas remote from several blood supplies (visual cortex), and (5) occlusion of ocular and visual cortical vessels produces visual deficits, while occlusion of equivalent-sized vessels elsewhere in the CNS is clinically silent.

Embolic theory. Emboli from extracranial vessels are believed to account for most episodes of TVL, based on several lines of evidence. In 1959, Fisher[30] described a patient with multiple attacks of monocular TVL and ipsilateral internal carotid stenosis in whom he observed "strikingly white and glistening" particles coursing through the retinal arterioles during an episode of visual loss. He suggested that these particles were emboli from the carotid artery. In 1961, Hollenhorst[44] observed "orange, yellow or copper-colored plaques at bifurcations of retinal arterioles." In some cases these plaques appeared during carotid endarterectomy. He postulated that they were "cholesterol crystals or liquid cholesterol dislodged from eroded atheromatous lesions in the aorta or the innominate, carotid, or opthalmic arteries." In 1963, David et al.[19] reported that bright intraluminal plaques observed in the retina after cervical carotid exploration proved at autopsy to be composed of cholesterol esters identical to those found in the carotid atheroma. Similar emboli were found in an occluded middle cerebral artery. McBrien et al.[63] noted whitish particles in the retinal arterioles after endarterectomy and patholgic examination disclosed platelet aggregates.

Further indirect support for the theory that the cervical carotid was the seat of cerebral emboli came from the observation of Gunning et al.[36] that patients with recent attacks of monocular blindness or hemispheric ischemia were found at endarterectomy to have carotid atheromas covered with a loose network of fibrin and platelets, while those whose TIAs had occurred at least 7 weeks prior to surgery had smooth atheromas.

The fact that cerebral angiography reveals carotid stenosis or occlusion in 85% to 97% of elderly patients with TVL adds further weight to the presumption that monocular TVL is caused by emboli from carotid atheroma.* Several authors[46,66,78] have documented the disappearance of monocular TVL after endarterectomy, although none of these studies has been adequately controlled.

There are several clinical facts that the embolic theory does not adequately explain. Emboli are not always observed in the retinal vessels during monocular TVL attacks. Dyll et al.[21] have observed the fundus of patients suffering transient monocular blindness and noted circulatory arrest with segmentation of venous blood without emboli. Hollenhorst[45] has described a perfectly normal fundus and an amaurotic pupil during an episode of monocular TVL. Furthermore it is difficult to explain how recurrent embolization would explain the fact that TVL (and other TIA) symptoms are frequently identical from episode to episode. Fisher[31] has noted that cardiac emboli do not cause stereotyped TIAs; instead, attacks produce varying symptoms corresponding to different CNS locations. This evidence suggests that, at least in some cases of extracranial atheromatous disease, transient ischemic symptoms may not result from emboli. An alternative explanation is that temporary vascular occlusion by platelet-fibrin thrombi occurs in an artery already compromised by atheroma.[52] The thrombus produces ischemic symptoms in the "distal field" of that artery. Symptoms are governed by the relative patency of smaller vessels in this distal field. As the thrombi are quickly dissolved or washed away, and adequate circulation restored, the symptoms disappear.

The embolic theory of TVL must also consider the fact that a substantial number of patients with TVL do not have atheromatous carotid artery disease. Fisher[29] reported 90 patients with recurrent TVL or other TIA symptoms with normal angiograms. All were over the age of 40, and 75% were over the age of 50. Pessin et al.[68] reported that of 33 patients who underwent angiography for monocular TVL, only 19 (57%) had hemodynamically significant carotid stenosis, and 8 (25%) patients had completely normal carotids. The description of the attacks of TVL was identical in patients with and without stenosing carotid atheroma. The finding of angiographically normal carotids in the presence of monocular TVL has led to the postulation that even when carotid atheroma is found in patients with TVL, it may not be the cause of the symptom, but merely a bystander. In fact, before the thromboembolic theory of TIAs gained preeminence, the conventional explanation for many of these episodes was vasospasm.[32] Vasospasm lost favor because structural damage to cerebral vessels from arteriosclerosis was believed to impair their reactivity. Angiographic studies of the coronary arteries in patients with variant (Prinzmetal) angina pectoris have recently disclosed vasospasm temporally linked to symptoms.[17] The vasospasm occurs both in normal and arteriosclerotic vessels. This new information reopens the question of whether vasospasm is contributory in the TVL suffered by patients with (or without) arteriosclerotic vascular disease.

Diagnosis. Retinal intraluminal plaques and carotid bruits are strong predictors of

---

*References 46, 55, 66, 71, and 75.

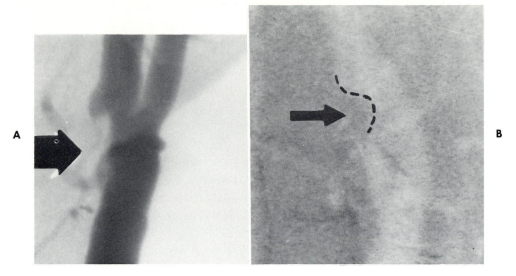

Fig. 2-4. A, Image of ulcerated plaque in internal carotid artery obtained by conventional arteriography. **B,** Same plaque demonstrated by digital subtraction angiography utilizing an intravenous injection of contrast material.

angiographically proven carotid stenosis. There is broad agreement[66,75] that the finding of a cholesterol (Hollenhorst) plaque indicates a greater than 90% chance of finding ipsilateral carotid atheromatous disease (high specificity). But plaques are only present in 10% to 20% of patients with angiographically proven carotid stenosis (low sensitivity).[55,66,71,75] Carotid bruits are also approximately 90% specific for stenosis and more sensitive (60%) than retinal plaques.[55,66,71,75]

The "noninvasive" carotid studies (in contrast to the "invasive" study: cerebral arteriography) are designed to measure cervical carotid contour and blood flow[2] and are currently used whenever there is a reasonable doubt that atheromatous carotid lesions will be found. The value of these studies is based on their reliability in excluding carotid wall lesions so that the morbidity and expense of cerebral angiography may be avoided. Of the noninvasive studies in widespread use the majority depend on finding (1) locally turbulent flow or alterations in acoustical impedance or (2) reduced distal flow or pressure in the ocular or orbital ciculation. Reliable results depend on considerable examiner skill and experience. Even under ideal conditions, none of the traditional noninvasive tests is better than 60% sensitive to carotid stenosis of less than 50%; even when stenosis is greater than 50%, sensitivity remains below 85%.[2,72]

Digital subtraction (intravenous) angiography[12] (DSA) (Fig. 2-4), a recently introduced noninvasive test, promises greater accuracy. It represents the melding of computer processing and intravenous angiography to produce a reasonably good contrast study of the thoracic and cervical arteries. Because this is an intravenous rather than an intraarterial injection study, risks are negligible. Imaging of intracranial vessels is still imperfect, however, and the expenses presently approach those of imaging by intraarterial injection.

Natural history. There are no satisfactory data on the natural (untreated) history of TVL. The only available prospective study[61] showed that of 80 patients with monocular

TVL followed for an average of 4.5 years, only 6% suffered a cerebral stroke and 11% a retinal infarction. This is a relatively low stroke rate compared to the 20% to 30% stroke rate reported for patients with hemispheric TIAs within the same follow-up period.[20] However, the results of this study may be misleading. Only 27 of the patients had undergone cerebral angiography, and 11 of these showed no abnormalities. Evidently patients with and without underlying atheromatous disease were mixed together in this study. Since the two groups probably have vastly different stroke prognoses, the aggregate data are not meaningful.

In the absence of better data it is most reasonable to presume that patients with TVL and carotid atheroma have a stroke prognosis equal to that of patients with retinal intraluminal plaques[69,76] or retinal stroke,[4,51,58,59] that is, 3% per year. This is slightly below the 5% per year stroke risk associated with other TIAs,[20,62] a discrepancy that may reflect the fact that ischemic events sufficient to interrupt vision are not as severe as those that interrupt other cerebral functions.

There is no information as to whether the threat of stroke in TVL is greatest within the first few months after the first event. This phenomenon has been observed for other TIAs, in which 20% of strokes will occur within 1 month and 50% within 1 year.[62] After that the stroke rate falls to 5% per year, still about five times greater than that for a control population.[62] The duration and frequency of TIAs have no prognostic value, except that some authors consider a sudden increase in frequency an ominous sign of impending stroke.[73]

The degree of carotid stenosis appears to predict likelihood of future stroke. Ziegler and Hassanein[87] have demonstrated that the risk of stroke in the presence of untreated extracranial atheromatous carotid disease is directly correlated with the degree of stenosis. Of 84 patients with less than 70% carotid stenosis, only seven (8%) developed a stroke within 3 years; of nine patients with 70% stenosis or more, four (44%) developed stroke within the same period. This information has led to a sense, though not a consensus, that endarterectomy should be limited to carotid stenosis of 50% of greater.[67] There is debate as to whether carotid ulceration is a separate risk factor.

There are no good data on the survivorship of patients with TVL. However, Pfaffenbach and Hollenhorst[69] found a 54% death rate after 7 years in patients with retinal intraluminal plaques, and Savino and Glaser[76] noted a 49% death rate after 7 years as compared to a 20% expected age-corrected death rate in a control population. This is comparable to the death rate in patients with other TIAs. Patients with TIAs occurring between age 55 and 64 have a 40% death rate after 5 years as compared to 5% for a control population.[35] The predominant cause of death is myocardial infarction, not stroke.[35,73] Patients 65 years or older at the time of onset of their first TIA have a death rate equal to that of a control population: 25% after 5 years.[35]

Risks and benefits of intervention. Therapy in patients with presumed atheromatous thromboembolism consists of endarterectomy and anticoagulation and platelet antiaggregant medications. The risks must also include those associated with cerebral angiography, which currently has an average morbidity of 0.25% and mortality of 0.1%.[82] However, in elderly patients with substantial atherosclerosis the risk may be higher.[82]

Endarterectomy. Many endarterectomy series report a surgical mortality of under 3%, but a weighted average of all reports from 1964 to 1973 was 4.7%.[38] In hospitals where surgeons perform fewer than two such operations per week, the complication rate may be much higher. In 228 consecutive endarterectomies performed from 1970 to 1976 in two 600-bed community hospitals, the overall stroke-mortality rate was 21%.[24] The procedures were performed by nine board-certified vascular surgeons and two neurosurgeons, all of whom had comparable complication rates. The stroke-mortality rate did not improve over time.

To justify these "up front" risks, endarterectomy must provide a significant reduction not only in TIAs but in stroke and stroke death. From 1961 to 1968 a multiinstitutional prospective trial randomized 316 TIA patients to undergo carotid endarterectomy (169) or receive anticoagulant treatment (147).[28] TIAs occurred in only 38% of the surgically treated group as compared to 55% of the medically treated group. In an average follow-up of 42 months, surgical patients had only 6 strokes (4%), while medical patients had 20 strokes (14%). However, 13 patients (7%) had postoperative strokes, and 6 (4%) died. Thus, if the perioperative outcomes are counted, surgical patients actually fared slightly worse. Careful statistical review indicates that endarterectomy would have had to yield a postoperative stroke-mortality rate of 2.9% or less in order to provide greater benefit than anticoagulation.[38] The collaborative study also revealed that patients with unilateral carotid stenosis fare better with surgery than those with bilateral stenosis. Recent-onset angina pectoris, congestive heart failure, hypertension, chronic obstructive pulmonary disease, obesity, and age over 70 increase the surgical morbidity of endarterectomy.[79]

Anticoagulants. If not monitored carefully, anticoagulants may increase the risk of cerebral hemorrhage.[41] But in a group of patients whose prothrombin times were assiduously controlled, warfarin anticoagulation did not significantly increase cerebral hemorrhage or mortality.[84] A review of the various randomized and nonrandomized studies reveals suggestive but no definitive evidence in favor of anticoagulation.[23]

Platelet antiaggregation agents. These agents have been used for the past decade to prevent stroke. They are without significant side effects, but of variable efficacy. Dipyridamole (Persantin) was found ineffective in reducing TIA, stroke, or death in one study.[1] Sulfinpyrazone (Anturane) did significantly reduce monocular TVL in one controlled study, but the cases were few, and follow-up was brief.[26] In two collaborative trials involving aspirin treatment, Fields et al.[27] found that aspirin (1300 mg per day) reduced TIAs but not stroke or death, while the Canadian Cooperative Study Group[11] showed a 48% reduction of stroke in males taking aspirin (1300 mg per day) but no therapeutic effect in females.

Management recommendations. In view of the limited state of our understanding of TIA and the problems associated with therapy, we advocate the following management: If history and examination suggest atheromatous vasculopathy and the patient reports monocular TVL, one must presume that carotid disease is causative (Chart 2-1, *E*). Only those patients suitable for endarterectomy should have cerebral angiography. Elderly patients ($\geq$70) with advanced cardiopulmonary disease are not good surgical risks and should be treated medically. Even if the patients are good surgical risks, they should be informed that endarterectomy entails at least a 1% to 3% risk of immediate stroke or death in return for the opportunity to reduce future stroke risk from 2% to 4% per year to 1% to 2% per year, without improvement in survival, which must be estimated at only 60% to 70% after 5 years.

Given that minimal carotid stenosis carries much less stroke risk than severe stenosis,[82] present (admittedly dated and inadequate) information supports endarterectomy only when there is 50% or greater stenosis with open distal circuits. Whether lesser degrees of stenosis or ulcerative plaques without stenosis are adequate indications remains controversial. Stenosis of the carotid siphon or complete cervical internal carotid occlusion are considered contraindications to endarterectomy, while external carotid stenosis is a debated indication. Under these constraints, Barnett estimates that "no more than 15% of stroke-threatened patients are eligible candidates (for) surgery."[8]

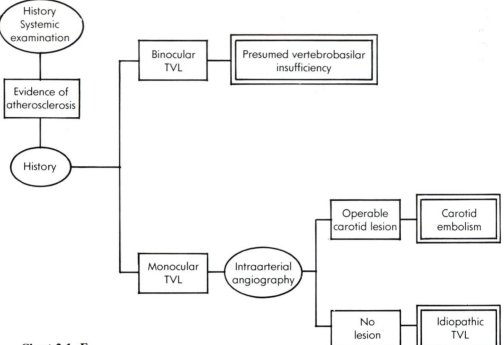

Chart 2-1, E

If patients with presumed atherosclerosis are certain that the TVL was binocular, either involving the entire field of both eyes, or the homonymous fields, then the diagnosis is likely to be VBI, and cerebral angiography and surgery are not indicated (Chart 2-1, E). There are no data to support the assertion that carotid endarterectomy is helpful in improving general cerebral perfusion in patients with vertebrobasilar ischemia.[39] Posterior circulation bypass and angioplasty procedures are now being performed, but their efficacy is unknown. We believe that patients with binocular TVL and evidence of atheromatous disease should be placed on aspirin (one tablet every other day). The exception is the patient presenting with a single attack of TVL and other brain stem symptoms or signs within the preceding 24 hours, who should be hospitalized promptly to rule out an evolving brain stem stroke, which requires immediate heparinization. Otherwise, these patients are also best managed with aspirin.

When there is no clinical evidence that monocular TVL is caused by atheromatous disease, as is so often the case in patients 40 or younger, we recommend DSA, a noninvasive investigation, because the likelihood of carotid disease is low (Chart 2-1, F). If DSA is normal, we consider the TVL to be idiopathic and either treat patients with aspirin or recommend no treatment. Patients of any age with binocular TVL and normal

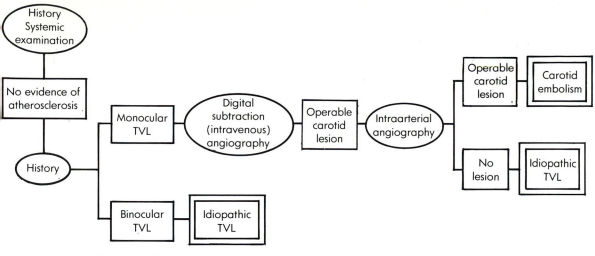

Chart 2-1, F

cardiac evaluation need not have DSA and may either be treated with aspirin or not be treated.

AN OVERVIEW

The essence of the TVL problem is that there are three populations:

1. An elderly population with widespread atherosclerosis
2. A small population of all ages with nonatherosclerotic diseases
3. A large nonelderly population with no demonstrable disease

For the first group, aggressive surgical treatment (endarterectomy) has been advised to forestall a high risk of future stroke. However, there is conflicting evidence as to whether the TVL population has the same or a slightly reduced stroke risk as compared to patients with other TIAs. Whatever the stroke risk, the therapeutic margin is slim in these patients, especially those with high surgical risk, because the best that surgery can promise is reduced TIA and stroke rate during a short residual lifetime. Platelet antiaggregants are a relatively safe and effective alternative in males but perhaps not in females.

For the second group, the patients with TVL and nonatherosclerotic disease, timely medical intervention may be of great value.

The large number of nonelderly patients with no demonstrable disease account for a large proportion of TVL cases. Their benign prognosis[22] makes it difficult to consider TVL equivalent to a cerebral or brain stem TIA. These patients should be minimally investigated, reassured, and not treated.

RETINAL ARTERY OCCLUSION

The considerations in managing patients with reversible ischemic visual deficits (TVL) apply in great measure to patients with completed retinal strokes. One must again ask the question: Is the patient at special risk of cerebral stroke? If so, what preventive measures should be undertaken?

Retrospective studies* of patients with retinal stroke suggest that the risk of cerebral

*References 4, 51, 58, 59, 69, and 76.

stroke is 2% to 3% per year—four to five times that of an age-matched population, but approximately half that of patients with hemispheric TIAs. Patients with both central retinal artery occlusion (CRAO) and branch retinal artery occlusion (BRAO) have reduced survivorship relative to age-matched controls. As with hemispheric TIA and stroke, the principal cause of death is myocardial infarction, not stroke.[69,76]

Evidently most patients with retinal stroke have widespread ischemic cardiovascular and cerebrovascular disease. Cohen[15] reviewed 25 cases of CRAO and found that 21 had arteriosclerotic risk factors, 11 had manifestations of arteriosclerotic vascular disease, 12 had substantial cervical carotid stenosis on angiography, and 8 developed infarctions within 9 months of follow-up. Appen et al.[4] found that of 44 patients over 40 years of age, the retinal stroke could be reasonably ascribed to arteriosclerosis in at least 20 (46%). Nonarteriosclerotic causes were diagnosed in 11 (25%), (5 with rheumatic heart disease, 2 with giant cell arteritis, 1 with lupus erythematosus, 1 with unspecified vasculitis, 1 with syphilis, and 1 with sickle-cell anemia). The rest remained idiopathic (13 [29%]). In this group, 18% developed strokes within 6 years.

There is, however, a youthful group of retinal stroke patients without atherosclerosis who have a much better prognosis. Among 10 patients under 40 years of age in the study of Appen et al.,[4] only 2 patients (20%) had arteriosclerotic disease (hypertension, 1; atrial fibrillation, 1). Retinal stroke was ascribed to nonarteriosclerotic disease in 3 (30%), including atrial myxoma (1), Marfan's with mitral valve insufficiency (1), orbital compression (1), and hypercoagulable state (1). In the remaining 5 (50%) the cause was never ascertained. In these 10 young patients, carotid angiography was normal, there were no risk factors or signs of arteriosclerosis, and no visible retinal emboli. With the exception of the patient with the atrial myxoma, there were no subsequent strokes in the average follow-up period of 6 years.

Wilson et al.[85] also found differences between the younger and older patient groups. In their series, 75% of the patients older than 50 who underwent angiography had operable lesions, as compared to only 15% of the younger patients.

Taken together, these data indicate that retinal stroke in patients more than 40 to 50 years old generally occurs in a setting of widespread arteriosclerotic disease. Nonarteriosclerotic causes are unusual but not unknown in this group and should be investigated when no arteriosclerotic risk factors or signs are present. The overall risk of stroke must, as with TVL, be viewed in the context of reduced longevity. On the other hand, the younger patients with retinal arterial occlusion rarely have arteriosclerosis, are not prone to stroke, and have normal survivorship. No single cause predominates, and many cases remain idiopathic.

The question of whether retinal strokes are principally embolic, thrombotic, or due to another mechanism cannot be settled with the present evidence. Although pathologic specimens are sparse, they suggest that either in situ thrombosis or embolism may be found in an occluded vessel.[88] Older patients with both CRAO and BRAO have a high probability of cervical carotid stenosis, but there is only circumstantial evidence that the carotid lesion is related to the retinal stroke, as with TVL.

Given these considerations, we believe that patients with retinal stroke should be managed just as one manages patients with TVL. Older patients with evidence of arteriosclerosis may indeed have a cervical carotid lesion as the source of the problem, but before one considers endarterectomy, one must bear in mind that the risk of stroke is not as great as with hemispheric TIAs. The more widespread the arteriosclerotic disease in the patient, the more unfavorable the patient is as a surgical candidate, both because of a high surgical risk and because of the reduced longevity. Consideration should be given to managing such patients with antiplatelet aggregation agents. Young patients must be carefully investigated for cardiac embolic and nonembolic causes. If none are found, DSA should be considered before cerebral angiography.

REFERENCES

1. Acheson, J, Danta, G, and Hutchinson, EC: Controlled trial of dipyridamole in cerebral vascular disease, Br Med J 1:614, 1969.
2. Ackerman, RH: A perspective on noninvasive diagnosis of carotid disease, Neurology (Minneap) 29:615, 1979.
3. Aita, JA: Systemic and nonarteriosclerotic causes of cerebral infarctions. In Vinken, PJ, and Bruyn, GW, editors: Handbook of clinical neurology, vol 11, Amsterdam, 1971, North Holland/American Elsevier, p 421.
4. Appen, RE, Wray, SH, and Cogan, DG: Central retinal artery occlusion, Am J Ophthalmol 79:374, 1975.
5. Barlow, JB, Pocock, WA, Marchand, P, and Denny, M: The significance of late systolic murmurs, Am Heart J 66:443, 1963.
6. Barnett, HJM: Cerebral ischemic events associated with prolapsing mitral valve, Arch Neurol 33:777, 1976.
7. Barnett, HJM: Pathogenesis of transient ischemic attacks. In Scheinberg, P, editor: Cerebrovascular diseases, Tenth Princeton Conference, New York, 1976, Raven Press, p 1.
8. Barnett, HJM: Progress towards stroke prevention: Robert Wortenberg Lecture, Neurology (Minneap) 30:1212, 1980.
9. Bartleson, JD, Swanson, JW, and Whisnant, JP: A migrainous syndrome with cerebrospinal fluid pleocytosis, Neurology (Minneap) 34:1257, 1981.
10. Boghen, D, and Glaser, JS: Ischaemic optic neuropathy. The clinical profile and natural history, Brain 98:689, 1975.
11. Canadian Cooperative Study Group (Barnett, HJM, et al): A randomized trial of aspirin and sulfinpyrazone in threatened stroke, N Engl J Med 299:53, 1978.
12. Christenson, PC, Ovitt, TW, and Fisher, HD: Intravenous angiography using digital video subtraction: intravenous cervicocerebrovascular angiography, Am J Neuroradiol. 1:379, 1980.
13. Cogan, DG: Blackouts not obviously due to carotid occlusion, Arch Ophthalmol 66:180, 1961.
14. Cogan, DG, and Wray, SH: Vascular occlusions in the eye from cardiac myxomas, Am J Ophthalmol 80:396, 1975.
15. Cohen, JL: The cardiovascular complications of retinal artery occlusion, Am J Cardiol 35:128, 1975.
16. Cohn, LH: Cardiac valve replacement with a stabilized gluteraldehyde porcine aortic valve: indications, operative results and follow-up, Chest 68:162, 1975.
17. Conti, CR, Pepine, CJ, and Curry, JC: Coronary artery spasm: an important mechanism in the pathophysiology of ischemic heart disease, Curr Probl Cardiol, vol 4, no 4, July 1979.
18. Dale, J: Arterial thromboembolic complications in patients with Bjork-Shiley and Lillehei-Kaster aortic disc valve prosthesis, Am Heart J 93:715, 1977.
19. David, NJ, Klintworth, GK, Friedberg, SJ, and Dillon, M: Fatal atheromatous cerebral embolism associated with bright plaques in retinal arterioles. Report of a case, Neurology (Minneap) 13:708, 1963.
20. Duncan, GW, Pessin, MS, Mohr, JP, and Adams, RD: Transient cerebral ischemic attacks, Adv Intern Med 21:1, 1976.
21. Dyll, L, Margolis, M, and David, NJ: Amaurosis fugax—funduscopic and photographic observations during an attack, Neurology (Minneap) 16:135, 1966.
22. Eadie, MJ, Sutherland, JM, and Tyrer, JH: Recurrent monocular blindness of uncertain cause, Lancet 1:319, 1968.
23. Easton, JD, and Byer, JA: Transient cerebral ischemia: medical management, Prog Cardiovasc Dis 22:371, 1980.
24. Easton, JD, and Sherman, DG: Stroke mortality rate in carotid endarterectomy: 228 consecutive operations, Stroke 8:565, 1977.
25. Ellenberger, C, Keltner, JL, and Burde, RM: Acute optic neuropathy in older patients, Arch Ophthalmol 28:182, 1973.
26. Evans, G: Effect of drugs that suppress platelet surface interaction on incidence of amaurosis fugax and transient cerebral ischemia, Surg Forum 23:239, 1972.

27. Fields, WS, Lemak, NA, Frankowski, RF, and Hardy, RJ: Controlled trial of aspirin in cerebral ischemia, Stroke 8:301, 1977.

28. Fields, WS, Maslenikov, V, Meyer, JF, Haff, WK, Remington, RD, and MacDonald, M: Joint Study of Extracranial Arterial Occlusion. V. Progress report of prognosis following surgical or non-surgical treatment for transient cerebral ischemic attacks and cervical carotid artery lesions, JAMA 211:1993, 1970.

29. Fisher, CM: Late-life migraine accompaniments as a cause of unexplained transient ischemic attacks, Can J Neurol Sci 7:9, 1980.

30. Fisher, CM: Observations of the fundus oculi in transient monocular blindness, Neurology (Minneap) 9:333, 1959.

31. Fisher, CM: Transient ischemic attacks—an update. In Scheinberg, P, editor: Cerebrovascular diseases, Tenth Princeton Conference, New York, 1976, Raven Press, p 50.

32. Fisher, CM: Transient monocular blindness associated with hemiplegia, Arch Ophthalmol 47:167, 1952.

33. Fox, IS, Spence, AM, Wheeles, RF, and Healey, LA: Cerebral embolism in Libman-Sacks endocarditis, Neurology (Minneap) 30:487, 1980.

34. Friedman, AP: Headache. In Baker, AB, and Baker, LH, editors: Clinical neurology, vol 2, Philadelphia, 1983, Harper & Row, Publishers, p 1.

35. Goldner, JC, Whisnant, JP, and Taylor, WF: Long-term prognosis of transient cerebral ischemic attacks, Stroke 2:160, 1971.

36. Gunning, AJ, Pickering, GW, Robb-Smith, AHT, and Russell, RR: Mural thrombosis of the internal carotid artery and subsequent embolism, Q J Med 33:155, 1964.

37. Hart, RG, and Easton, JD: Mitral valve prolapse and cerebral infarction, Stroke 13:429, 1982.

38. Hass, WK: Caution: falling rock zone: an analysis of the medical and surgical management of threatened stroke, Proc Inst Med Chic 33:80, 1980.

39. Heilbrun, P: Transient cerebral ischemia: surgical considerations, Prog Cardiovasc Dis 22:378, 1980.

40. Henkind, P, Charles, NC, and Pearson, J: Histopathology of ischemic neuropathy, Am J Ophthalmol 69:78, 1970.

41. Heyman, A, Nefziger, MD, and Acheson, RM: Epidemiologic study of the relationship of anticoagulant therapy to mortality from intracranial hemorrhage, Trans Am Neurol Assoc 97:152, 1972.

42. Hinton, RC, Kistler, JT, Fallon, JT, Friedlich, AL, and Fisher, CM: Influence of etiology of atrial fibrillation on incidence of systemic embolism, Am J Cardiol 40:509, 1977.

43. Hollenhorst, RW: Embolic retinal phenomena. In Symposium on neuro-ophthalmology. Transactions of the New Orleans Academy of Ophthalmology, St Louis, 1976, The CV Mosby Co, p 168.

44. Hollenhorst, RW: Significance of bright plaques in the retinal arterioles, JAMA 178:23, 1961.

45. Hollenhorst, RW. The neuro-ophthalmology of strokes. In Smith, JC, editor: Neuro-ophthalmology Symposium of the University of Miami and the Bascom Palmer Eye Institute, vol 1, St Louis, 1965, The CV Mosby Co, p 109.

46. Hooshmand, H, Vines, FS, Lee, HM, and Grindal, A: Amaurosis fugax: diagnostic and therapeutic aspects, Stroke 5:643, 1974.

47. Hoyt, WF: Ocular signs and symptoms. In Wylie, EJ, and Ehrenfield, WK, editors: Extracranial occlusive cerebrovascular disease, Philadelphia, 1970, WB Saunders Co, p 72.

48. Hulse, JA, Taylor, DSI, and Dillon, MJ: Blindness and paraplegia in severe childhood hypertension, Lancet 1:553, 1979.

49. Hutchinson, EC, and Stock, JP: Paroxysmal cerebral ischemia in rheumatic heart disease, Lancet 2:653, 1963.

50. Jellinek, EH, Painter, M, Prineas, J, and Ross-Russell, R: Hypertensive encephalopathy with cortical disorders of vision, Q J Med 130:239, 1964.

51. Karjalainen, K: Occlusion of the central retinal artery and retinal branch arterioles. A clinical, tonographic and fluorescein angiographic study of 175 patients, Acta Ophthalmol [Suppl] (Copenh) 109:1, 1971.

52. Kistler, JP, and Ropper, AH: Therapy of cerebrovascular disease. In Harrison's principles of internal medicine, update #1, New York, 1981, McGraw-Hill Book Co, p 69.

53. Kline, LB, and Kelly, CL: Ocular migraine in a patient with cluster headaches, Headache 20:253, 1980.

54. Knopman, DS, Anderson, DC, Asinger, RW, et al: Indications for echocardiography in patients with ischemic strokes, Neurology (Minneap) 32:1005, 1982.

55. Lemak, NA, and Fields, WS: The reliability of clinical predictors of extracranial artery disease, Stroke 7:377, 1976.

56. Lessell, S: Disorders of higher visual function. In Glaser, JS, and Smith, JL, editors: Neuro-ophthalmology Symposium of the University of Miami and the Bascom Palmer Eye Institute, vol 8, St Louis, 1975, The CV Mosby Co, p 5.

57. Lieberman, A: Intracranial hemorrhage and infarction in anticoagulated patients with prosthetic heart valves, Stroke 9:18, 1978.

58. Liversedge, LA, and Smith, VH: Neuromedical and ophthalmic aspects of central retinal artery occlusion, Trans Ophthalmol Soc UK 82:571, 1962.
59. Lorentzen, SE: Occlusion of the central retinal artery: a follow-up, Acta Ophthalmol 47:690, 1969.
60. Lovett, JC, Sandok, BA, Guiliani, ER, and Nasser, FN: Two-dimensional echocardiography in patients with focal cerebral ischemia, Ann Intern Med 95:1, 1981.
61. Marshall, J, and Meadows, S: The natural history of amaurosis fugax, Brain 91:419, 1968.
62. Matsumoto, N, Whisnant, JP, Kurland, LT, et al: Natural history of stroke in Rochester, Minnesota, 1955-1969: an extension of a previous study, Stroke 4:20, 1973.
63. McBrien, DJ, Bradley, RD, and Ashton, N: The nature of retinal emboli in stenosis of the internal carotid artery, Lancet 1:697, 1963.
64. McDowell, FH: Cerebral embolism. In Vinken, PJ, and Bruyn, GW, editors: Handbook of clinical neurology, vol 11, Amsterdam, 1972, North Holland/American Elsevier, p 386.
65. Meyer, JS, Charney, JZ, Rivera, VM, and Matthew, N: Cerebral embolization: prospective clinical analysis of 42 cases, Stroke 2:541, 1971.
66. Mungas, JE, and Baker, WH: Amaurosis fugax, Stroke 8:232, 1977.
67. Ojemann, RG, Crowell, RM, Roberson, GH, and Fisher, CM: Surgical treatment of extracranial carotid occlusive disease, Clin Neurosurg 22:214, 1975.
68. Pessin, MS, Duncan, GW, Mohr, JP, and Poskanzer, DC: Clinical and angiographic features of carotid transient ischemic attacks, N Engl J Med 296:358, 1977.
69. Paffenbach, DD, and Hollenhorst, RW: Morbidity and survivorship of patients with embolic cholesterol crystalization in the ocular fundus, Am J Ophthalmol 75:66, 1973.
70. Pomerance, A, and Davies, MG: Strokes: a complication of mitral leaflet prolapse, Lancet 2:1186, 1977.
71. Ramirez-Lassepas, M, Sandok, BA, and Burton, RC: Clinical indicators of extracranial carotid artery disease in patients with transient symptoms, Stroke 4:537, 1973.
72. Sanborn, GE, Miller, NR, Langham, ME, and Kumar, AJ: An evaluation of currently available, noninvasive tests of carotid artery disease, Ophthalmology 87:435, 1980.
73. Sandok, BA, Furlan, AJ, Whisnant, JP, and Sundt, TM: Guidelines for the management of transient ischemic attacks, Mayo Clin Proc 53:665, 1978.
74. Sandok, BA, and Guiliani, ER: Cerebral ischemic events in patients with mitral valve prolapse, Stroke 13:452, 1982.
75. Sandok, BA, Troutmann, JC, Ramirez-Lassepas, M, Sundt, TM, and Houser, OW: Clinical-angiographic correlations in amaurosis fugax, Am J Ophthalmol 79:137, 1975.
76. Savino, P, and Glaser, JS: Retinal stroke, Arch Ophthalmol 95:1185, 1977.
77. Silverstein, A, Gilbert, H, and Wasserman, LR: Neurologic complications of polycythemia, Ann Intern Med 57:909, 1962.
78. Slepyan, DH, Rankin, RM, Stahler, C, and Gibbons, GE: Amaurosis fugax: a clinical comparison, Stroke 6:493, 1975.
79. Sundt, TM, Sandok, BA, and Whisnant, JP: Carotid endarterectomy: complications and preoperative assessment of risk, Mayo Clin Proc 50:301, 1975.
80. Swash, M, and Earl, CJ: Transient visual obscurations in chronic rheumatic heart disease, Lancet 2:324, 1970.
81. Troost, BT, and Newton, TH: Occipital lobe arteriovenous malformations: clinical and radiologic features in 26 cases with the differentiation from migraine, Arch Ophthalmol 93:250, 1975.
82. Vitek, JJ: Femorocerebral angiography. Analysis of 2,000 consecutive examinations: special emphasis on carotid catheterization in older patients, Am J Roentgenol 118:633, 1973.
83. Waters, WE: Prevalence of migraine, J Neurol Neurosurg Psychiatry 38:613, 1975.
84. Whisnant, JP, Matsumoto, N, and Elveback, LR: The effect of anticoagulant therapy on the prognosis of patients with transient cerebral ischemic attacks in a community: Rochester, Minnesota, 1955 through 1969, Mayo Clin Proc 48:844, 1973.
85. Wilson, IA, Warlon, CP, and Ross-Russell, RW: Cardiovascular disease in patients with retinal arterial occlusion, Lancet 1:292, 1979.
86. Wolter, SR, and Burchfield, WJ: Ocular migraine in a young man resulting in unilateral transient blindness and retinal edema, J Pediatr Ophthalmol 8:173, 1971.
87. Ziegler, DK, and Hassanein, RS: Prognosis in patients with transient ischemic attacks, Stroke 4:666, 1973.
88. Zimmerman, LE: Embolism of central retinal artery secondary to myocardial infarction with mural thrombosis, Arch Ophthalmol 73:822, 1965.

CHAPTER 3

Abnormal optic disc

The abnormal optic disc may represent acquired disease or a congenital anomaly. We have divided optic disc abnormalities into those with and those without disc elevation.

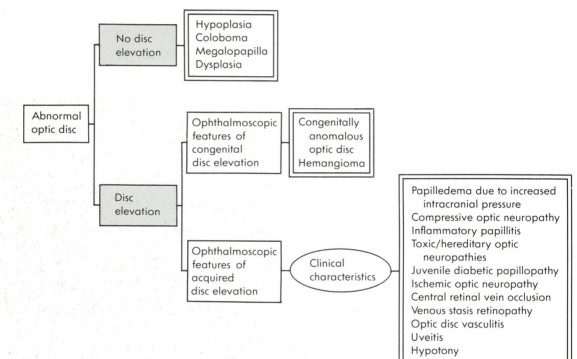

Chart 3-1

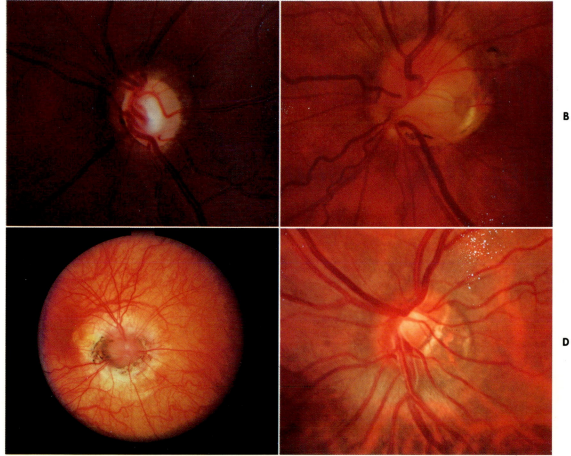

Plate 6. Congenitally anomalous optic discs without elevation. **A,** Hypoplasia: disc is smaller than normal, but vessels are of normal caliber. Rim of depigmentation (double ring sign) is evident, especially nasally. There is attrition of retinal nerve fiber layer. **B,** Optic pit: excavation at inferotemporal portion of left disc. **C,** Dysplasia: disc is larger than normal and is dysplastic. **D,** Tilted disc: disc is obliquely inserted into globe with a crescent being present inferotemporally.

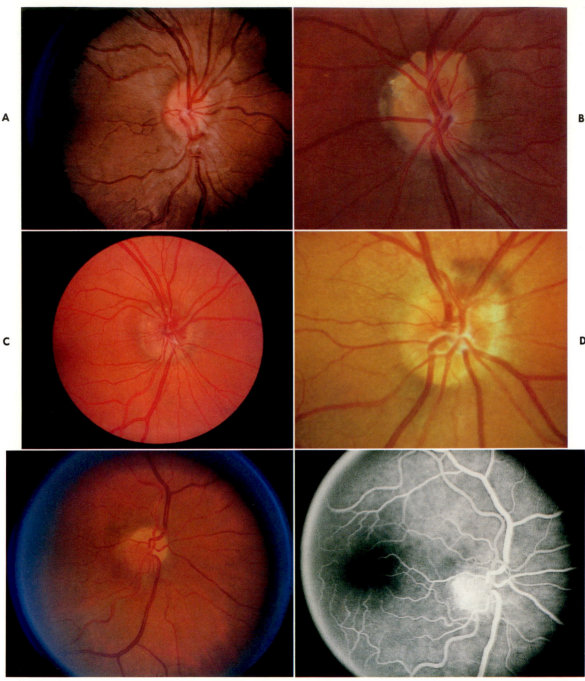

Plate 7. Congenitally anomalous optic discs with elevation. **A,** Without hyalin bodies: elevated disc without a cup showing abnormal branching pattern of large disc vessels. **B,** Hyalin bodies: note crystalline appearance of superior portion of disc. **C,** Hemorrhages on congenitally anomalous disc with obvious intrapapillary hyalin bodies. **D,** Subretinal-subRPE hemorrhage at superior pole of a congenitally anomalous disc. **E,** Hemangioma: reddish elevation may simulate sector swelling of ischemic optic neuropathy. Fluorescein angiography, **F,** delineates extent of this vascular malformation of disc.

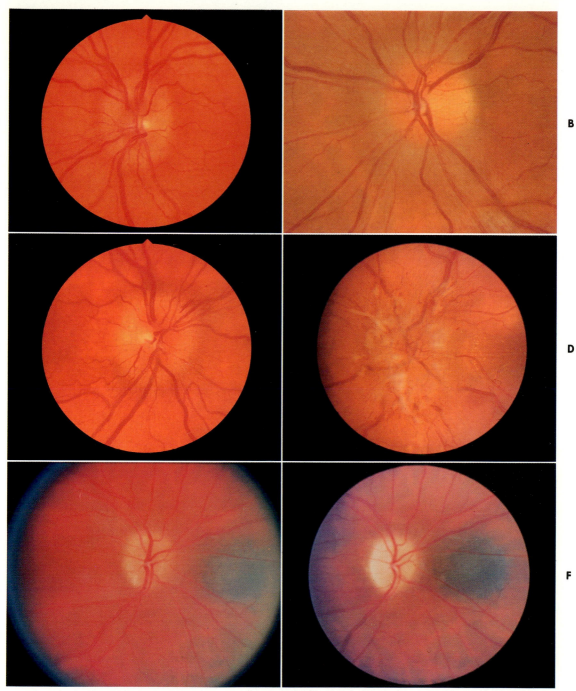

Plate 8. Stages of papilledema. **A,** Early: hyperemia due to engorgement of disc capillaries. **B,** Early: opacification of peripapillary nerve fiber layer obscures detail of disc margin. **C,** Fully developed: peripapillary nerve fiber layer hemorrhages appear. **D,** Fully developed: nerve fiber layer infarcts further obscure disc details. **E,** Chronic: disc is pale without hemorrhages. Crystalline deposits presumably of chronically stagnant axoplasm appear at 7 o'clock (pseudodrusen). **F,** Atrophic: disc is flat and pale. Pseudodrusen have disappeared.

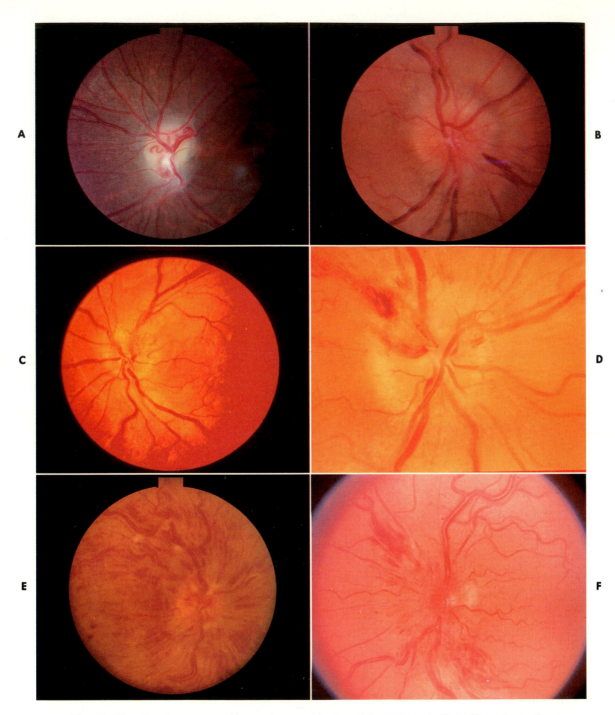

Plate 9. Disc elevation not secondary to increased intracranial pressure. **A,** Optociliary shunt: disc atrophic in patient with optic nerve sheath meningioma. **B,** Papillitis: disc hyperemic with blurred margins. A nerve fiber layer hemorrhage is present at 4 o'clock. **C,** Diabetic papillopathy: segmental swelling of right optic nerve with dilatation of radial capillary net in asymptomatic, insulin-dependent juvenile diabetic patient with 20/20 vision and normal visual field. **D,** Ischemic optic neuropathy: superior sector of disc is elevated and pale. Hemorrhage appears in this sector as well. **E,** Central retinal vein occlusion: disc margins blurred with nerve fiber layer infarcts at disc margin. Extensive nerve fiber layer hemorrhages beyond peripapillary area indicate primary retinal venous problem. **F,** Papillophlebitis: hemorrhages extend off the elevated disc but not to periphery as in **E.**

☐ **Optic disc anomalies without elevation** (Chart 3-1, *A*)
☐ **Hypoplasia**

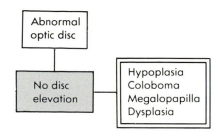

Chart 3-1, A

Complete absence of the optic disc and retinal vessels (optic disc aplasia) is rare. However, optic disc hypoplasia, where the optic nerve head is smaller than normal, is recognized as a relatively frequent cause of visual dysfunction. Optic disc hypoplasia may be unilateral or bilateral. The diagnosis is an ophthalmoscopic one; the optic disc appears smaller than its fellow or smaller than normal. The diagnosis is not difficult to make when the disc is severely hypoplastic. However, a spectrum of hypoplasia exists such that ophthalmoscopically subtle hypoplasia may be associated with severe visual deficits. While attempts have been made to measure optic nerve heads photographically, this is a cumbersome and largely unnecessary exercise. The small optic nerve head is often surrounded by two rings of pigmentation constituting the double-ring sign (Plate 6, *A*). The outer ring represents the junction between sclera and lamina cribrosa where the choroid is discontinuous, while the inner ring represents the termination of the retinal pigment epithelium.[52] Ophthalmoscopic evaluation of the retina usually reveals a decrease in the plushness of nerve fiber layer.[20]

The exact cause of optic disc hypoplasia is not known, although several hypotheses have been advanced. Hypoplasia may represent a primary failure of differentiation of retinal ganglion cells, but it may also be caused by secondary degeneration of ganglion cells and their fibers.[52] Contributing etiologic factors are a young maternal age and the use of anticonvulsants or hallucinogens during the gestational period.[32,66]

Visual acuity in patients with optic nerve hypoplasia may be normal or depressed. Even with normal acuity, visual field defects of an arcuate, altitudinal, or nasal sector variety may exist.[5,19] It is important to recognize the disorder so that unnecessarily prolonged occlusion of the contralateral eye is not undertaken because of the mistaken impression that amblyopia alone is the cause of decreased vision. However, a short trial of occlusion in the appropriate age group is indicated since associated amblyopia may be present. If vision does not improve within 2 weeks, patching should be discontinued.

Bilateral optic disc hypoplasia may be associated wtih central nervous system (CNS) and neuroendocrinologic disorders. Septo-optic dysplasia is a syndrome that includes optic disc hypoplasia, agenesis of the septum pellucidum and hypothalamus, and malformations of the optic chiasm resulting in a bitemporal hemianopia. The presence of optic disc hypoplasia and bitemporal hemianopia should prompt neuroradiologic investigation with CT scanning to document fusion of the lateral ventricles anteriorly. Patients with hypoplasia may have a growth hormone deficiency. Their short stature is reversible if treatment with growth hormone is instituted before epiphyseal closure occurs. Therefore these patients should be referred for endocrinologic evaluation.

☐ Coloboma

Colobomas are dysplastic excavations of the disc that can extend to involve the retina and choroid or be limited to the disc (optic pit). Pits are small, incomplete colobomas that routinely occupy the temporal, usually inferior, portion of the optic disc (Plate 6, *B*). They are nonprogressive lesions often associated with arcuate visual field defects that correspond to the location of the pits. Acuity remains normal unless serous detachment of the macula occurs. The point of origin of this serous fluid is probably the vitreous cavity.[8]

☐ Megalopapilla

Certain optic discs are larger than normal (megalopapilla). This abnormality is encountered much less frequently than hypoplasia. Megalopapilla also may be associated with cerebral defects. A large dysplastic optic disc (Plate 6, *C*) may occur with midline facial or skull abnormalities.[25] The complete syndrome includes midline cranial defects, such as hypertelorism, a broad, flat nasal root, cleft lip, and basal encephaloceles. Patients with megalopapilla require CT scanning of the base of the skull to demonstrate any midline bony defects with encephaloceles (Fig. 3-1).

☐ Other dysplasias

Some congenitally abnormal discs do not conveniently fit into any category. This spectrum of disc anomalies includes tilted discs, congenital crescents, situs inversus, and other oddly shaped discs that defy classification.

The *tilted optic disc* results from an oblique instead of a direct insertion of the optic nerve into the globe. As a result the disc appears oval with its vertical axis being directed obliquely, with a resulting inferior depression and relative superior elevation of the disc margin. Often there is nasal sweeping of the retinal vessels (situs inversus) with a rim of sclera visible inferiorly *(crescent)*. The inferior nasal fundus is often hypopigmented because of scleral thinning or a localized ectasia of the inferior fundus[70] (Plate 6, *D*).

These patients may be referred for neurosurgical evaluation because of visual field loss, which may resemble a bitemporal hemianopia. The scotoma, however, does not respect the vertical meridian on perimetry but tends to cross to the nasal side, thus distinguishing it from a true chiasmal visual field defect.

Field loss in some of these patients may be due to an exaggerated myopic astigmatism at an oblique axis. When perimetry is performed with an appropriate astigmatic lens in place, the scotoma often disappears.

☐ Optic disc anomalies with elevation

When the optic disc is found to be elevated, a critical distinction must be made between a static, congenital and a progressive, acquired disc elevation. This distinction may almost always be made on the basis of ophthalmoscopic criteria alone.

Congenital disc elevations include optic disc drusen and other dysplasias, while acquired entities include papilledema due to increased intracranial pressure, inflammatory

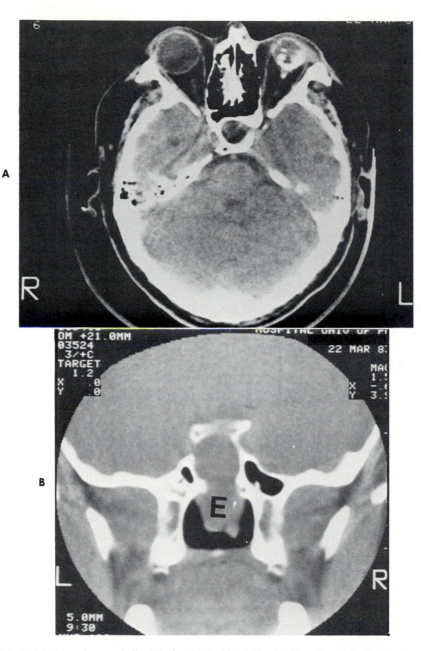

Fig. 3-1. Axial, **A,** and coronal, **B,** CT of patient with midline cleft syndrome (patient's disc shown in Plate 6, *C*). The sella is round with a scooped out appearance. Encephalocele, *E,* is seen extending through midline defect into sphenoid sinus.

papillitis, ischemic optic neuropathy, compressive optic neuropathy, ocular hypotony, and retinal venous stasis anomalies.

☐ **Ophthalmoscopic features of congenitally elevated optic disc** (Chart 3-1, *B*)

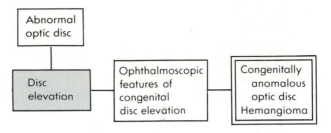

Chart 3-1, B

The congenitally elevated disc has a monotonously consistent appearance. It has no optic cup, and the retinal vessels appear to originate at the central core of the disc. In acquired disc elevation the central cup is generally preserved unless the swelling is marked, in which case other signs of acquired disc edema will be present.

The vascular pattern of the large optic disc vessels is abnormal in one third of patients with congenital disc elevation. These abnormalities consist of arterial and venous trifurcations or quadrifurcations as well as loops or coils on the optic disc (Plate 7, *A*). The large-vessel anomalies are distinctly different from small-vessel changes of telangiectasia or neovascularization of acquired disc swelling. Spontaneous venous pulsations are often present in congenital disc elevation but absent in acquired disc swelling because of increased intracranial pressure. The ophthalmoscopic detection of glistening hyalin bodies (drusen) within the optic nerve head indicates a congenital cause of disc elevation. Congenitally anomalous discs due to buried hyalin bodies are usually bilateral, being unilateral in approximately one third of patients.[59] Hyalin bodies are found almost exclusively anterior to the lamina cribrosa and tend to enlarge, becoming more visible with age (Plate 7, *B*).

Hemorrhage on or around the disc may occur rarely with intrapapillary hyalin bodies (Plate 7, *C*). The hemorrhages may be in the superficial nerve fiber layer or in the subretinal space. The deeper hemorrhages may lie beneath the retinal pigment epithelium (RPE) or between this layer and Bruch's membrane[68] (Plate 7, *D*). The subRPE hemorrhages can produce peripapillary pigment alterations with areas of loss of RPE at times alternating with pigment hypertrophy. Approximately one third of patients with intrapapillary hyalin bodies show these pigment changes,[59] suggesting that subRPE hemorrhages are more frequent than presently appreciated. Subretinal neovascular membranes may develop and cause bleeding into the subretinal space. Bleeding may uncommonly extend into the vitreous.[62] Because of the rare association of hemorrhage with hyalin bodies of the disc however, the appearance of peripapillary hemorrhage in or around an elevated optic disc should suggest *acquired* disc elevation.

Obscuration of the nerve fiber layer is an important sign that helps distinguish acquired from congenital disc elevation. The underlying mechanism by which acquired disc elevation occurs is swelling of the nerve fiber layer axons secondary to interruption or stagnation of axoplasmic flow. Since there is no axoplasmic stasis in the congenitally elevated optic disc, the nerve fiber remains clear.

There is, unfortunately, no single ophthalmoscopic feature that reliably separates acquired from congenital optic disc elevation. It is essential to examine all the features of the optic disc to make an ophthalmoscopic checklist or balance sheet. To recapitulate, following are the characteristics that should be evaluated:

1. The optic cup: absence of an optic cup with no other signs of florid disc edema is strongly suggestive of a congenitally anomalous disc.
2. The optic disc vasculature: large vessel trifurcations, loops, or coils indicate a congenitally anomalous elevated disc, whereas abnormalities of the smaller vessels with telangiectasia, new vessel formation, or optociliary shunt vessels suggest acquired elevation.
3. Spontaneous venous pulsations: their presence is further evidence against increased intracranial pressure, but their absence is not necessarily indicative of elevated intracranial pressure.[43]
4. Peripapillary hemorrhages: the presence of nerve fiber layer hemorrhages strongly suggests an acquired disc elevation, although in some patients, drusen of the optic disc can produce hemorrhages indistinguishable from those of true papilledema.
5. The nerve fiber layer: opacification due to axoplasmic damming is a sign of acquired disc elevation; a clear nerve fiber layer suggests congenital disc elevation.

Even with the utilization of this checklist the distinction between congenital and acquired disc elevation may not be obvious. It is often helpful to examine family members of such patients because congenital anomalous disc elevation may be familial. The presence of congenital disc elevation in a parent or sibling is good circumstantial evidence that the disc in question is congenitally anomalous. In these instances and in the absence of any focal neurologic signs, it is appropriate to obtain photographs of the optic disc. The patient is reexamined in 2 to 3 days, and if there is no change in the disc appearance, the patient is reexamined within a week. If the disc elevation is acquired, there will be ophthalmoscopic changes, whereas if the elevation is congenital, there will be no change.

Certain congenital vascular anomalies of the optic disc and retina may cause progressive visual loss and may therefore be confused with acquired disc elevation. Capillary hemangiomas are examples of such lesions. They are usually reddish in color, and upon close inspection the vascular nature of the lesions can be appreciated (Plate 7, *E*). Fluorescein angiography will reveal early filling and late dye leakage (Plate 7, *F*). Most hemangiomas are isolated abnormalities, but they may be associated with the von Hippel-Lindau disease.[22,63]

☐ **Ophthalmoscopic features of acquired disc elevation** (Chart 3-1,*C*)
☐ **Papilledema**

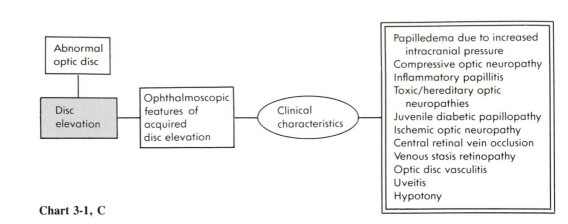

Chart 3-1, C

Most neuro-ophthalmologists reserve the term papilledema for optic disc elevation due to increased intracranial pressure. However, the term papilledema itself is to a certain extent a misnomer. Light and electron microscopy have shown that disc elevation primarily is due to axonal swelling and degeneration. Some interstitial edema is present, but the glial cells show no sign of intracellular edema.[65] The exact mechanism producing papilledema is still debated. It appears that there must be transmission of the increased pressure to the optic nerves along their meningeal sheaths since surgical opening of the perioptic meninges will result in detumescence of the disc[21] without decreasing the increased intracranial pressure.[36] This increased perineural pressure results in a damming of the slow component of axoplasmic flow at the lamina cribrosa. This process is believed to produce disc swelling and nerve fiber layer opacification. The fast component of axoplasmic flow is also involved, but this is probably a secondary phenomenon.

Papilledema is almost invariably a bilateral phenomenon if both optic discs were previously normal. If one disc is atrophic, nerve fiber layer edema cannot develop. For example, the papilledema seen in Foster Kennedy's syndrome is truly unilateral, because one optic disc has become atrophic from chronic compression of the optic nerve by a subfrontal tumor.[40] On rare occasions, strictly unilateral papilledema may occur with a normal appearing contralateral optic disc. It is suggested that the increased intracranial pressure is not transmitted to the optic nerve subarachnoid space because of an optic nerve sheath anomaly.[41] However, the patient who has unilateral optic disc swelling with a normal appearing fellow optic disc is unlikely to have papilledema (disc swelling due to increased intracranial pressure). In this instance it is prudent to look for a local ocular or orbital process as the cause of the disc elevation.

The ophthalmoscopic appearance of papilledema will vary depending on the duration of the disc swelling. Hoyt and Beeston[33] described the following staging of papilledema:

1. Early papilledema: shows minimal hyperemia of the disc, early opacification of the nerve fiber layer, and the absence of spontaneous venous pulsations (Plate 8, *A* and *B*).
2. Acute (fully developed) papilledema: the addition of hemorrhage or exudation to the signs of early papilledema (Plate 8, *C* and *D*).

3. Chronic papilledema: there is a paucity of hemorrhages or exudates, but there is capillary telangiectasia on the disc surface. Small, refractile, drusenlike bodies may appear on the disc surface, but they may disappear should the disc swelling abate[56] (Plate 8, *E*). Optociliary shunt vessels also develop at this stage.
4. Atrophic papilledema: characterized by optic disc pallor with nerve fiber bundle visual field defects (Plate 8, *F*).

We do not advocate the use of fluorescein angiography as an aid in the diagnosis of papilledema. In fully developed papilledema fluorescein angiography is unnecessary. In incipient papilledema if the ophthalmoscopic diagnosis is uncertain, fluorescein angiography is likely to be equivocal.

The patient with papilledema may complain of transient obscurations of vision. These may occur in one or both eyes and typically last only for seconds. They may occur as the patient moves from a sitting to standing position or may be independent of any postural change. Obscurations occur only with well-developed papilledema and are probably caused by compression of the blood vessels at the optic nerve itself.[12] The occurrence of obscurations does not appear to be a sign of impending infarction of the optic disc,[15] although infarction does occur rarely in papilledema.[26]

Visual acuity is normal in acute papilledema unless there is concomitant macular edema. Preretinal or subRPE macular hemorrhages, exudates in a star figure, or choroidal folds extending through the macula may decrease central acuity in acute papilledema.[51]

Perimetry will reveal only enlargement of the blind spots in the early stages of papilledema. In the more chronic forms visual field defects will appear, the most frequent being inferior nasal nerve fiber bundle defects identical to those seen in glaucoma.[15,28] Visual acuity loss is a late finding.

The diagnosis of papilledema constitutes a medical emergency (Chart 3-1, *D*). The patient should be admitted to the hospital immediately and a CT scan performed. If a mass lesion is discovered, further testing to determine its nature and appropriate treatment is indicated. If no mass is detected and the ventricles are not dilated, lumbar puncture is performed to measure the cerebrospinal fluid (CSF) pressure and to exclude meningitis. If the spinal fluid is normal, except for increased pressure, the patient probably has pseudotumor cerebri.

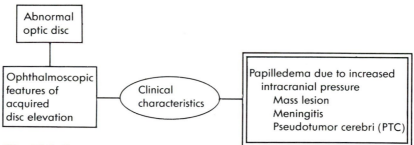

Chart 3-1, D

☐   **Pseudotumor cerebri (PTC)**

1. Signs of increased intracranial pressure usually but not invariably[64,69] manifested by papilledema.
2. The absence of neurologic signs with the exception of sixth cranial nerve paresis.
3. A normal or small ventricular system on computerized tomography (CT) scan[30] and no evidence of an intracranial mass lesion. An empty sella may be seen in up to 25% of patients.[15]
4. Normal CSF except for increased pressure.

Etiology of PTC. The syndrome of PTC may be produced by a variety of conditions or agents, or it may be idiopathic:

Intracranial (dural) venous sinus thrombosis. Dural sinus thrombosis may occur following head trauma, suppurative otitis media or mastoiditis,[34] and obstruction of the superior vena cava or jugular vein. Dural sinus thrombosis decreases the pressure differential across the arachnoid villi, causing decreased absorption of CSF.[35] CT scan may reveal a hyperdensity within one of the dural sinuses with a lucent defect in the torcular Herophili, but arteriography is most often necessary to establish this diagnosis.[6] The thrombosed sinus usually recanalizes, with resultant resolution of the PTC.

Exogenous agents. Drugs such as tetracycline,[23] nalidixic acid,[14] and nitrofurantoin,[53] corticosteroid use or withdrawal,[67] or hypervitaminosis A[44] may cause PTC. The dose of vitamin A necessary to induce PTC varies from 25,000 to 60,000 IU daily.[18]

Endocrinologic abnormalities. Endocrinologic abnormalities appear to play an important role in the PTC syndrome. Most patients are obese young women who frequently have menstrual irregularities. No consistent endocrine abnormality has been detected in these patients. A mild hypothalamic-hypophyseal insufficiency was documented in five patients with PTC, but this may be an effect of chronically increased intracranial pressure and not its cause.[3] Pseudotumor cerebri has also been reported in patients with Turner's syndrome,[17] hypoparathyroidism, and adrenal adenoma.[7] Because of the infrequency of definable endocrinologic abnormalities in PTC, we recommend that no endocrinologic studies be performed in these patients unless relevant clinical signs are present.

Systemic disorders. Rarely, certain systemic disorders such as systemic lupus erythematosus,[11] chronic respiratory insufficiency, or iron-deficiency anemia may be associated with PTC.

Idiopathic PTC. Johnston and Paterson[34] were able to identify a cause for PTC in 44% of their 110 patients. Rush,[61] however, found a cause in only about 15% of his 63 patients. Our experience is that most patients with PTC are obese women in the third decade of life with the idiopathic variety of the disorder.[15] In our collective experience a cause for PTC is usually identified in less than 5% of patients.

In its idiopathic form, PTC may be a self-limiting disorder that resolves within months.[34] However, recurrence of PTC may occur in up to 40% of patients.[61]

Pathogenesis of PTC. The exact mechanism by which PTC is produced remains unknown. The theory most often advanced is that there is increased arachnoid resistance to CSF drainage.[1,47] Other theories support an abnormality of the cerebral microvasculature causing increased cerebral blood volume. Proponents of this theory claim that incracranial hypertension is produced by brain tissue swelling due to increased water content.[58]

Hypersecretion of CSF usually results in hydrocephalus, but this mechanism may explain the occurrence of PTC, especially in obese young women.[16] Supporters of the hypersecretion theory point to the low CSF protein concentration as evidence of the dilution effect of hypersecretion.

Symptoms of PTC. Headache is the most frequent symptom, being reported in 75% to 99% of patients. *Diplopia,* due to sixth nerve paresis, is a nonspecific sign of increased intracranial pressure (ICP). Visual disturbances include transient obscurations of vision, visual field defects, or decreased acuity.[9,34,61]

The persistence of intracranial hypertension in PTC appears to have no consequences other than those resulting from the visual morbidity of chronic atrophic papilledema. Blinding visual loss or severe visual impairment was found in 14 of 57 patients with PTC observed for up to 41 years.[15] Duration of papilledema does not appear to be a critical factor in the development of visual field loss. Progressive visual field defects may appear in weeks or may not occur even after years of chronic papilledema.[15,61] The only risk factor to vision in the series by Corbett et al.[15] was systemic hypertension. The characteristic visual field defects are optic nerve related, for example, enlarged blind spots, nasal arcuate defects, generalized constriction, and, less commonly, cecocentral scotomas. The appearance or progression of one of these field defects on sequential perimetry necessitates the institution or intensification of treatment.

Treatment of PTC. The presence of papilledema in PTC is not in itself an indication for treatment. Some patients may tolerate years of papilledema with no visual consequences. Patients who develop signs of visual loss from chronic papilledema or those with intractable headache should be treated. Treatment will vary, depending on the identification of a cause of the increased ICP.

Increased venous pressure. Since thrombosed venous sinuses producing PTC will usually recanalize, the papilledema is usually transient and as a rule does not produce permanent visual disability. If progressive visual loss occurs in the setting of prolonged papilledema, systemic corticosteroids should be given. Continued deterioration of vision despite this treatment is an indication for lumboperitoneal shunt or optic nerve sheath decompression (see below). Dehydrating agents should be avoided in this syndrome because they will aggravate the thrombosis.

PTC induced by exogenous agents. The withdrawal of any ingested agent that has produced PTC will result in resolution of the papilledema.

PTC associated with systemic diseases. In those rare instances of PTC associated with systemic disease (lupus, anemia), treatment of the associated disorder should be undertaken simultaneously with the treatment of PTC.

Idiopathic PTC. The treatment of idiopathic PTC is controversial, and a variety of medical and surgical regimens have been advocated:

1. Repeated lumbar puncture: Because the CSF volume removed by lumbar puncture is re-formed within less than 24 hours, we cannot advocate this form of therapy for the treatment of a chronic disorder. Lumbar puncture is also uncomfortable for the patients, who often fail to return for follow-up treatment.
2. Dehydrating agents: The oral dehydrating agents (glycerol and isosorbide) are rapidly metabolized, and their pressure-lowering effect is short lived, lasting only 4 hours. Oral glycerol is nauseatingly sweet and often results in poor patient compliance. It is also difficult to recommend in morbidly obese patients who are often diabetics.
3. Carbonic anhydrase inhibitors: Acetazolamide (4 g daily) has been shown to

decrease ICP in two patients with PTC who underwent continuous ICP recording.[29] This dose is often poorly tolerated because of the side effects of numbness and tingling of the hands and feet, anorexia, malaise, a tinlike taste, and fatigue. If side effects result, methazolamide (Neptazane) may be substituted. Although no data are available, we have used this drug successfully in the treatment of PTC. Diurectics such as furosemide and hydrochlorothiazide also have been utilized in the treatment of PTC.

4. Corticosteroids: The administration of oral corticosteriods will decrease ICP and promote the resolution of papilledema. However, PTC tends to be a chronic disorder, and chronic corticosteroid administration to already obese patients may aggravate this aspect of their problem.

5. Weight reduction: Loss of weight alone or in combination with other medical therapy may be beneficial in the treatment of PTC.[54] We urge weight reduction in all our obese patients with PTC.

6. Surgical treatment: A variety of surgical procedures will relieve the chronic intracranial hypertension of PTC. Since the ventricles are not enlarged, shunting procedures are more easily performed via the lumboperitoneal route. These shunts may cease to function, and reoperation for shunt revision is often necessary. Subtemporal decompression is rarely performed today since the advent of lumboperitoneal shunting operations. Relief of papilledema may be attained by incision of the sheath surrounding the intraorbital portion of the optic nerve.[21] While this will effectively provide local relief to the optic nerve, it does not lower the increased ICP.[36] Findings from isolated case reports leave little doubt that disc elevation subsides and visual field loss may reverse following sheath decompression.[10,39] To date, however, no series has appeared that outlines indications, complications, or long-term effects of optic nerve sheath decompression. Therefore this mode of treatment may be recommended only with caution.

Management of PTC. In addition to visual acuity measurement, color vision testing (with Ishihara or similar plates) at each visit is mandatory. A progressing acquired dyschromatopsia is compelling evidence of a developing optic neuropathy.[55] Visual field examination with particular attention to the arcuate areas is performed at each visit.

Our recommendations for the management of patients with PTC are as follows:

1. The patient who has papilledema with no symptoms and an otherwise normal ophthalmologic examination requires no treatment to lower the increased ICP. This patient must be reexamined monthly initially to detect signs of early optic nerve compromise. If visual function remains normal for 3 months, the periodic reexaminations may be extended (2 to 3 months). We emphatically urge weight loss and place all obese patients on a weight reduction regimen.

2. The patient with papilledema who has transient visual obscurations or signs of optic nerve dysfunction is begun on acetazolamide. The initial dose is 1 g daily but is increased to higher doses (2 to 4 g daily) depending on the patient's tolerance of the drug. The patient is reexamined every 2 to 3 weeks for signs of progressive optic nerve compromise.

3. The patient with papilledema who develops a progressive optic neuropathy while taking therapeutic doses of acetazolamide (or metazolamide) requires more aggressive treatment to lower the ICP. Corticosteroids at a dose of 80 to 100 mg

of prednisone daily will lower the ICP. The difficulties with chronic steroid administration in this patient population have been outlined.

Other treatment alternatives include repeat lumbar puncture, lumboperitoneal shunt, or optic nerve sheath decompression. If the patient has no headache and the only signs or symptoms are visual, we would recommend sequential bilateral optic nerve sheath decompression. The presence of nonvisual symptoms attributable to increased ICP is an indication for a lumboperitoneal shunt.

☐ Compressive optic neuropathy

Optic disc elevation and decreased acuity may be associated with optic nerve tumors (meningioma or glioma), cysts, or with a variety of orbital tumors causing optic nerve compression. Orbital inflammation (pseudotumor or dysthyroid orbitopathy) may cause compression of the optic nerve with resultant decreased acuity and disc edema. Inflammatory orbital disease usually is associated with proptosis or diplopia so that the optic disc elevation is only one part of an overall constellation of signs and is rarely, if ever, an isolated finding (see Chapter 9). Optic nerve tumors are usually slow growing, and because they are intradural, they strangle the optic nerve, causing chronic optic disc elevation. The presence of optociliary shunt vessels is another sign of chronic, progressive constriction or infiltration of the optic nerve (Plate 9, A). However, these shunt vessels may be seen with chronic disc elevation from any cause. Chronic meningitis caused by infection (cryptococcosis) or neoplasm (carcinomatous meningitis, leukemia) may produce disc swelling either by causing elevation of ICP or infiltration of the optic nerves. CSF findings (cells, protein, cryptococcal antigen) should establish the correct diagnosis.

☐ Inflammatory papillitis

Disc elevation and decreased acuity may be caused by optic neuritis (Plate 9, B). Optic neuritis may rarely produce bilateral simultanous swollen discs. The correct diagnosis is made by the typical visual field abnormalities.

☐ Toxic and hereditary optic neuropathy

The presence of symmetric bilateral cecocentral scotomas with disc swelling usually implies a toxic or hereditary cause. However, most toxic or hereditary optic neuropathies do not have disc elevation. An agent that produces a toxic optic neuropathy with disc edema is chloramphenicol.[24] Since this drug is often used in children with cystic fibrosis, the presence of a papillitis-like syndrome should suggest chloramphenicol toxicity. Vision recovers upon drug withdrawal. Patients with Leber's optic neuropathy may appear to have disc swelling, but this is really a telangiectasia of the peripapillary region (see Chapter 1, Part II).

☐ Juvenile diabetic papillopathy

Another rare cause of acquired disc swelling is the disc edema that occurs in juvenile diabetics (Plate 9, C). This entity may present with few symptoms, or there may be a host of visual findings including central scotomas, arcuate visual field defects, and afferent pupillary defects. Disc edema is usually bilateral but may be unilateral. Acuity routinely improves within a 3-month period, although the disc edema itself may take a year to resolve.

The visual prognosis is generally, but not uniformly, favorable. All eight patients in one study had 20/20 vision without optic atrophy after 3 months of follow-up. One patient, however, had a constricted visual field, a relative afferent pupillary defect, and "mild optic atrophy."[57] The vision in 6 of 21 eyes reported by Barr et al.[4] did not return to normal. One patient had amblyopia, with vision never being better than 20/400; a second patient's vision improved to 20/50, but he had been observed for only 3 months at the time of the report. Four patients experienced deterioration of vision during the follow-up period, but two had proliferative retinopathy with vitreous hemorrhage; one developed a central retinal vein occlusion; the fourth had macular edema. Four additional patients had a permanent visual field defect and optic atrophy.[4]

The exact mechanism producing the disc swelling remains obscure. Fluorescein angiography does not show ischemia at the optic disc.[57] Barr et al.[4] speculate that optic nerve damage may result from relative anoxia secondary to failure of glucose utilization.

☐ Ischemic optic neuropathy

Acquired optic disc elevation with an altitudinal or arcuate visual field defect suggests infarction of the optic disc (Plate 9, *D*). Visual acuity may be normal or severely depressed (see Chapter 1, Part II).

☐ Central retinal vein occlusion and venous stasis retinopathy

Optic disc elevation, in one or both eyes, may be caused by central retinal vein occlusion (CRVO) or other anomalies of the retinal venous circulation (Plate 9, *E*). There are two major clinical forms of CRVO: ischemic (hemorrhagic) and nonischemic. Both forms present with an elevated optic disc and intraretinal hemorrhages. The distinction between the two is the presence of capillary nonperfusion on fluorescein angiography, which identifies the ischemic form. The ischemic type is more likely than the nonischemic form to lead to neovascular glaucoma.[46]

Kearns and Hollenhorst[38] described a form of optic disc edema associated with peripheral retinal hemorrhages and dilated retinal veins in patients with carotid occlusive disease. They named this condition *venous stasis retinopathy,* a term unfortunately later used by Hayreh[31] to describe a form of retinal vein occlusion. One of the important factors distinguishing between the two conditions is that the retinal artery pressure in the retinopathy of carotid disease is always decreased, while it is normal in this form of vein occlusion.[37]

CRVO may signify the presence of a variety of disorders. The most frequently associated diseases are arterial hypertension, diabetes mellitus, and cardiovascular disease.[48,60] Kohner et al.[42] reviewed 191 consecutive patients with CRVO and found the following percentages of intercurrent disease: hypertension 44%, elevated serum urea 25%, diabetes mellitus 15%, elevated triglycerides 40%, and cholesterol 30%. They also recommended an erythrocyte sedimentation rate and packed cell volume to detect hyperviscosity syndromes. The visual outcome was independent of the associated medical condition or its treatment. Chronic open-angle glaucoma is the ocular condition most frequently associated with CRVO, as it is found in approximately one third of all patients with CRVO.[27,46]

We recommend that the patients with CRVO have a medical evaluation that includes the following tests:

- Blood pressure determination
- 2-hour postprandial blood sugar
- Electrocardiogram
- Complete blood count
- Lipid profile
- Serum protein electrophoresis
- Serum viscosity

Optic disc vasculitis

Some patients may present a picture similar to CRVO or venous stasis retinopathy, but pathologic examination will reveal inflammation of the retinal veins.[2,13] Most instances of phlebitis will resolve without permanent visual sequelae. This may be identical to that form of disc swelling called papillophlebitis (Plate 9, *F*), which is encountered in young patients.[45]

A similar or possibly identical form of self-limiting, benign disc elevation seen in young, otherwise healthy individuals has been termed the *big blind spot syndrome*.[49] The only positive clinical findings are an elevated optic disc with venous overfilling, occasional retinal hemorrhages, and enlargement of the blind spot on visual field testing. The etiology remains obscure, but this syndrome may represent optic neuritis without involvement of central acuity or a mild form of venous occlusive disease.[50]

Uveitis/ocular hypotony

Optic disc elevation is often seen in patients with uveitis. There is often an accompanying diffuse posterior uveitis (posterior scleritis) or a peripheral uveitis (pars planitis). The optic disc will also be elevated in the hypotonous eye. The combination of uveitis and hypotony makes disc elevation a frequent finding in ocular inflammation.

REFERENCES

1. Aisenberg, RM, and Rottenberg, DA: The pathogenesis of pseudotumor cerebri, J. Neurol Sci 48:51, 1980.
2. Appen, RE, deVenecia, G, and Ferwerda, J: Optic disk vasculitis, Am J. Ophthalmol 90:352, 1980.
3. Barbar, SG, and Garvan, N: Is "benign intracranial hypertension" really benign? J Neurol Neurosurg Psychiatry 43:136, 1980.
4. Barr, CC, Glaser, JS, and Blankenship, G: Acute disc swelling in juvenile diabetes. Clinical profile and natural history of 12 cases, Arch Ophthalmol 98:2185, 1980.
5. Bjork, A, Laurell, CG, and Laurell, U: Optic nerve hypoplasia with normal visual acuity, Am J Ophthalmol 86:524, 1978.
6. Brant-Zawadzki, M, Chang, GY, and McCarty, GE: Computed tomography in dural sinus thrombosis, Arch Neurol 39:446, 1982.
7. Britton, C, Boxhill, C, Brust, JCM, et al: Pseudotumor cerebri, empty sella syndrome, and adrenal adenoma, Neurology (Minneap) 30:292, 1980.
8. Brown, GC, Shields, JA, Patty, BE, et al: Congenital pits of the optic nerve head, I. Experimental studies in collie dogs, Arch Ophthalmol 97:1341, 1979.
9. Bulens, C, DeVries, AEJ, and Van Crevel, H: Benign intracranial hypertension. A retrospective and follow-up study, J Neurol Sci 40:147, 1979.
10. Burde, RM, Karp, JS, and Miller, RN: Reversal of visual defect with optic nerve decompression in long-standing pseudotumor cerebri, Am J. Ophthalmol 77:770, 1974.
11. Carlow, TJ, and Glaser, JS: Pseudotumor cerebri syndrome in systemic lupus erythematosus, JAMA 228:197, 1974.
12. Cogan, DG: Blackouts not obviously due to carotid occlusion, Arch Ophthalmol 66:180, 1961.
13. Cogan, DG: Retinal and papillary vasculitis, In Cant, JS, editor: The William Mackenzie Centenary Sympsoium on the Ocular Circulation in Health and Disease, St. Louis, 1969, The CV Mosby Co, p 249.

14. Cohen, DN: Intracranial hypertension and papilledema associated with nalidixic acid therapy, Am J. Ophthalmol 76:680, 1973.

15. Corbett, JJ, Savino, PJ, Thompson, HS, et al: Visual loss in pseudotumor cerebri. Follow-up of 57 patients from five to 41 years and a profile of 14 patients with permanent severe visual loss, Arch Neurol 39:461, 1982.

16. Donaldson, JO: Pathogenesis of pseudotumor cerebri syndromes, Neurology (Minneap) 31:877, 1981.

17. Donaldson, JO, and Binstock, JL: Pseudotumor cerebri in an obese woman with Turner syndrome, Neurology (Minneap) 31:758, 1981.

18. Edmunds, C, Behrens, M, Lewis, L, and Lennon, R: Pseudotumor cerebri and low vitamin-A intake, JAMA 226:674, 1973.

19. Frisén, L: Visual field defects due to hypoplasia of the optic nerve, Doc Ophthalmol 19:81, 1979.

20. Frisén, L, and Holmegaard, L: Spectrum of optic nerve hypoplasia, Br J Ophthalmol 62:7, 1978.

21. Galbraith, JEK, and Sullivan, JH: Decompression of the perioptic meninges for relief of papilledema, Am J. Ophthalmol 76:687, 1973.

22. Gass, JD, and Braunstein, R: Sessile and exophytic capillary angiomas of the juxtapapillary retina and optic nerve head, Arch Ophthalmol 98:1790, 1980.

23. Giles, CL, and Soble, AR: Intracranial hypertension and tetracycline therapy, Am J. Ophthalmol 72:981, 1971.

24. Godel, V, Nemet, P, and Lazar, M: Chloramphenicol optic neuropathy, Arch Ophthalmol 98:1417, 1980.

25. Goldhammer, Y, and Smith, JL: Optic nerve anomalies in basal encephalocele, Arch Ophthalmol 93:115, 1975.

26. Green, GJ, Lessell, S, and Loewenstein, JI: Ischemic optic neuropathy in chronic papilledema, Arch Ophthalmol 98:502, 1980.

27. Green, WR, Chan, CC, Hutchins, GM, et al: Central retinal vein occlusion: a prospective histopathologic study of 29 eyes in 28 cases, Retina 1:27, 1981.

28. Grehn, F, Knorr-Held, S, and Kommerell, G: Glaucomatouslike visual field defects in chronic papilledema, Albrecht Von Graefes Arch Klin Exp Ophthalmol 217:99, 1981.

29. Gucer, G, and Viernstein, L: Long-term intracranial pressure recording in the management of pseudotumor cerebri, J. Neurosurg 49:256, 1978.

30. Hahn, FJ, and McWilliams, FE: The small ventricle in pseudotumor cerebri: demonostration of the small ventricle in benign intracranial hypertension by computed tomography, CT 2:249, 1978.

31. Hayreh,SS: Central retinal vein occlusion: differential diagnosis and management, Trans Am Acad Ophthalmol Otolaryngol 83:OP379, 1977.

32. Hoyt, CS, and Billson, FA: Maternal anticonvulsants in optic nerve hypoplasia, Br J. Ophthalmol 62:3, 1978.

33. Hoyt, WF, and Beeston, D: The ocular fundus in neurologic disease, St. Louis, 1966, The CV Mosby Co, p 2.

34. Johnston, I, and Paterson, A: Benign intracranial hypertension. I. Diagnosis and prognosis, Brain 97(2):289, 1974.

35. Johnston, I, and Paterson, A: Benign intracranial hypertension. II. CSF pressure and circulation, Brain 97(2)301, 1974.

36. Kaye, AH, Galbraith, JEK, and King, J: Intracranial pressure following optic nerve decompression for benign intracranial hypertension, J Neurosurg 55:453, 1981.

37. Kearns, TP: Differential diagnosis of central retinal vein obstruction, Ophthalmology 90:475, 1983.

38. Kearns, TP, and Hollenhorst, RW: Venous-stasis retinopathy of occlusive disease of the carotid artery, Mayo Clin Proc 38:304, 1963.

39. Keltner, JL, Albert, DM, Lubow, M, et al: Optic nerve decompression: a clinical pathologic study, Arch Ophthalmol 95:97, 1977.

40. Kennedy, F: Retrobulbar neuritis as an exact diagnostic sign of certain tumors and abscesses in the frontal lobes, Am J Med Sci 42:355, 1911.

41. Kirkham, TH, Sanders, MD, and Sapp, GA: Unilateral papilledema in benign intracranial hypertension, Can J Ophthalmol 8:533, 1973.

42. Kohner, EM, Laatikainen, L, and Oughton, J: The management of central retinal vein occlusion, Ophthalmology 90:484, 1983.

43. Levin, BE: The clinical significance of spontaneous pulsations of the retinal vein, Arch Neurol 35:37, 1978.

44. Lombaert, A, and Carton, H: Benign intracranial hypertension due to A-hypervitaminosis in adults and adolescents, Eur Neurol 14:340, 1976.

45. Lonn, LI, and Hoyt, WF: Papillophlebitis. A cause of protracted yet benign optic disc edema, Ear Nose Throat 45:62, 1966.

46. Magargal, LE, Brown, GC, Augsburger, JJ, et al: Neovascular glaucoma following central retinal vein obstruction, Ophthalmology 88:1095, 1981.

47. Mann, JD, Johnson, RN, Butler, AB, and Bass, NH: Impairment of cerebrospinal fluid circulatory dynamics in pseudotumor cerebri and response to steroid treatment, Neurology (Minneap) 29:550, 1979.

48. McGrath, MA, Wechsler, F, Hunyor, ABL, et al: Systemic factors contributory to retinal vein occlusion, Arch Intern Med 138:216, 1978.

49. Miller, NR: The big blind spot syndrome: unilateral optic disc edema without visual loss or increased intracranial pressure. In Smith, JL, editor: Neuro-ophthalmology update, New York, 1977, Masson Publishing USA, p 163.

50. Miller, NR, editor: Walsh and Hoyt's clinical neuro-ophthalmology, ed. 4, Baltimore, 1982, The Williams & Wilkins Co, p 223.

51. Morris, AT, and Sanders, MD: Macular changes resulting from papilloedema, Br J. Ophthalmol 64:211, 1980.

52. Mosier, MA, Lieberman, MF, Green, WR, et al: Hypoplasia of the optic nerve, Arch Ophthalmol 96:1437, 1978.

53. Mushet, GR: Pseudotumor and nitrofurantoin therapy, Arch Neurol 34:257, 1977.

54. Newborg, B: Pseudotumor cerebri treated by rice-reduction diet, Arch Intern Med 133:802, 1974.

55. Nikoskelainen, E, and Falck, B: Do visual evoked potentials give relevant information to the neuro-ophthalmological examination in optic nerve lesions? Acta Neurol Scand 66:42, 1982.

56. Okun, E: Chronic papilledema simulating hyaline bodies of the optic disc, Am J Ophthalmol 53:922, 1962.

57. Pavan, PR, Aiello, LM, Wafai, Z, et al: Optic disc edema in juvenile–onset diabetes, Arch Ophthalmol 98:2193, 1980.

58. Raichle, ME, Grubb, RL, Jr, Phelps, ME, et al: Cerebral hemodynamics and metabolism in pseudotumor cerebri, Ann Neurol 4:104, 1978.

59. Rosenberg, MA, Savino, PJ, and Glaser, JS: A clinical analysis of pseudopapilledema. I. Population, laterality, acuity, refractive error, ophthalmoscopic characteristics and concident disease, Arch Ophthalmol 97:65, 1979.

60. Rubinstein, K, and Jones, EB: Retinal vein occlusion: long-term prospects—10 years follow-up of 143 patients, Br J Ophthalmol 60:148, 1976.

61. Rush, JA: Pseudotumor cerebri clinical profile and visual outcome in 63 patients, Mayo Clin Proc 55:541, 1980.

62. Sanders, TE, Gay, AJ, and Newman, M: Hemorrhagic complications of drusen of the optic disk, Am J Ophthalmol 71:204, 1971.

63. Schindler, RF, Sarin, LK, and MacDonald, PR: Hemangiomas of the optic disc, Can J Ophthalmol 10:305, 1975.

64. Spence, JD, Amacher, AL, and Willis, NR: Cerebrospinal fluid (CSF) pressure monitoring in the management of benign intracranial hypertension without papilledema, Neurology (Minneap) (abstr) 29:551, 1979.

65. Tso, MO, and Hayreh, SS: Optic disc edema in raised intracranial pressure. III. A pathologic study of experimental papilledema, Arch Ophthalmol 95:1448, 1977.

66. Van Dyk, HJL, and Morgan, KS: Optic nerve hypoplasia and young maternal age, Am J Ophthalmol 89:879, 1980.

67. Walker, AE, and Adamkiewicz, JJ: Pseudotumor cerebri associated with prolonged corticosteroid therapy, JAMA 188:779, 1964.

68. Wise, GN, Henkind, P, and Alterman, M: Optic disc drusen and subretinal hemorrhage, Trans Am Acad Ophthalmol Otolaryngol 78:212, 1974.

69. Wolfe, R, and Bird, AC: Fundus. In Lessell, S, and van Dalen, JTW, editors: Neuro-ophthalmology, Amsterdam, 1980, Excerpta Medica, vol 2, p 9.

70. Young, SE, Walsh, FB, and Knox, DL: The tilted disk syndrome, Am J Ophthalmol 82:16, 1976.

CHAPTER 4

Gaze and vergence disturbances

Abnormalities of ocular motor function can exist in isolation or as part of more widespread central nervous system (CNS) disease without visual symptoms. Such abnormalities involve either the supranuclear gaze centers and their connections or the extraocular muscles themselves. Recognition of these relatively asymptomatic ocular movement disorders is helpful in characterizing and classifying the underlying disease.

Definitions

The ocular motor system in man has but one purpose, to place the image of regard upon both foveas simultaneously and to maintain this physiologic state in all gaze positions until the individual decides to look at something else. The ocular motor system may be conceptualized in many ways. Functionally, there appear to be five distinct supranuclear systems[3]: (1) saccadic system, (2) pursuit system, (3) vergence system, (4) position maintenance fixation system, and (5) vestibular system. These supranuclear systems are defined by the stimuli that activate the movement and by the response characteristics of the ocular movements initiated (Table 4-1). Some of these supranuclear systems have been identified with particular cortical substrates (Table 4-1). With the exception of the vestibular system these supranuclear systems have a supratentorial control center that projects to a subservient, but still supranuclear, brain stem center. The function of the brain stem center is modulated by the cerebellum and the vestibular complex.

Supranuclear systems specify the action of coordinated muscle groups and not of individual muscles. Destruction of supranuclear centers results in a loss of gaze function, not in diplopia. The output of these supranuclear systems is translated into action in one of three modes[17]: (1) rapid eye movements, 400° to 600°/s, (2) slow eye movements, up to 40°/s, and (3) vergence movements, up to 20°/s.

Supranuclear mechanisms

Fast movement or saccadic supranuclear system. Command, random eye movements and involuntary movements toward visual and auditory stimuli are always fast or saccadic. The corrective fast phases of all types of jerk nystagmus, rapid eye movements seen during sleep, and corrective movements during pursuit exceeding 40°/s are also saccadic. With the exception of foveational movements in response to visual stimuli, all saccades probably originate in the contralateral frontal eye fields (Brodmann's areas 8 alpha and gamma). Saccades to visual stimuli are probably initiated in the general area of the occipitoparietal junction. Whether they are mediated through the frontal eye fields or the superior colliculus is unknown. Recent evidence[34,42] suggests that the ipsilateral

Table 4-1. Supranuclear control mechanism

	Position maintenance	Pursuit	Saccadic	Vergence	Nonoptic reflex (vestibular)
Function	Maintain eye position vis-à-vis target	Maintain object of regard near fovea; matches eye and target	Place object of interest on fovea rapidly	Align visual axes to maintain bifoveal fixation	Maintain eye position with respect to changes in head and body posture
Stimulus	Visual interest and attention (?)	Moving object near fovea	Object of interest in peripheral field	Retinal disparity	Stimulation of semicircular canals, utricle, and saccule
Latency (from stimulus to onset of eye movement)		125 ms	200 ms	160 ms	Very short
Velocity	Both rapid (flicks, microsaccades) and slow (drifts)	To 100°/s, accurately to 30°/s	To 400°/s	Around 20°/s	To 300°/s*
Feedback		Continuous	Sampled data		
Substrate	Occipitoparietal junction	Occipitoparietal junction	Frontal lobe; occipitoparietal junction; superior colliculus(?)	Unknown	Vestibular apparatus: muscle receptors in neck → cerebellum(?)

From Burde, RM: The extraocular muscles. In Moses, RA, editor: Adler's physiology of the eye, ed 7, St Louis, 1981, The CV Mosby Co, p 122.
*Slow phase only. The fast phase, although initiated in the pontine reticular formation, is discharged via the saccadic mechanism.

frontal cortex is capable of initiating ipsilateral saccades when the contralateral hemisphere has been damaged.

The frontobulbar projection arises in the frontal eye fields and courses dorsomedially to pass through the anterior limb of the internal capsule near its knee adjacent to the globus pallidus. Here the fibers separate into two bundles:

1. Major pathway: courses dorsomedially along the ventrolateral surface of the thalamus through the zona incerta and the fields of Forel. In the rostral midbrain these fibers are situated in the dorsal aspect of the corticospinal tract as part of the corticobulbar projection and decussate in the lower midbrain and upper pons to end up in the paramedian pontine reticular formation (PPRF) at the level of the abducens nuclei.
2. Secondary pathway: continues ipsilaterally rather than decussating before turning dorsally to enter the pontine tegmentum.

The pathways subserving saccadic movements initiated in the occipitoparietal region remain unknown. Disorders affecting this part of the saccadic system have not yet been recognized clinically.

The PPRF acts as the brain stem center subserving conjugate ipsilateral horizontal gaze movements of all types. In addition the PPRF sends projection pathways to the mesencephalon that subserve vertical gaze. Büttner-Ennever et al.[5] and Pierrot-Deseilligny et al.[31] have presented evidence that the secondary centers for vertical gaze in the mesencephalon are the rostral interstitial nuclei of the medial longitudinal fasciculi (riMLF). Each nucleus lies dorsomedial to the anterior pole of the red nucleus, rostral to the interstitial nucleus of Cajal, and lateral to the nucleus of Darkshevich. There is agreement that the medial and lateral areas of the riMLF subserve either upgaze or downgaze but disagreement as to which part of the riMLF is responsible for which function. Straight up and down movements from the primary position require bilateral cortical input.

Slow movement or pursuit supranuclear system. The pursuit supranuclear system is used for tracking targets moving in a fairly regular fashion across the environment. This system can maintain foveal fixation on targets with speeds of 30° to 40°/s. There is general agreement[4] that the center for smooth pursuit is located in the broad region of the occipitoparietal junction. Although the pathways subserving smooth pursuit projecting to the PPRF are unknown, a double decussation is postulated.[15] Clinically, supranuclear dysfunction of this system is best understood in terms of ipsilateral control; that is, the right occipitoparietal junction controls smooth pursuit to the right, and the left junction to the left.[15]

Vergence system. Disjunctive eye movements enable the subject to fixate bifoveally at all points in space from infinity to the near point of convergence. This flexibility calls for active convergence or divergence, the supranuclear substrates of which are unknown. Vergence movements have a maximum velocity of approximately 20°/s. Under normal conditions the act of convergence is associated with pupillary miosis and accommodation.

Position maintenance fixation supranuclear system. This supranuclear system works to maintain the object of regard on the foveas once it is placed there by a foveation movement. Robinson[33] has added weight to the separation of this supranuclear system from that of the pursuit supranuclear system.

Fixation is a relative term. The eyes are never absolutely still, even under laboratory conditions. Three types of movement[32] may be seen during fixation, but their combined effect results in an amplitude of eye movement that is usually less than 10 minutes of arc.

Vestibular system. The vestibular apparatus, including the peripheral labyrinth (utriculus, sacculus, and semicircular canals) and its central connections, is intimately involved with coordinating tone of the body musculature, including the extraocular muscles, in response to gravitational and accelerational changes. This system is discussed in greater detail in Chapter 6.

Disorders involving supranuclear control pathways

Since supranuclear centers specify the action of coordinated muscle groups, dysfunction results, for the most part, in gaze abnormalities, not in diplopia. The patients often are either not aware of their gaze deficits or relate the symptoms, such as blurring of vision in spasm of the near reflex or their inability to see the food on their plates in progressive supranuclear palsy, to a deficiency in their glasses. These disorders will be discussed first in terms of dysfunction of the supranuclear centers and then in terms of more diffuse CNS or extraocular muscle disease.

Disorders of saccadic movements. Such disorders can be caused by lesions anywhere from the frontal eye fields to the PPRF.

Unilateral pathology. Saccadic palsy can be produced by large lesions involving the frontal eye fields. Acutely, when these patients are stuporous, their eyes will be deviated toward the side of the lesion. At this time the doll's head maneuver of passive head turning or caloric stimulus will produce a full range of ocular movements. The saccadic corrective phase will be absent in the direction contralateral to the lesion during caloric testing. As these patients regain consciousness, their eyes assume the straight-ahead position, but they are unable to make volitional or fixational movements to the side contralateral to the lesion. Reflex stimuli ordinarily used to cause corrective fast phase nystagmus in the direction contralateral to the lesion will produce a tonic deviation of the eyes toward the side of the lesion.

With time there is improvement from saccadic palsy through paresis to what appears as clinically normal saccades if the contralateral hemisphere is intact. As the saccadic palsy begins to improve, the eyes will move eccentric to the midline, but the eccentric gaze position cannot be held, and a coarse gaze-paretic nystagmus develops with a drift toward the midline followed by a corrective saccade in the eccentric direction. Over weeks or months these saccadic movements become more and more normal with a concomitant disappearance of the gaze-paretic nystagmus. Similar recovery will be seen in reflexly induced fast movements. If the contralateral frontal lobe has been damaged, the patient may remain with a global saccadic palsy.

Bilateral pathology. Bilateral dysfunction of the frontomesencephalic system produces a loss of saccadic function in all directions of gaze with maintenance of pursuit and oculocephalic and tonic vestibular deviations. Depending on the processes, vertical saccades are affected variably.

Ocular motor apraxia

Congenital form. Although apraxia is defined as the loss of a previously acquired ability to perform intricate skilled acts,[18] there is no evidence that the patients defined as having congenital ocular motor apraxia by Cogan and Adams[9] ever had normal saccadic function. This disorder is characterized by the inability of patients to make normal voluntary horizontal saccades when their heads are immobilized. These patients use head thrusts to induce compensatory eye movements by the vestibular system. That is, if they want to look at an object off to the right, the following typical sequence ensues:

1. Closure of the lids to break fixation.
2. A rapid head thrust to the right driving the eyes tonically to the left, the head thrust overshooting the target and placing the image of regard on the foveas of each eye in left gaze.
3. The object is held fixated by each eye, and the head is slowly rotated to the left until the eyes are in midposition.

Most of these patients have normal vertical saccades and pursuit movements.[8] In addition these patients have severe defects in the production of the fast phase of optokinetic and caloric nystagmus.[9] Head thrusts become less apparent with age as these patients develop some degree of saccadic function.[8] Although this is usually a benign familial disorder, it may be associated with pigmentary retinopathy, Gaucher's disease, spinocerebellar degeneration, and Pelizaeus-Merzbacher disease.[10]

Zee et al.[45] have reported three patients who had what is apparently a forme fruste of the complete syndrome. With the head immobilized, these individuals showed delayed initiation and hypometria of voluntary saccades. The fast phase of both optokinetic and vestibular nystagmus were almost normal. These patients utilized head thrusts to boost or trigger the saccadic movement.

Acquired forms. There are a variety of forms of acquired volitional saccadic palsy. The saccadic deficit varies from a global loss of volitional or fixational saccadic movements to delayed initiation and hypometria of voluntary saccades. Some of these patients maintain random saccadic movements.[9,15] Patients may or may not have deficits in the fast phases of induced nystagmus. Others have minimal pursuit deficits. As Cogan has pointed out, "The paradoxical maintenance of random eye movements with loss of purposeful eye movements often gives rise to the erroneous impression of hysterical blindness."[6] Many of these patients have associated difficulty with initiating head movements and sometimes movements of the arms and legs. This is not surprising, as head and limb movements are programmed in areas contiguous to eye movement centers in the prefrontal eye fields.

Huntington's chorea. Huntington's chorea is an autosomally dominant genetic disease with an insidious onset, usually in the late thirties. The ocular abnormality is a marked loss of saccadic velocity.[38] Initially, dysarthria and choreic movements, most notable in the face and distal extremities, are seen, which steadily become worse. Mental deterioration begins a few years after the onset of the involuntary movements and progresses inexorably to total dementia. Late in the course of the disease there are no fast movements during attempted voluntary gaze, optokinetic stimulation, vestibular testing, reading, and REM (rapid eye movement) sleep. In addition, there is an absence of random eye movements. Other findings include intermittent, nonstereotypical spasm of the facial muscles accompanied by periods of eyelid closure and periods during which the lids remain wide open.

Miscellaneous. Saccadic paralysis has been reported in multiple sclerosis, Wilson's disease, lipidosis, and spinocerebellar degenerations.[16]

Disorders of smooth pursuit. Disorders of smooth pursuit may be caused by lesions involving the occipitoparietal junction, the projection pathways to the PPRF, and the brain stem itself. The normal smooth pursuit movement is replaced by a series of small saccades. Similarly, certain cerebellar diseases cause saccadic pursuit.

Unilateral pursuit paresis. Unilateral pursuit paresis is most often caused by lesions in the posterior cortical hemisphere or in the hemisphere of the cerebellum. In cortical disease there is a loss of ipsilateral pursuit, which is usually accompanied by Cogan's sign of spasticity of gaze. To demonstrate this phenomenon the patient is instructed to squeeze his eyes closed, and the examiner forcibly opens the lids. The globes will be displaced to the side opposite the lesion instead of assuming the up and out position of Bell's phenomenon. Such lesions are associated with contralateral homonymous visual field defects and an asymmetry of the optokinetic response. Hemispheric cerebellar lesions produce ipsilateral pursuit deficits without producing the other signs that are found in cortical disease.

Bilateral pursuit deficits. The presence of bilateral saccadic pursuit can be produced by diffuse posterior hemispheric, cerebellar, or brain stem disease. In the latter case the saccadic pursuit movements are seen in the setting of more global deficits such as those associated wtih Parkinson's disease or progressive supranuclear palsy. Many sedative drugs lower the maximum velocity at which smooth pursuit movements can be generated. Thus even when tracking slow targets, affected patients will demonstrate intermittent superimposed ''catch-up'' saccades.

Disorders of the vergence system

Divergence paralysis and convergence paralysis. Patients with either of these disorders usually present with the complaint of diplopia and therefore are discussed in Chapter 5.

Spasm of the near reflex. The major complaint of patients with spasm of the near reflex is a general blurring of their vision. A smaller number will note diplopia, and an even smaller number will note crossing of their eyes. The diagnosis is based on the finding of a variable esotropia associated with varying pupillary size. Similar changes in accommodation can be demonstrated with sequential measurements of the near point of accommodation. Spasm of the near reflex is most often associated with some sort of psychic stress such as puberty or studying for college examinations. Some patients can voluntarily cross their eyes and use this ability to feign illness. Although in most cases the spasm disappears spontaneously, at times it may be necessary to use ''tricks'' to alleviate the patient's symptoms. This can be accomplished in a number of different ways. We suggest using the following sequence of maneuvers.

1. Saccadic gaze movements: Instruct the patient to look to the right, to the left, up, and down in rapid sequence either by direction or by providing a target in the various gaze positions.

2. Grasp the patient's hand and ask him to follow his thumb. Move the hand slowly in all gaze directions.

3. If both of these maneuvers fail to interrupt the spasm, use an optokinetic target and have the patient count the targets out loud. Slowly increase the speed of the optokinetic stimulus. In the vast majority of cases the spasm will be interrupted.

4. At this point, if the patient still cannot relax his eyes to normal alignment, irrigation of the external auditory canals (after otoscopic examination to exclude middle ear pathology) with cold water (50 ml, 4°C) will induce caloric nystagmus, breaking the spasm. Recurrent bouts of spasm of the near reflex may require the use of 2% to 5% homatropine once or twice a day for a short period of time.

Disorders of the position maintenance fixation system. Abnormalities of this subsystem may be the underlying defect in afferent system and congenital nystagmus (see Chapter 6). Fixation instability often accompanies cerebellar disease, for example, ocular dysmetria, flutter, and opsoclonus, which may represent lack of cerebellar modulation over the brain stem input from this system.

Disorders of the vestibular system. Since vestibular dysfunction generally produces nystagmus, disease states affecting the vestibular system are discussed in Chapter 6.

Gaze abnormalities

Gaze palsies are defined[16] as an inability to move the eyes either by saccades or smooth pursuit in a given direction. They can be caused by lesions anywhere from the cerebral cortex, where they must be diffuse involving both the frontal and occipitoparietal centers, to the PPRF. Lesions may be more localized when involving the projection pathways, especially within the midbrain, but the effects produced are rarely limited to a gaze palsy.

Isolated horizontal gaze deficit. There is a group of patients who have familial congenital paralysis of horizontal gaze.[44] In this group all horizontal conjugate eye movements are absent. Vertical movements and optokinetic nystagmus, as well as convergence, are variably affected. It is postulated that these patients have a developmental anomaly affecting motor neurons and interneurons in the abducens and paraabducens nuclei.

Vertical gaze palsies

Downgaze. Isolated paralysis of downgaze has been reported in a number of cases of pretectal disease.[5,31] Büttner-Ennever et al.[5] reviewed six pathologic cases of isolated paralysis of downgaze that had been reported, while Pierrot-Deseilligny et al.[31] reported the pathologic findings in an additional two cases. These patients all had lesions involving the riMLF just rostral to the third nerve nucleus and dorsomedially to the red nucleus in the pretectum.

Upgaze. Büttner-Ennever et al.,[5] as well as Pierrot-Deseilligny et al.,[31] note that isolated upgaze paralysis is associated wtih lesions contiguous to the posterior commissure. Both groups suggest that involvement of the riMLF or its projections are necessary for upgaze paresis. Thames et al.[40] describe a man with upgaze paralysis who had a single lesion of the brain stem confined to the periaqueductal gray matter between the levels of the superior and inferior colliculi. They suggest that the upgaze paresis was due to interruption of fiber pathways going to or away from the riMLF.

Parinaud's syndrome (sylvian aqueduct syndrome, dorsal midbrain syndrome). Patients with Parinaud's syndrome generally present initially with a paresis of saccadic upgaze. The first complaint is often related to difficulty with playing a sport at which they had previously excelled, such as baseball or basketball. Upon attempting upward saccades (exaggerated by using an optokinetic stimulus in the downward direction[36]), both eyes will be seen to make a convergence movement while simultaneously being retracted into the orbits. This movement is produced by cofiring of muscles supplied by the third nerve nucleus.[22] Diplopia is often recognized due to the concomitant presence of a partial third or fourth cranial nerve palsy or secondary to a skew deviation. These patients may also complain of transient obscurations of vision secondary to the papilledema. Other common findings include middilated (4 to 5 mm) pupils that demonstrate

---

OCULAR SIGNS AND SYMPTOMS OF PARINAUD'S SYNDROME

Common

1. Loss of saccadic upgaze
2. Light-near dissociation of the pupillary reflexes (pupils are 4 to 5 mm in diameter)
3. Papilledema
4. Convergence-retraction nystagmus elicited by the use of an optokinetic tape in the downward direction

Less common

1. Third cranial nerve paresis
2. Fourth cranial nerve paresis
3. Skew deviation
4. Spontaneous convergence-retraction movements elicited by upgaze movements
5. Loss of upgaze pursuit

Infrequent

1. Peduncular hallucinosis
2. Precocious puberty

---

light-near dissociation, convergence paresis, lid retraction (Collier's sign),[11] convergence spasm, downgaze paresis, and corectopia.

Precocious puberty and peduncular hallucinosis have also been reported as part of this syndrome but must be rare. The sylvian aqueduct syndrome is most frequently caused by aqueductal stenosis and tumors of the pineal gland, but it has also been reported with infiltrating tumors in the region of the aqueduct and the superior colliculus as well as with neurosyphilis, multiple sclerosis, trauma, and stroke.[7]

Monocular elevation paresis. Monocular elevation paresis is a rare acquired disorder in which there is an interruption of supranuclear input from the presumed vertical upgaze center in the pretectum to the oculomotor complex.[25,29] The characteristic findings are listed:

1. Acute onset.
2. Diplopia on upward gaze due to limitation of elevation in one eye.
3. No vertical anomaly on cover test in the primary position or in general on looking down, but occasionally there may be weakness of ipsilateral depression.
4. The elevating muscles of the other eye appear normal.
5. Bell's phenomenon is reduced to the degree of paresis.
6. No ptosis, lid retraction, or enophthalmos are present.
7. There may be associated pupillary abnormalities including anisocoria, sluggish light reactions, and light-near dissociation.
8. Occasionally there may be convergence weakness.
9. Forced duction testing and the Tensilon test are both negative.

Jampel and Fells[25] postulate a discrete ischemic lesion in the pretectum as the cause in their patients. Lessell[29] adds credence to their postulate in his report of a patient with bronchiogenic carcinoma who lost the ability to elevate his left eye voluntarily and who was found to have a metastatic lesion in the right pretectum at postmortem examination. Although no long-term follow-up is reported in the cases of Jampel and Fells, in our experience this tends to be a long-lasting problem.

Upgaze and downgaze paresis. Progressive supranuclear palsy and Parkinson's disease are two other entities in which the pathology is primarily supranuclear but which show involvement of the ocular motor nuclei as well. Another disease, chronic progressive external ophthalmoplegia (CPEO), may mimic both progressive supranuclear palsy and Parkinson's disease. Whether CPEO is a neurologic disease or myopathic disease remains unresolved at the present time.

Progressive supranuclear palsy. Progressive supranuclear palsy, or Steele-Richardson-Olszewski syndrome,[39] is a degenerative disease of the CNS characterized by progressive supranuclear palsy initially affecting voluntary downgaze, accompanied by dystonia of the neck. Thus the loss of the ability to move the eyes downward is compounded by the inability of the patients to bend their necks, and they present with various complaints reflecting this downgaze difficulty (e.g., ''inability to read,'' ''can't see the food on my plate,'' ''can't walk downstairs''). The ophthalmoplegia progresses with some regularity of order to loss of voluntary upgaze and horizontal gaze followed by pursuit deficits. During this time the patients may develop ocular misalignment due to involvement of the ocular motor nuclei, and over time there is a loss of facial expression (masked face) with dystonia of the trunk muscles and progressive dementia developing as well. Late in the disease, when the neck dystonia has progressed to the point where the head is almost immobile, caloric stimulation will demonstrate the integrity of nuclear and infranuclear pathways. Caloric stimulation will produce a tonic deviation of the eyes. Very late in the evolution of the disease process the nuclear pathways may become affected, and the eyes will no longer move to caloric stimuli.

The disease has an equal sex distribution, and for the most part is found in patients

---

OCULAR SIGNS OF PARKINSON'S DISEASE

1. Lid dysfunction.
   a. Blepharospasm
   b. Decreased blinking and weakness
2. Conjugate gaze abnormalities. Early cogwheel saccades followed by loss of volitional saccadic upgaze, followed by down and horizontal gaze deficits, producing a picture that may mimic CPEO. In addition, smooth pursuit is often absent, being replaced by microsaccadic movements. Oculocephalic maneuvers produce smooth movements with full excursions in all directions.
3. Convergence paresis with diplopia at near is not an infrequent complaint.
4. Seborrheic dermatitis and blepharitis may produce ocular discomfort.
5. Oculogyric crisis is a spasmodic upward deviation of the eyes associated with fixed-dilated pupils. The head is usually thrown back, and the mouth is open. Frequently the attack is accompanied by painful sensations. These attacks may last seconds to hours and may recede gradually or suddenly.[43]

in the sixth and seventh decades. These patients usually have an inexorably progressive downhill course, with death ensuing in 8 to 10 years.

Parkinson's disease. Parkinson's disease is characterized by the triad of tremor, rigidity, and akinesia. Early in the course of the disease conjugate saccadic movements become hypometric, producing so-called cogwheel saccades. Masked facies, involuntary laughing, drooling, and difficulty swallowing mark the progression of the disease. It is a degenerative disease of the extrapyramidal system in which there is an imbalance at a biochemical level between the dopaminergic and cholinergic systems within the basal ganglia. The complaint of diplopia in these cases is most often associated with near tasks due to convergence paresis. A list of the ocular signs of Parkinson's disease is found in the box on p. 140.

Internuclear ophthalmoplegia

Internuclear ophthalmoplegia (INO) is a sign of intrinsic brain stem disease involving the medial longitudinal bundle between the abducens and the oculomotor nuclei (Fig. 4-1). The hallmark of INO is a lag of the agonist medial rectus muscle in a conjugate gaze movement, adduction lag. Although often the most striking clinical finding to the casual observer, the presence of abducting nystagmus is not mandatory to make the diagnosis of an INO. The adduction lag in a patient with an INO can be made more obvious by having the patient make repeated saccadic movements in the field of action of the involved medial rectus muscle, for example, optokinetic stimulus moving toward the side of the lesion.[37] The patient may complain of transient diplopia during the induced saccadic movement or nondescript visual discomfort in the presence of the abducting nystagmus.

Unilateral or bilateral INO in a young adult is most likely to be due to multiple sclerosis, whereas a unilateral INO in a patient over the age of 50 years is most likely to represent brain stem vascular occlusive disease. INO is often accompanied by vertical upbeat nystagmus in upgaze and a skew deviation.[24] Although much has been made of classifying INO into anterior and posterior varieties, the accompanying signs localize the lesion independent of the presence of the INO.

INO produced by a mesencephalic lesion is usually bilateral and is marked by an absence of convergence. This form of INO has been called an anterior INO. In addition, if the patient is exotropic (WEBINO syndrome[15]), it is impossible to exclude involvement of the medial rectus subnuclei as well as the medial longitudinal bundles.

Lesions in the pons in the region of the sixth nerve nuclei can produce certain distinctive syndromes involving internuclear pathways. Small lesions may produce INO of abduction,[28] sometimes called a posterior INO. In this entity there is a decrease in the speed of the abducting eye during a conjugate gaze movement to the ipsilateral side. There is full lateral movement, and no deviation is present in any position of gaze, differentiating this entity from a sixth nerve palsy. During the abduction lag in the conjugate gaze movement the patient may experience transient diplopia.

Pontine gaze paralysis

Lesions in the PPRF produce an ipsilateral gaze paresis that may be permanent. Defects rostral to the abducens nuclei spare the vestibuloocular reflexes, whereas those at the level of the abducens nuclei or caudal to it obliterate all ipsilateral horizontal movement.[13]

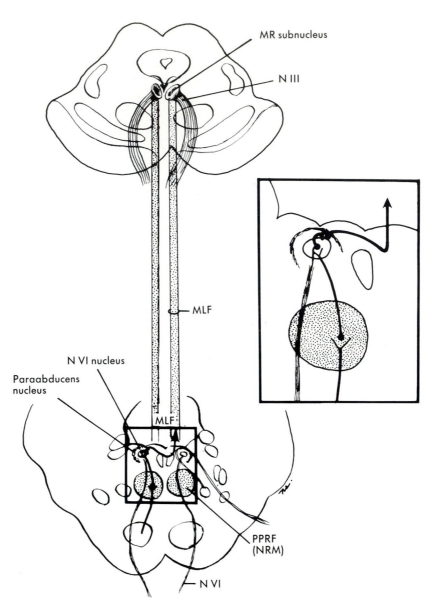

Fig. 4-1. Pathway for conjugate eye movements. Impulse arrives at PPRF from supranuclear centers. Fibers project from PPRF to ipsilateral abducens nucleus. From abducens nucleus (1) interneuron arises that projects to ipsilateral paraabducens nucleus, from which fibers arise to cross midline dorsally and enter contralateral MLF to eventually terminate in MR subnucleus of oculomotor nerve, driving contralateral eye to side ipsilateral to originating PPRF and (2) fibers enter ipsilateral sixth cranial nerve. *MR*, medial rectus; *MLF*, medial longitudinal fasciculus; *PPRF*, paramedian pontine reticular formation; *NRM*, nucleus reticularis magnocellularis.

Larger lesions in this region of the brain stem can produce a one-and-one-half syndrome.[21] This syndrome is characterized by a total paralysis of horizontal gaze toward the side of the lesion due to involvement of the ipsilateral PPRF or abducens and para-abducens nuclei as well as failure of the eye ipsilateral to the lesion to make a contralateral conjugate gaze movement due to involvement of the ipsilateral MLF. Thus the eye on the side of the lesion will be immobile during conjugate gaze movements in either direction, while the contralateral eye will abduct appropriately but will float back toward the midline in response to a conjugate gaze demand ipsilateral to the lesion.

Ocular myopathies

Chronic progressive external ophthalmoplegia (CPEO). The term CPEO, as generally used, includes a number of different entities that have in common the development of a slowly progressive, generally symmetric, external ophthalmoplegia. The symmetry of the ophthalmoplegia makes these patients appear to have multidirectional gaze palsies similar to those seen in progressive supranuclear palsy. Progressive supra-nuclear palsy is differentiated from CPEO by the maintenance of full ocular rotations to oculocephalic maneuvers.

Berenberg et al.[2] have emphasized that the Kearns-Sayre syndrome* can be separated as a distinct entity from the large group of patients with CPEO. Kearns-Sayre syndrome is characterized by the clinical triad of progressive external ophthalmoplegia, atypical pigmentary degeneration of the retina, and heart block. The cerebrospinal fluid (CSF) protein is almost universally elevated, exceeding 100 mg/dl. The onset of the disease is before age 20. The sequence of manifestations may vary, and the cardiopathy may be delayed for many years. Patients with ophthalmoplegia, pigmentary degeneration of the retina (atypical retinitis pigmentosa, i.e., salt-and-pepper pigmentary changes without bone spicule formation involving the periphery or macula), and elevated CSF protein content are at risk to develop progressive cardiac conduction defects. The severity of cardiac involvement varies from those patients with a normal electrocardiogram (ECG) to those with intraventricular conduction defect, bundle branch block, bifascicular disease, and finally to complete heart block. These patients must be followed with annual ECG recordings and the family prepared for the possible need to implant a pacemaker.

Rowland[35] has offered an inclusive classification of patients with progressive ophthalmoplegia (see Box, p. 144), pointing out that the disorder may occur in isolation, with weakness of other cranial and limb muscles, or with a variety of other neurologic abnormalities.

Often there is other evidence of widespread neurologic disease affecting specific areas, including the cerebellum, auditory and vestibular pathways, skeletal muscle, and less often, intellectual function. The patients tend to be short and have delayed sexual maturation. The syndrome usually appears sporadically without a family history. Biopsy of skeletal or ocular muscle in these patients, as well as in those with other forms of progressive external ophthalmoplegia, often will reveal ragged red fibers (i.e., giant mitochondria)[1] or other morphologic mitochondrial changes.[2] Histopathologic postmortem studies of brain specimens characteristically will show spongiform degeneration.[2,14]

There is a form of CPEO that may exist in isolation, that is, limited to the extraocular

*References 12, 14, 19, 20, 26, 27, and 35.

CLASSIFICATION OF PROGRESSIVE OPHTHALMOPLEGIA[35]

1. Site uncertain
   a. Ophthalmoplegia and ptosis, congenital and late forms, sporadic and genetic
      (1) Ophthalmoplegia alone
      (2) Ptosis alone
2. Ocular myopathies
   a. Ocular and other cranial muscles
      (1) Oculopharyngeal muscular dystrophy (genetic)
      (2) Oculopharyngeal myopathy (sporadic)
   b. Ocular and proximal limb muscles
   c. Ocular and distal limb muscles
   d. Myotonic muscular dystrophy
   e. Myotubular or centronuclear myopathy
   f. Ophthalmoplegia, glycogen storage, and abnormal mitochondria
   g. Ophthalmopathy of Graves' disease (euthyroid, hypothyroid, hyperthyroid)
   h. Ocular myositis (orbital pseudotumor)
   i. Congenital myopathic ptosis or ophthalmoplegia
      (1) Limb weakness
      (2) Anomalous insertion of ocular muscles
      (3) Some cases of Möbius syndrome
3. Disorders of neuromuscular junction
   a. Curare-sensitive ocular myopathy
   b. Myasthenia gravis
4. Neural ophthalmoplegias
   a. Nuclear and supranuclear abnormalities
      (1) Congenital: Möbius syndrome; isolated ophthalmoplegia
      (2) Ophthalmoplegia with central myelopathy or encephalopathy of later onset: mental retardation, hereditary ataxias, hereditary spastic paraplegia, hereditary multisystem disease, dystonia musculorum deformans, abetalipoproteinemia (Bassen-Kornzweig), progressive supranuclear bulbar palsy (Steele-Richardson-Olszewski)
      (3) Ophthalmoplegia with motor neuron disease: infantile spinal muscular atrophy (Werdnig-Hoffmann), juvenile spinal muscular atrophy simulating muscular dystrophy (Wohlfart-Kugelberg-Welander)
      (4) Ophthalmoplegia, retinitis, cardiopathy, and neural disorder (Kearns-Sayre)
   b. Peripheral neuropathies

muscles and lid, an oculofacial form in which the facial muscles are involved, and an oculofacial-pharyngeal form in which bulbar musculature is involved with associated temporalis wasting. Isolated CPEO and the oculofacial-pharyngeal form appear to be hereditary. The isolated form tends to have its onset earlier in each succeeding generation.[7]

Lid crutches offer at best a temporary solution to the problem of the ptosis, but one must be wary of performing ptosis surgery in these individuals because with the loss of upgaze (no Bell's phenomenon) there is danger of developing exposure keratitis with subsequent corneal ulceration.

Myotonic dystrophy. Myotonic dystrophy may be difficult to differentiate from CPEO, at least initially. It is a rare disorder that classically produces a symmetric external ophthalmoplegia, again mimicking gaze paresis. In addition to the ophthalmoplegia, these patients may have ptosis, lack of smooth ocular pursuit, orbicularis weakness, and myotonia of lid closure and gaze holding.[23] Occasionally diplopia may be a complaint.[30] Thompson et al.[41] have noted that these patients have sluggishly reactive pupils. These patients also have polychromatic cataracts, pigmentary changes of the retina including the macula, testicular atrophy, and frontal balding.

REFERENCES

1. Adachi, M, Torii, J, Volk, BW, Briet, P, Wolintz, A, and Schneck, L: Electron microscopic and enzyme histochemical studies of cerebellum, ocular and skeletal muscles in chronic progressive ophthalmoplegia, Acta Neuropathol (Berl) 23:300, 1973.
2. Berenberg, RA, Pellock, JM, DiMauro, S, Schotland, DL, Bonilla, E, Eastwood, A, Hays, A, Vicale, CT, Behrens, M, Chutorian, A, and Rowland, LP: Lumping or splitting? "Ophthalmoplegia-plus" or Kearns-Sayre syndrome? Ann Neurol 1:37, 1977.
3. Burde, RM: Control of eye movements. In Moses, RA, editor: Adler's physiology of the eye, ed 7, St Louis, 1981, The CV Mosby Co, pp 122-165.
4. Burde, RM: Control of eye movements. In Moses, RA, editor: Adler's physiology of the eye, ed 7, St Louis, 1981, The CV Mosby Co, p 143.
5. Büttner-Ennever, JA, Büttner, U, Cohen, B, and Baumgartner, G: Vertical gaze paralysis and the rostral interstitial nucleus of the medial longitudinal fasciculus, Brain 105:125, 1982.
6. Cogan, DG: Neurology of the ocular muscles, Springfield, Ill, 1956, Charles C Thomas, Publisher, p 106.
7. Cogan, DG: Neurology of the ocular muscles, Springfield, Ill, 1956, Charles C Thomas, Publisher, p 123.
8. Cogan, DG: Congenital ocular motor apraxia, Can J Ophthalmol 1:253, 1966.
9. Cogan, DG, and Adams, RD: A type of paralysis of conjugate gaze (ocular motor apraxia), Arch Ophthalmol 50:434, 1953.
10. Cogan, DG, Chu, FC, and Reingold, D: Notes on congenital ocular motor apraxia: associated abnormalities. In Glaser, JS, editor: Neuro-ophthalmology Symposium of the University of Miami and the Bascom Palmer Eye Institute, vol 10, St Louis, 1980, The CV Mosby Co, pp 171-179.
11. Collier, J: Nuclear ophthalmoplegia. With special reference to retraction of the lids and ptosis and to lesions of the posterior commissure, Brain 50:488, 1927.
12. Daroff, RB: Chronic progressive external ophthalmoplegia: a critical review, Arch Ophthalmol 82:845, 1969.
13. Daroff, RB: Ocular motor manifestations of brainstem and cerebellar dysfunction. In Smith, JL, editor: Neuro-ophthalmology, vol 5, Hallandale, Fla, 1970, Huffman, p 104.
14. Daroff, RB, Solitaire, GB, Pincus, JH, and Glaser, GH: Spongiform encephalopathy with chronic progressive external ophthalmoplegia. Central ophthalmoplegia mimicking ocular myopathy, Neurology (Minneap) 16:161, 1966.
15. Daroff, RB, and Hoyt, WF: Supranuclear disorders of ocular control systems in man. Clinical, anatomical, and physiological correlations—1969. In Bach-y-Rita, P, Collins, CC, and Hyde, JE, editors: The control of eye movements, New York, 1971, Academic Press, pp 175-235.
16. Daroff, RB, and Troost, BT: Supranuclear disorders of eye movements. In Glaser, JS, editor: Neuro-ophthalmology, Hagerstown, Md, 1978, Harper and Row, Publishers, pp 201-218.
17. Dell'Osso, LF, and Daroff, RB: Eye movement characteristics and recording techniques. In Glaser, JS, editor: Neuro-ophthalmology, Hagerstown, Md, 1978, Harper & Row, Publishers, pp 185-200.
18. Dorland's illustrated medical dictionary, ed 25, Philadelphia, 1974, WB Saunders Co, p 124.
19. Drachman, DA: Ophthalmoplegia plus: the neurodegenerative disorders associated with progressive external ophthalmoplegia, Arch Neurol 18:654, 1968.
20. Drachman, DA, Wetzel, N, and Wasserman, M: Experimental pathology of the ocular muscles and the syndromes of "ocular myopathy," Neurology (Minneap) 19:282, 1969.
21. Fisher, CM: Some neuro-ophthalmologic observations, J Neurol Neurosurg Psychiatry 30:383, 1967.
22. Gay, AJ, Brodkey, J, and Miller, JE: Convergence retraction nystagmus. An electromyographic study, Arch Ophthalmol 70:456, 1963.
23. Glaser, JS, editor: Neuro-ophthalmology, Hagerstown, Md, 1978, Harper & Row, Publishers, p 280.
24. Gonyea, EF: Bilateral internuclear ophthalmoplegia, Arch Neurol 31:168, 1974.
25. Jampel, RS, and Fells, P: Monocular elevation paresis caused by a central nervous system lesion, Arch Ophthalmol 80:45, 1968.

26. Kearns, TP: External ophthalmoplegia, pigmentary degeneration of the retina, and cardiomyopathy: a newly recognized syndrome, Trans Am Ophthalmol Soc 63:559, 1965.

27. Kearns, TP, and Sayre, GP: Retinitis pigmentosa external ophthalmoplegia and complete heart block, Arch Ophthalmol 60:280, 1958.

28. Kommerell, G: Internuclear ophthalmoplegia of abduction, Arch Ophthalmol 93:531, 1975.

29. Lessell, S: Supranuclear paralysis of monocular elevation, Neurology (Minneap) 25:1134, 1975.

30. Lessell, S, Coppeto, J, and Samet, S: Ophthalmoplegia in myotonic dystrophy, Am J Ophthalmol 71:1231, 1971.

31. Pierrot-Deseilligny, C, Chain, F, Gray, F, Serdaru, M, Escourolle, R, and Lhermitte, F: Parinaud's syndrome. Electro-oculographic and anatomical analyses of six vascular cases with deductions about vertical gaze organization in the premotor structures, Brain 105:667, 1982.

32. Ratliff, F, and Riggs, LA: Involuntary motions of the eye during monocular fixation, Nature 162:25, 1948.

33. Robinson, DA: Oculomotor unit behavior in the monkey, J Neurophysiol 33:393, 1970.

34. Robinson, DA, and Fuchs, AF: Eye movements evoked by stimulation of the frontal eye fields, J Neurophysiol 32:637, 1969.

35. Rowland, LP: Progressive external ophthalmoplegia. In Vinken, PJ, Bruyn, GW, and DeJong, JMBV, editors: System disorders and atrophies, Part II. Handbook of clinical neurology, vol 22, New York, 1975, American Elsevier Publishing Co, pp 177-202.

36. Smith, JL, Zieker, F, Gay, AJ, and Cogan, DG: Nystagmus retractorius, Arch Ophthalmol 62:864, 1959.

37. Smith, JL, and David, NJ: Internuclear ophthalmoplegia: two new clinical signs, Neurology (Minneap) 14:307, 1964.

38. Starr, A: A disorder of rapid eye movements in Huntington's chorea, Brain 90:545, 1967.

39. Steele, JC, Richardson, JC, and Olszewski, J: Progressive supranuclear palsy, Arch Neurol 10:333, 1964.

40. Thames, PB, Trobe, JD, and Ballinger, WE: Upgaze paralysis caused by a lesion of the periaqueductal grey matter, Arch Neurol 41:437, 1984.

41. Thompson, HS, Van Allen, MW, and von Noorden, GK: The pupil in myotonic dystrophy, Invest Ophthalmol 3:325, 1964.

42. Troost, BT, Weber, RB, and Daroff RB: Hemispheric control of eye movements. II. Quantitative analysis of refixation saccades in a hemispherectomy patient, Arch Neurol 27:449, 1972.

43. Walsh, FB, and Hoyt, WF: Clinical neuro-ophthalmology, vol 2, Baltimore, 1969, The Williams & Wilkins Co, pp 1321-1322.

44. Yee, RD, Duffin, RM, Baloh, RW, and Isenberg, SJ: Familial, congenital paralysis of horizontal gaze, Arch Ophthalmol 100:1449, 1982.

45. Zee, DS, Yee, RD, and Singer, HS: Congenital ocular motor apraxia, Brain 100:581, 1977.

CHAPTER 5

Diplopia

True diplopia is the awareness of seeing the same object located in two different places in visual space. This sensory experience is produced when the object of regard (the object at which the individual is looking) stimulates the fovea in one eye while simultaneously stimulating extrafoveal retina in the other eye. When this situation occurs, there is immediate foveal suppression in the nonfixing eye, presumably to avoid the totally unacceptable sensory experience of seeing two different images superimposed upon one another (''visual confusion'').

As we have defined it, true diplopia implies misalignment of the eyes. Many patients use the term ''double vision'' to describe another sensory experience occurring with normal ocular alignment. For the most part this experience is produced by a lack of uniformity of the various refractive surfaces and media within one or both eyes producing multiple images on the retina(s). This experience is best described as an overlapping of imagery similar to ''ghosting'' on a television set.

Some patients will not report diplopia even when the eyes are misaligned, either because vision is poor in one eye or both, because suppression of the nonfixing eye has occurred, or because they fail to appreciate the symptom. A patient with a subtle internuclear ophthalmoplegia (INO) will frequently fail to describe diplopia during the dissociative period when there is a lag of adduction due to failure of appropriate innervation to the agonist medial rectus muscle. Similarly, these patients cannot verbalize the illusory to-and-fro movement of the environment that must occur during the period of nystagmus of the abducting eye. Patients with a subtle, incomplete sixth cranial nerve palsy may not describe diplopia as such but will be acutely aware of visual difficulty when the eyes move into the direction of gaze of the involved muscle. These patients generally complain of ''blurring of vision,'' and even with careful questioning this experience cannot be better defined.

147

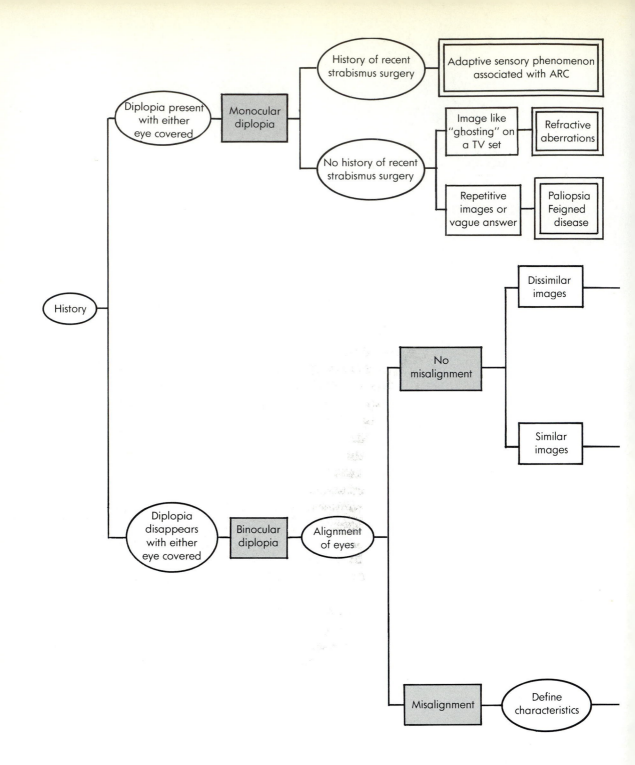

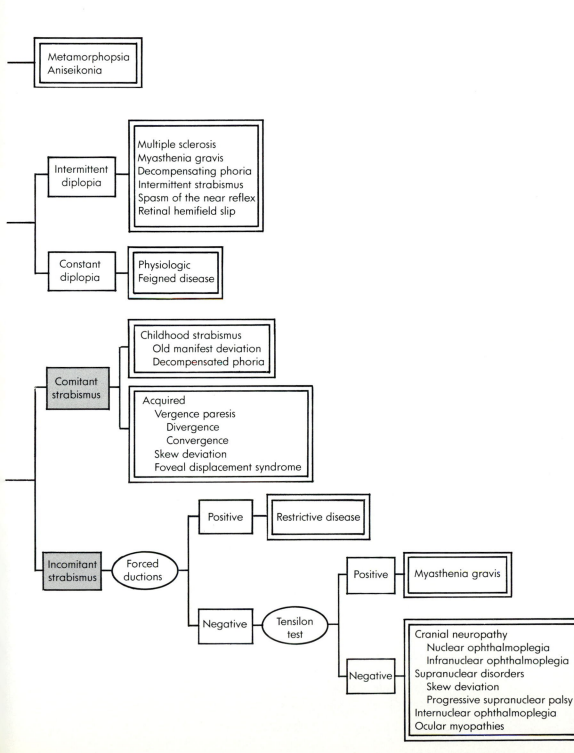

Metamorphopsia
Aniseikonia

Intermittent diplopia
- Multiple sclerosis
- Myasthenia gravis
- Decompensating phoria
- Intermittent strabismus
- Spasm of the near reflex
- Retinal hemifield slip

Constant diplopia
- Physiologic
- Feigned disease

Comitant strabismus
- Childhood strabismus
  - Old manifest deviation
  - Decompensated phoria
- Acquired
  - Vergence paresis
    - Divergence
    - Convergence
  - Skew deviation
  - Foveal displacement syndrome

Incomitant strabismus — Forced ductions
- Positive — Restrictive disease
- Negative — Tensilon test
  - Positive — Myasthenia gravis
  - Negative —
    - Cranial neuropathy
      - Nuclear ophthalmoplegia
      - Infranuclear ophthalmoplegia
    - Supranuclear disorders
      - Skew deviation
      - Progressive supranuclear palsy
    - Internuclear ophthalmoplegia
    - Ocular myopathies

CAUSES OF DIPLOPIA AND SIMILAR SENSORY EXPERIENCES

I. Diplopia
  A. No misalignment of the eyes
    1. Monocular
      a. Following strabismus surgery in a patient with abnormal retinal correspondence[1]
      b. Feigned
    2. Binocular
      a. Foveal displacement syndrome
      b. Physiologic
      c. Feigned
  B. Misalignment of the eyes
    1. Supranuclear
      a. Skew deviation
      b. Convergence paresis
      c. Divergence paresis
      d. Convergence accommodative spasm (spasm of the near reflex)
      e. Convergence retraction nystagmus
    2. Internuclear
    3. Nuclear (III, IV, VI)
    4. Infranuclear
      a. Fascicle
      b. Nerve
      c. Myoneural junction—myasthenia gravis
      d. Extraocular muscle
        (1) Restrictive disease
        (2) Degenerative disease
    5. Following strabismus surgery with normal or abnormal retinal correspondence
II. Sensory experiences that mimic diplopia
  A. No misalignment—''monocular diplopia'' or ghosting
    1. Refractive abnormalities
      a. Corneal abnormalities
        (1) Astigmatism
        (2) Keratoconus
        (3) Cornea plana
        (4) Irregular astigmatism
          (a) Intrinsic corneal disease
          (b) Extrinsic pressure, e.g., chalazion
      b. Iris abnormalities
        (1) Polycoria
        (2) Large, relatively nonreactive pupils in association with astigmatic refractive error or nuclear sclerosis
      c. Lens abnormalities
        (1) Nuclear sclerosis
        (2) Subluxated lens
    2. Paliopsia
  B. Misalignment of the eyes
    1. Hemifield slip
    2. Internuclear ophthalmoplegia
    3. Minimal ocular motor palsies
    4. Superior oblique myokymia
    5. Convergence retraction nystagmus

PART I

Diagnostic approach

The approach to a patient with the complaint of diplopia deviates from the classic format of the complete elucidation of a history followed by the performance of a physical examination. Each question or step in the ordered examination of a patient with diplopia is structured to provide information upon which subsequent steps are based (Chart 5-1). The initial question, "Is the diplopia present with one eye closed?" is of such critical importance that if, as is often the case, the patient is unable to answer this question (having failed to cover one eye or the other), the patient should be instructed at this point to cover one eye and then the other and thus to provide this information.

☐ **Monocular diplopia** (Chart 5-1, *A)*

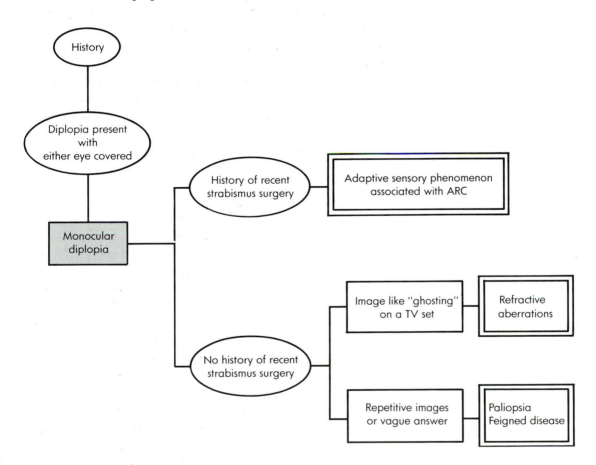

If diplopia is still present with one eye covered, the patient has monocular diplopia, a problem of different etiologic significance and, for the most part, of less serious consequence than that of binocular diplopia. With few exceptions monocular diplopia reflects optical aberrations within the refracting media of the eye.

☐ **Adaptive sensory phenomenon associated wtih ARC.** Once it is determined that the diplopia is monocular (although it may be experienced with each eye), the next step is to exclude the presence of a rare adaptive sensory phenomenon that may follow extraocular muscle surgery in patients with abnormal retinal correspondence (ARC) in which two retinal points in one eye function simultaneously. This sensory state is transient (weeks to months), but it has been known to persist.[4] The finding represents a cortical failure of immediate sensory readaptation to motor realignment. Recent extraocular muscle surgery should suggest the presence of this peculiar phenomenon. In patients with ARC the fovea of the deviating eye appears to be able to shift its subjective visual direction depending upon the testing situation. Thus in certain patients with ARC, if the extraocular muscle surgery has failed to place the fovea in the appropriate anatomical position, the patient may experience monocular diplopia with binocular triplopia.

☐ **Aberrations of refracting media.** If there is no history of childhood strabismus and recent muscle surgery, then one most likely is dealing with optical aberrations within the refracting media of the eye. Optical aberrations are associated with an overlapping of images similar to ghosting on television. The most common cause of this symptom is myopic astigmatism. Patients with myopic astigmatism are most acutely aware of this experience in dim illumination. Since these individuals have lived with this sensory experience all their lives, they rarely pay attention to it.

The most common cause of monocular diplopia that is clinically bothersome is the development of early nuclear sclerotic changes in the lens producing a lamellarlike refractive effect. Such a lens can be likened to an onion cut in cross section, with a slightly different refractive effect occurring at each interface. The wider the pupillary aperture, the greater the chance of paraxial rays being differentially refracted, thus producing a secondary, superimposed, blurred image. As with the ghosting of myopia, the ghosting of nuclear sclerosis is exaggerated in dim illumination and often is not present in bright light. Other structural or pathologic changes in the integrity of the cornea, iris, or lens can produce monocular diplopia by forming multiple refractive images. The elimination of the ghost image by the use of a pinhole confirms the suspected diagnosis of a refractive aberration. The changes in the ocular media may be so minimal that the only objective physical finding will be a subtle alteration of the retinoscopic reflex. Ghosting is so characteristic of alterations in the refractive media that if the patient sees two distinct images with one eye rather than overlapping images, one is dealing with feigned disease.

☐ **Palinopsia.** Critchley[5] defined palinopsia as "visual perseveration in time." The patient is unable to erase cortical images and sees one scene superimposed on another, not two images of the same scene. It is a rare finding that occurs with severe cortical (occipital lobe) disease.[12] It is doubtful that a patient with palinopsia will be seen in an outpatient setting.

☐ **Feigned disease.** If all the possible causes of monocular diplopia have been excluded, the only diagnosis left to the clinician is that of feigned diplopia. In these litigious times feigning of diplopia should not be surprising. We use the broad generic term "feigned disease" to include both hysterical conversion reactions (unconscious dissembling) and malingering (conscious dissembling).

☐ **Binocular diplopia**

○ **Ocular alignment.** If covering each eye alleviates the diplopia, one is dealing with a binocular sensory experience. The next step is to determine if the eyes are misaligned. This may be done subjectively, utilizing the red glass test or objectively utilizing the

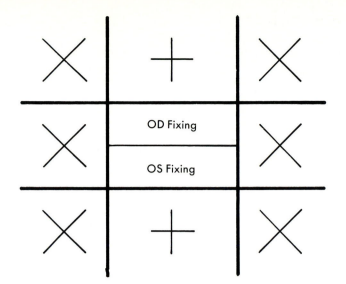

Fig. 5-1. The clinically important gaze positions in acquired strabismus are the primary position, right and left eye fixing in turn, and those marked by an *X*. The measurements in the straight up and down position (+) are important in comitant strabismus (A and V patterns).

cover-uncover test in the cardinal positions of gaze with distance and near fixation (Fig. 5-1).

Red glass test. A red glass is placed in front of the right eye, identifying the image perceived by the right eye as it will appear red. In addition a green filter can be placed in front of the left eye, thus making this image more easily identifiable than if no filter were used. The use of a combination red and green filter more clearly identifies the images of the right and left eyes and improves the accuracy of the subjective responses. The patient is asked to look first at a fixation light at 20 feet (6 m) and then at a fixation light at 14 inches (35 cm). The patient is simply asked if during fixation at distance or near he or she sees two lights separated in space, one red and one white (or green if a green filter has been used). The presence or absence of misalignment is then determined at distance and near in the cardinal positions of gaze. The recognition of two separate images is indicative of ocular misalignment.

Cover-uncover test. This test is the objective counterpart of the red glass test. The patient should be wearing an appropriate refractive correction and instructed to fixate on a letter or object that he or she can identify first at 20 feet and then at 14 inches. First one eye is covered, and the other eye is observed to see if it moves to pick up fixation. If the eye moves to pick up fixation, then a manifest deviation (tropia) is present. If there is no movement of the opposite eye, then that eye is fixing on the target appropriately. The occluder is then removed, and the eye that was covered is observed to see if it moves to pick up fixation, suggesting the presence of a latent deviation (phoria). The sequence is then repeated covering the other eye, ultimately testing the patient in the cardinal positions of gaze with both distance and near fixation.

No misalignment (Chart 5-1, *B*)

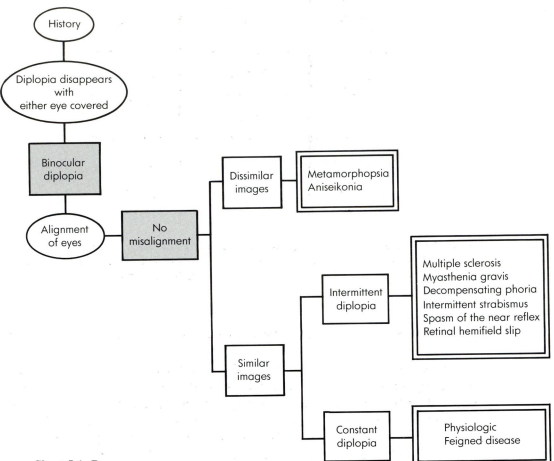

Chart 5-1, B

If no misalignment is found, the patient is told to cover one eye at a time and is asked whether the images perceived are the same.

☐   **Dissimilar images.** If the imagery is dissimilar, the problem is either metamorphopsia (implying retinal disease) or aniseikonia due to a corrected or uncorrected refractive error. If the patient has metamorphopsia, the image perceived by the involved eye is distorted, and this can be confirmed subjectively by the use of an Amsler grid. If the patient has aniseikonia, there will be a distinct difference in image size between eyes, but both images will be distinct.

☐   **Similar images with intermittent diplopia.** If the image seen by each eye is similar and there is no obvious misalignment on examination, it is important to determine if the patient's symptoms are intermittent. A series of questions should be interposed to extract specific historical data in an attempt to elucidate the circumstances under which the diplopia occurs. For example, patients with multiple sclerosis may experience transient blurring of vision, diplopia, or nystagmus with a rise in core body temperature of as little as 0.1° C. This can be produced by hot baths, hot showers, or exercise. Depending upon the degree of demyelination, even walking upstairs or across the street can make the patient symptomatic. Whether it is the rise in body temperature or a change in the electrolytic milieu that produces the reversible conduction block is unknown; the patient's susceptibility depends on a change in myelination of axons. This transient change in the functioning of the afferent or efferent visual system is commonly termed Uhthoff's sign.[7] Rarely it may be seen in patients with collagen vascular disease. If the patient relates his or her symptoms to exercise, an attempt can be made to reproduce the symptoms by having the patient run up and down three or four flights of stairs. Similar results have been obtained by increasing the core body temperature with an electric blanket. If these environmental manipulations reproduce the symptoms, one can be sure there are demyelinated segments of nerves.

Patients with early congestive endocrine ophthalmopathy will tend to have greater difficulty maintaining single binocular vision in the morning, whereas patients with myasthenia gravis or a decompensating phoria will tend to have diplopia later in the day. If the diplopia is worse later in the day, specific note should be made of ptosis, which is a characteristic finding in at least 75% to 80% of patients with myasthenia gravis. During the examination of such a patient, attempts should be made to fatigue the extraocular muscles, including the levator, in an effort to produce either ptosis or diplopia. Arrangements may need to be made to examine the patient later in the day.

A history of childhood strabismus, of having worn glasses or a patch as a child, or of squinting one eye in bright sunlight (intermittent exotropia) suggests decompensation of a longstanding heterophoria. Supportive evidence would include the presence of consistent head tilt or head turn, especially if photographs can show it to have been present for a long period of time. Patching one eye for an hour may unmask an intermittent strabismus. The finding of large vertical fusional amplitudes (15 to 20 prism diopters) is almost diagnostic of a large latent deviation, for example, congenital superior oblique palsy.

The association of double vision and concurrent visual blurring during periods of stress (e.g., studying for exams) suggests the presence of spasm of the near reflex. In general, spasm of the near reflex is not associated with organic disease. There is a marked overaction of the components of the near synkinesis. Overconvergence produces diplopia. The accommodative spasm produces a blur for all objects remote to the near point. This blurring of vision, rather than the recognition of diplopia, is generally the complaint that prompts the patient to seek help. Pupillary constriction is an obligate component of the near reflex, and it is the miosis that helps differentiate this entity from bilateral or unilateral lateral rectus paresis. Some individuals have learned to use the near synkinesis to mimic a lateral rectus muscle(s) palsy and use it to feign an actual muscle paresis.

A rare cause of intermittent diplopia is retinal hemifield slip, which occurs only when there is a complete or nearly complete bitemporal hemianopia, and thus no corresponding retinal areas to lock the eyes together in normal alignment (Fig. 5-2). Intermittently there may be ocular convergence with a blank space between the vertical meridians (Fig. 5-2, *C3*) as they "slip" inward, divergence with overlapping of the vertical meridians as the eyes "slip" apart (Fig. 5-2, *C2*), or vertical sliding (Fig. 5-2, *D*).[7] For the most part, complete bitemporal hemianopia is produced by large mass lesions in and around the chiasm. Thus patients with hemifield slip should be questioned to determine if there are any symptoms to suggest hypothalamic or pituitary dysfunction.

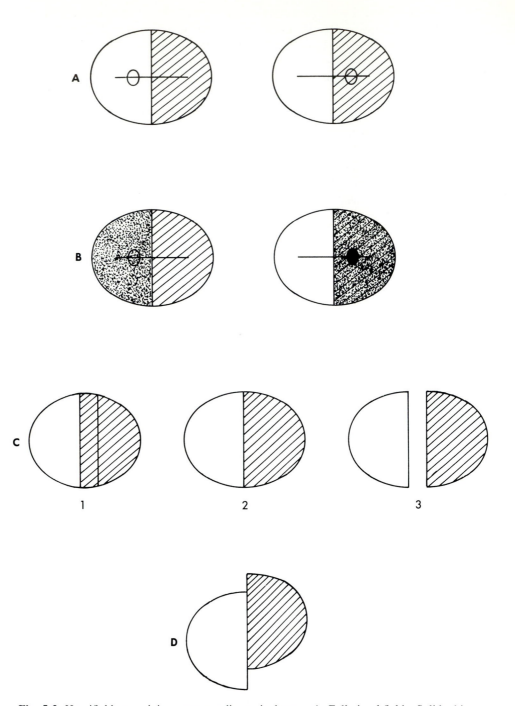

Fig. 5-2. Hemifields containing corresponding retinal areas. **A,** Full visual fields. Solid white areas and cross-hatched areas represent fields containing corresponding retinal areas. **B,** Bitemporal field loss (dark areas) superimposed on hemifields containing corresponding retinal areas. **C,** Retinal slip cyclopean view: *1*, divergence; *2*, fusion, *3*, convergence. **D,** Retinal vertical slip cyclopean view.

☐   **Similar images with constant diplopia.** If the diplopia is definitely present and objective findings are negative at the time of examination, it is necessary to determine if the patient has simply become aware of physiologic diplopia. In this case the patient will see one clear image with two blurred images. The examiner should demonstrate physiologic diplopia at near and distance. The patient is instructed to look at a pencil point held at about 14 inches (35 cm) and to note if there is doubling of the background behind the examiner and if this reproduces the symptoms. The patient is then instructed to fixate on a distant target and to place his or her two forefingers end-to-end and hold them in his or her line of sight. The patient is asked if the overlapping images of his or her forefingers reproduce the sensory experience. If the patient's sensory experience has not been reproduced, then having excluded physiologic diplopia, the examiner must conclude that "the patient's symptoms are not compatible with the objective findings" and represent feigned diplopia.

☐ **Ocular misalignment** (Chart 5-1, C)

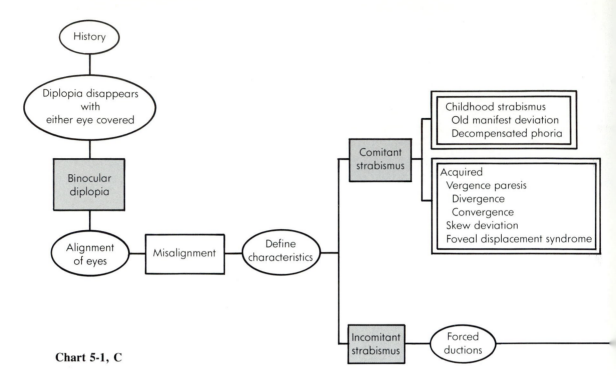

Chart 5-1, C

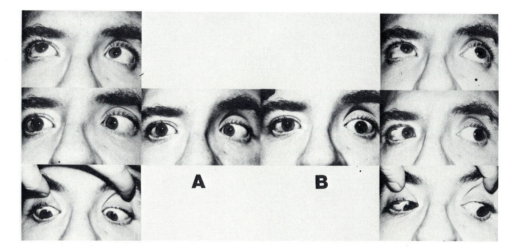

Fig. 5-3. This man sustained a right sixth cranial nerve palsy in an accident. **A,** Secondary deviation with right eye (paretic) fixing; there is marked increase in the esotropia as compared to **B,** primary deviation with nonparetic left eye fixing. **C** and **D,** Demonstrate variation in alignment with different gaze positions.

Once it has been determined by rapid screening with the subjective and objective tests mentioned previously that there is ocular misalignment, it is necessary to have an appropriate quantitative testing sequence that will determine whether the deviation is comitant or incomitant. The patients should be carefully observed to determine whether they consistently adopt a given head posture[14] or whether other signs of neurologic or systemic diseases are present. In the great majority of cases of incomitant strabismus a compensatory head posture is adopted to obtain binocular single vision. In those cases in which binocular single vision cannot be achieved by compensatory head postures the patient may assume a head position in which the diplopia is less bothersome. The patient may place his or her eyes in such a position that the deviating eye is occluded by the nose or in a position that will exaggerate the deviation, making the diplopic image easier to ignore. Old photographs are of immeasurable importance in marking the chronicity of the problem. If not available at the time of the initial examination, a series of sequential

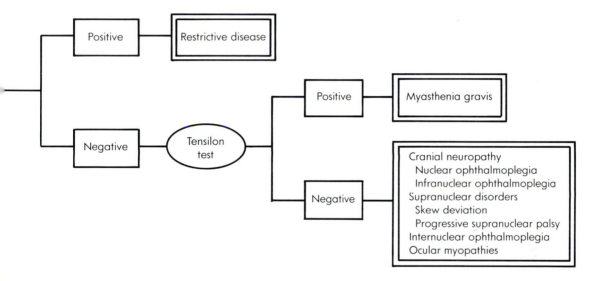

photographs dating back to childhood should be obtained. With a +14 diopter lens or by using the slit lamp[17] adequate magnification is readily available to study the photographs in order to document the presence of an ocular deviation or suggestive head position dating back a number of years.

○ **Define characteristics.** Incomitant deviations are differentiated from comitant deviations by the presence of (1) a variation of the angle of misalignment in different gaze directions (incomitance) and (2) a difference in the degree of misalignment, depending on which eye is used for fixation (primary and secondary deviation[3,10,11]) (Figs. 5-3 and 5-4).

Comitance. At this point it is important to determine the type of misalignment and its alteration in various gaze positions, including head tilt maneuvers. First establish whether the deviation is horizontal, vertical, or oblique.

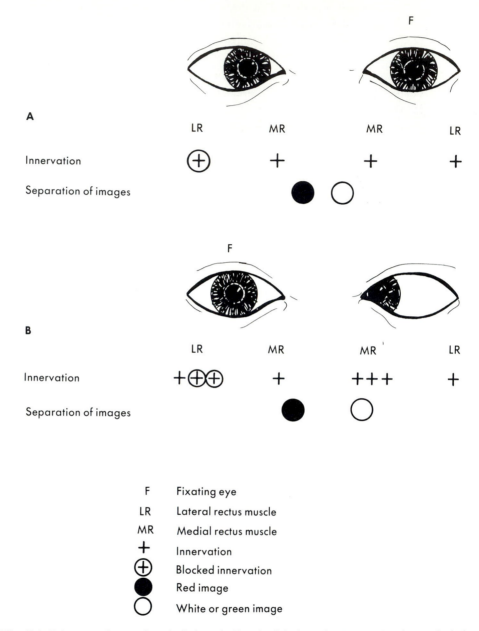

Fig. 5-4. Primary and secondary deviation. **A,** Paretic right lateral rectus *(+)*, primary deviation. Left eye fixing *(F)* in straight-ahead gaze. Equal innervation to all four horizontal rectus muscles. Since right lateral rectus muscle cannot respond normally to input designated by + signs, right eye will be deviated medially a given amount, *X.* Subjective deviation is demonstrated. **B,** Paretic right lateral rectus muscle, secondary deviation. Right eye fixing in straight-ahead position. Since greater input to right lateral rectus muscle is required to maintain eye in straight-ahead position, greater innervation is sent to yoke of left medial rectus (Hering's law), and result is a greater absolute deviation and a greater subjective separation of images.

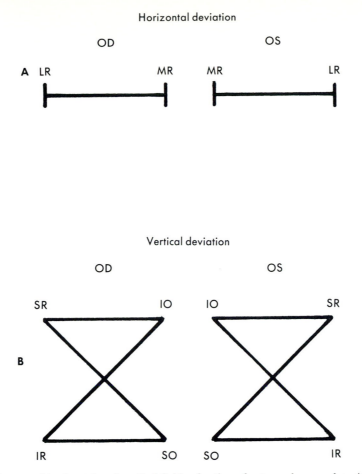

Fig. 5-5. Separated horizontal and vertical fields of action of extraocular muscles. **A,** If deviation is horizontal, one of four muscles is involved. **B,** If deviation is vertical, vertical rectus or oblique muscles are involved. *OD,* right eye; *OS,* left eye; *LR,* lateral rectus muscle; *MR,* medial rectus muscle; *SR,* superior rectus muscle; *IR,* inferior rectus muscle; *SO,* superior oblique muscle; *IO,* inferior oblique muscle.

With the red glass in front of the right eye instruct the patient to use his fingers to show you how far apart the images are. By doing this the patient will demonstrate whether the image separation is (1) horizontal (horizontal rectus muscles) or (2) vertical or "diagonal" (vertical rectus or oblique muscles). If the separation is horizontal, one of four muscles is involved (Figs. 5-5, *A,* and 5-6). If the separation is vertical or diagonal, there may be involvement of the vertical and horizontal as well as the oblique muscles. If the deviation is mainly vertical, usually a vertical rectus or oblique muscle is affected (Fig. 5-5, *B*).

Identification of involved muscle(s) in horizontal deviations (Fig. 5-6). If the patient has a horizontal deviation, ask him if the red image is to the left or right of the white image. If the red image is to the left of the white image (i.e., crossed diplopia), the eyes are relatively exotropic, and one of the medial rectus muscles is not working. Conversely, if the red image is to the right of the white image (i.e., uncrossed diplopia),

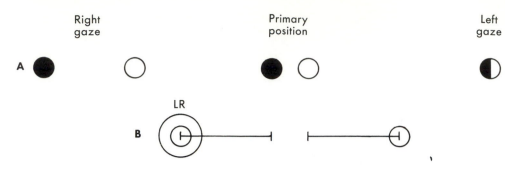

Fig. 5-6. Horizontal deviation with uncrossed diplopia present; that is, red image (solid circle) is to right of white image, **A;** therefore one of lateral rectus muscles is not working, and a circle can be placed around each of these muscles, **B.** Take the test target first into left and then right gaze and have patient use his fingers to demonstrate how deviation changes. If deviation increases in right gaze, **A,** a second circle can be placed around muscle that acts in right gaze, **B.** Two circles identify the involved muscle in horizontal deviations, **A.**

the eyes will be esotropic, and one of the lateral rectus muscles is paretic. The misalignment will be greater in the field of action of the paretic muscle. Since one medial rectus muscle and one lateral rectus muscle act in right gaze and the other medial and lateral rectus muscle pair act in left gaze, the number of involved muscles can be reduced to two determining in which gaze position the deviation is greatest. If the diplopia is crossed, the medial rectus muscle is paretic, and if the diplopia is uncrossed, the lateral rectus muscle is paretic (Fig. 5-6). Although restrictive disease may mimic a neurogenic paresis, identification of the presence of such mechanical limitation will be made subsequently by forced duction testing. In cases of comitant (nonparalytic) squint the deviation should be determined in the straight up and down position (A or V pattern) as well as at near.

Identification of involved muscle(s) in vertical deviations. When examining the patient who complains of vertical or oblique diplopia, ask if the red image is higher or lower, or have him point to the red light (Fig. 5-7). The hypertropic eye always produces the lower image. If the patient has a right hypertropia, the involved muscles are either the depressors of the right eye or the elevators of the left eye, and vice versa for a left hypertropia.

The number of muscles involved can again be reduced to two by determining whether the deviation is greater in right or left gaze (Fig. 5-8). It is apparent from these diagrams that of the two possible involved muscles one has its field of action in upgaze and the other in downgaze (Fig. 5-9); thus the final step is to determine if the deviation is greater in right or left upgaze and downgaze, identifying the paretic muscle.

An absence of a differential deviation in upgaze and downgaze occurs with chronicity in vertical deviations. This lack of a differential deviation is due to an adaptive phenomenon postulated to be caused by "inhibitional palsy of the contralateral antagonist."[11] This type of adaptation is termed *spread of comitance,* and its presence signifies chronicity. In these patients additional information can be obtained by using the Bielschowsky head tilt test* (Fig. 5-10). The measured vertical deviation increases when the head is tilted

*References 2, 3, 8, 9, 15, and 16.

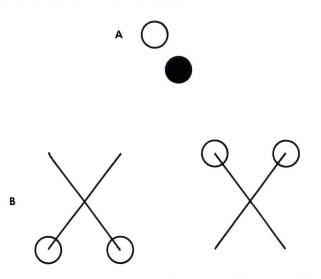

Fig. 5-7. Where is the red image? Images patient sees are demonstrated in **A.** This response indicates that right eye is hypertropic or higher eye. Involved muscles are either depressors on right or elevators on left. Therefore a circle can be placed around these muscles, reducing the possibilities from eight involved muscles to four, **B.** Solid circle = red image.

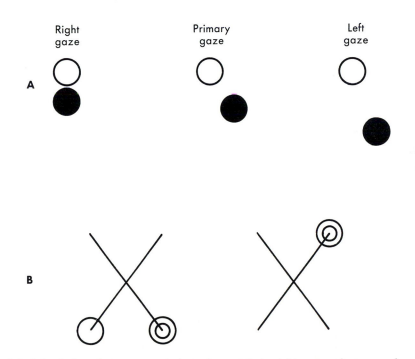

Fig. 5-8. It is obvious that one muscle in each eye acts in right gaze and one muscle acts in left gaze. Images patient sees are demonstrated in **A.** Patient is instructed to demonstrate change in image separation when target is placed first in right gaze and then in left gaze. Deviation is greater in left gaze, and therefore a circle can be placed around the two muscles that act in left gaze, **B.** Solid circle = red image.

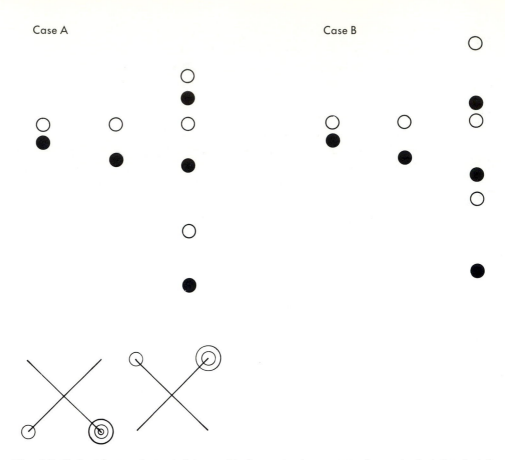

Fig. 5-9. Patient is now instructed to use his fingers to demonstrate change in deviation in left upgaze and left downgaze. It is obvious from the diagram that of the possible involved muscles, one acts in upgaze and one acts in downgaze. Images the patient sees are shown. In case *A,* patient has a greater deviation in downgaze, and a third circle can be placed around muscle that has its major vertical action in downgaze. In vertical or oblique deviations three circles are diagnostic. In case *B* there is no vertical incomitance and a further step is needed—the Bielschowsky head tilt test (see Fig. 5-10).

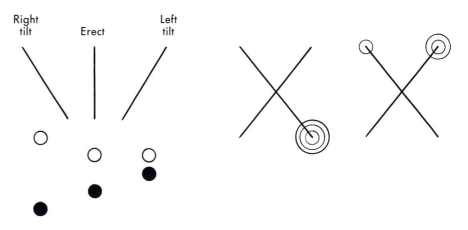

Fig. 5-10. Vertical deviation for superior muscles, that is, intorters, increases when head is tilted toward paretic side. In this case a third circle is placed around involved muscle in right eye.

toward the involved side if intorting superior muscles (superior rectus, superior oblique) are paretic and increases when the head is tilted to the opposite side when extorting inferior muscles (inferior rectus, inferior oblique) are paretic. Misleading results can be obtained in the Bielschowsky test if the eyes are not maintained in the primary (straight-ahead) position.

Primary and secondary deviations. The presence of a primary and secondary deviation is helpful, but the results of testing may be equivocal late in the evolution of many cranial nerve palsies, especially those of great chronicity such as "congenital superior oblique palsies."[11] The primary deviation is defined as the deviation noted when the nonparetic eye is fixating. A secondary deviation is defined as the deviation noted when the paretic eye is fixating. Thus with the red filter in front of the right eye and no filter or a green filter in front of the left eye, the patient is instructed to look at the red image, fixating with the right eye. The patient is asked to show you, using his fingers, how far apart the images are. Then the patient is told to look at the white (green) image (left eye fixing) and again demonstrate with his fingers how far apart the images are. A subjective difference when fixating with one eye versus the other, as witnessed by the change in finger separation, indicates nuclear or infranuclear pathology. The larger deviation occurs when the paretic eye is fixing (secondary deviation). The secondary deviation is always larger than the primary deviation (Figs. 5-3 and 5-4).

If the greater separation of the images occurs when the patient is looking at the red image, the right eye is subserved by the paretic muscle, and if it is greater when looking at the white (green) image, the left eye has the paretic muscle (Fig. 5-4). The eye with the paretic muscle determined during comitance testing should demonstrate a secondary deviation, especially in the acute phase of a paresis.

Torsional diplopia or aberrations. Many patients with paresis of oblique muscles (rarely with vertical rectus muscles) experience torsional diplopia with tilting of one or both images. This symptom may be accompanied by dizziness and nausea. Some patients experience a peculiar perception of the entire environment leaning in a particular direction. Torsional symptoms may occur without vertical misalignment.[13]

The demonstration of a torsional deviation is helpful in isolating a paretic vertical muscle when "spread of comitance" and inhibitional palsies have developed. The presence of a torsional misalignment is best demonstrated using double Maddox rods[18] (Fig. 5-11). The rods are placed in the front cells of a trial frame with the bars parallel to the 0° to 180° axis. The appropriate spherical correction for distance is placed in the back cell. The patient's head is placed in the erect position, and the patient is told to look at a distance fixation light. He is then instructed to turn the control knob until the two linear images are parallel and perpendicular to the horizon (straight up and down) (Fig. 5-12). The induced torsion secondary to the paresis is read in degrees from the cylinder axis marker on the trial frame. This test is invaluable for determining the presence of a torsional misalignment without vertical misalignment and for following the progression or regression of fourth cranial nerve palsy. The presence of any amount of torsion in a symptomatic patient is pathologic, and if the measured deviation exceeds 10°, the diagnosis of bilateral superior oblique palsies is strongly suggested.

Quantitating changes in the deviation over time. Repeatable quantitation of either the progression or regression of an extraocular muscle palsy is most easily achieved using the binocular single vision test adapted to the bowl perimeter by Feibel and Roper-Hall.[6]

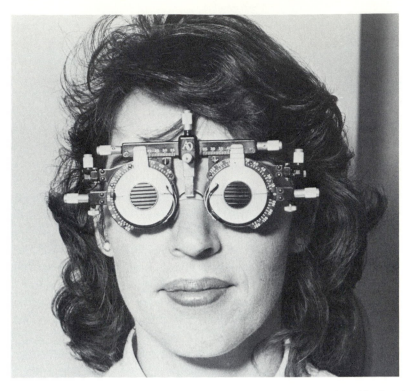

Fig. 5-11. Patient wearing double Maddox rod. The two Maddox rods are placed in the trial frame in such a manner that both lines formed are perpendicular to the horizon.

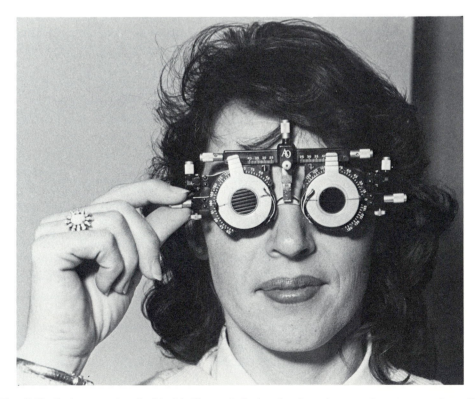

Fig. 5-12. Patient wearing double Maddox rod. Patient has been instructed to turn anterior cells to set linear images perpendicular to horizon and parallel to each other. The amount of induced cyclotorsion is then read in degrees of arc directly from the trial frame.

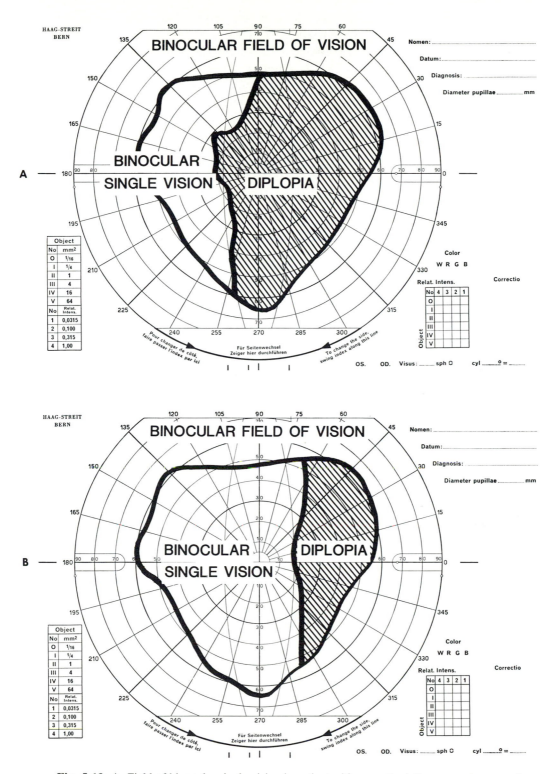

Fig. 5-13. A, Field of binocular single vision in patient with an acute sixth nerve palsy secondary to trauma. **B,** Field of binocular single vision 3 months following field in **A.**

In this test the patient is seated at a bowl perimeter (kinetic variety) with both eyes open, the head erect and centered, and the chin and head rest adjusted so the fixation target is centered at eye level. The III$_4$e test target is placed within the patient's field of binocular single vision, and the patient is instructed to follow the light with his eyes. The light is moved radially outward in all directions, and the patient is asked to report the onset of diplopia. The test quantitatively produces an outline of the area of binocular single vision (Fig. 5-13), can be performed in less than 10 minutes, and over time determines the stability of a given paresis (Fig. 5-13). Similar results can be obtained with the use of a Hess or Lees screen.

REFERENCES

1. Bielschowsky, A: Über monokuläre Diplopie ohne physikalische Grundlage nebst Bemerkungen über das Sehen Schielender, Albrecht Von Graefes Arch Klin Ophthalmol 46:143, 1898.
2. Bielschowsky, A: Lectures on motor anomalies, Hanover, NH, 1943, Dartmouth College Publications.
3. Burde, RM: The extraocular muscles. Part I:Anatomy, physiology, and pharmacology. In Moses, RA, editor: Adler's physiology of the eye, ed 7, St Louis, 1981, The CV Mosby Co, pp 84-121.
4. Burian, HM, and von Noorden, GK: Binocular vision and ocular motility, St Louis, 1974, The CV Mosby Co, pp 260-261.
5. Critchley, M: Types of visual perseveration: "paliopsia" and "illusory visual spread," Brain 74:267, 1951.
6. Feibel, RM, and Roper-Hall, G: Evaluation of the field of binocular single vision in incomitant strabismus, Am J Ophthalmol 78:800, 1974.
7. Goldstein, JE, and Cogan, DG: Exercise and the optic neuropathy of multiple sclerosis, Arch Ophthalmol 72:168, 1964.
8. Haagedorn, A: A new diagnostic motility scheme, Am J Ophthalmol 25:726, 1942.
9. Hardesty, HH: Diagnosis of paretic vertical rotators, Am J Ophthalmol 56:811, 1963.
10. Hering, E: Die Lehre vom binocularen Sehen, Leipzig, 1868, Engelmann.
11. Hering, E: Dr. Raumsin und die Bewegungen der Auges. In Hermann, L: Handbuch der Physiologie, vol 3 (pt 1), 1879; English translation by CA Radde, Baltimore, 1942, American Academy of Optometry.
12. Lessell, S: Higher disorders of visual function: positive phenomenon. In Glaser, JS, and Smith, JL, editors: Neuro-ophthalmology Symposium of the University of Miami and the Bascom Palmer Eye Isntitute, vol 8, St Louis, 1975, The CV Mosby CO, pp 27-44.
13. Metz, HS, and Lerner, H: The adjustable Harada-Ito procedure, Arch Ophthalmol 99:624, 1981.
14. Nachtigäller, H, and Hoyt, WF: Störungen des Seheindruckes bei bitemporaler Hemianopsie und Verschiebung der Sehachsen, Klin Monatsbl Augenheilkd 156;821, 1970.
15. Parks, M: Isolated cyclovertical muscle palsy, Arch Ophthalmol 60:1027, 1958.
16. Roper-Hall, G, and Burde, RM: The extraocular muscles. Part 3: Clinical analysis of extraocular muscle paralysis. In Moses, RA, editor: Adler's physiology of the eye, ed 7, St Louis, 1981, The CV Mosby Co, pp 166-183.
17. Safran, AB, and Roth, A: Using a slit lamp for the neuro-ophthalmologic evaluation of old photographs, Am J Ophthalmol 95:558, 1983.
18. von Noorden, G, and Maumenee, AE: Atlas of strabismus, ed 2, St Louis, 1967, The CV Mosby Co, p 140.

PART II

Comitant strabismus

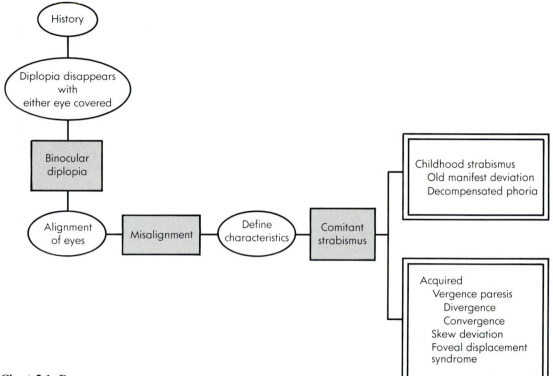

Chart 5-1, D

If the examination fails to reveal any change in the measurement of the ocular misalignment in different gaze positions, then by definition the patient has a comitant strabismus. The largest group of patients with comitant deviations are those we categorize as having childhood strabismus. Childhood strabismus includes those cases of congenital and acquired deviations dating from childhood that may be due to accommodative or nonaccommodative vergence abnormalities that remain to be defined. Whether most of these individuals are born with a miswiring of the visual system or with an innate lack of cortical fusional abilities is a topic that cannot be addressed within the confines of this text.

☐ Childhood strabismus

If the deviation is comitant (Chart 5-1, D) and there is no ocular history to suggest the diagnosis of a childhood deviation, helpful signs to establish the presence of early-onset ocular misalignment would include the finding of amblyopia, absence of normal stereoacuity, dissociated hyperphorias, latent nystagmus, or a positive 4-diopter baseout prism test.

Evidence helpful in making the diagnosis of decompensation of a latent deviation is an adaptive head posture and the presence of large fusional amplitudes. The measurement of fusional amplitudes can be easily accomplished with loose prisms, prism bar, or

Table 5-1. Normal vergence amplitudes

	Convergence	Divergence	Sursumvergence
Distance	16^Δ*-20^Δ	6^Δ-8^Δ	2^Δ-4^Δ
Near	26^Δ-30^Δ	12^Δ-14^Δ	2^Δ-4^Δ

*Δ = Diopters of prism.

rotatory prism starting from the point of neutralization of the tropia. The patient is seated and told to fixate on either a distance or near target. A sequence of prisms is introduced in front of one eye to produce the desired fusional movement, for example, baseout prism for convergence, and the prism strength is increased until the patient reports that the fixation object appears double. When the patient reports insuperable diplopia, the required amount of prism is noted, and this represents the vergence amplitude for that particular movement. (See Table 5-1 for normal ranges.)

Decompensation of a childhood squint (either a horizontal phoria or compensated superior oblique palsy) has been associated with febrile illness, head trauma, and changing refractive needs such as increasing myopia (esotropia) or presbyopia requiring plus lenses (exotropia). In most cases, however, there is no clear precipitating event.

☐ **Acquired comitant deviation**

If childhood strabismus is excluded, there are two diagnostic possibilities: vergence paresis or skew deviation.

☐   **Vergence paresis**

Divergence paralysis. Divergence paralysis is a supranuclear paresis heralded by the sudden onset of esotropia accompanied by diplopia. There is full excursion of both lateral rectus muscles on conjugate gaze. The deviation is horizontally comitant for all gaze positions. As the object of regard approaches the patient, there is a small range in which fusion takes place. At more proximal points a relative convergence insufficiency may be present. There is some debate whether this entity really exists or whether the findings represent a mild symmetric binocular lateral rectus paresis.[8] It is our opinion that it is an entity distinct from bilateral sixth cranial nerve palsies, convergence spasm, and decompensating latent esotropia of the divergence insufficiency type. If this condition is present in isolation, that is, without any other neurologic findings, no further evaluation is indicated. In our experience most often it is benign and self-limited, and we have seen it following head trauma, lumbar puncture, epidural anesthetic blocks, and presumed viral illnesses, as well as in an idiopathic form.

There are occasional reports associating divergence paralysis with encephalitis, demyelinating disease, neurosyphilis, trauma, and tumors in and around the cerebellum.[4] In these cases other focal neurologic signs will be found.

Convergence paralysis. Convergence paralysis is another type of supranuclear gaze failure. These patients complain of diplopia for near objects. They can fully adduct their eyes during conjugate gaze movements. The deviation is comitant across the field of gaze for a given distance. This diagnosis must be made with caution, since the amplitude of convergence is, among other things, dependent upon patient effort. Because of the need for patient cooperation this condition may be feigned easily. Pupillary miosis is a good objective sign of attempted convergence, being an obligate part of the near synkinesis.

Unfortunately, in many patients pupillary and accommodative functions are disturbed as well, and the absence of miosis does not necessarily imply feigned disease. The diagnosis is then dependent upon consistency of objective findings during successive examinations. An appropriate accommodative target should be employed to attempt to produce convergence.

Although convergence paresis is known to occur with structural disease, such as ischemic infarction or demyelination, it has been our experience that it often occurs in isolation as a sequela of a flu syndrome. In the latter case it may be transient or permanent. When convergence paralysis exists in isolation, that is, without accommodative or pupillary involvement or evidence of central nervous system disease, it may be difficult to differentiate from convergence insufficiency. A history that implies chronicity of complaints such as asthenopic symptoms of long duration associated with near fixation is most consistent with a diagnosis of convergence insufficiency. If the symptoms are recent in onset, they may be related to a change in accommodative need, such as the correction of hypermetropia or myopia of 5 or 6 diopters[3] or an initial presbyopic correction. The diagnosis of convergence insufficiency is based on the finding of a remote near point of convergence and decreased fusional convergence at near fixation. Because a partial paralysis of convergence shares these findings, differentiation of convergence paralysis from convergence insufficiency can only be established easily if the patient has a sudden onset of reading difficulty.

☐   **Skew deviation.** If one cannot identify or isolate an offending extraocular muscle or muscles in the presence of a vertical deviation, the possibility of a skew deviation must be entertained. Skew deviation may appear as a comitant or incomitant deviation but is not associated with the presence of a primary and secondary deviation.

The presence of a skew deviation implies posterior fossa disease, and the search for other signs and symptoms involving this broad area should be instituted. In our experience skew deviation never occurs without other neurologic signs and symptoms. However, the associated findings may be subtle and may involve only disorders of ocular movement, that is, saccadic pursuit or nystagmus. The only time that a skew deviation has localizing significance with respect to the side of a brain stem lesion is when it is accompanied by an internuclear ophthalmoplegia. In this circumstance the adduction lag points to the side of the lesion.

Alternating skew deviation[7] is a noncomitant form of skew deviation in which the right eye is hypertropic in one field of gaze, and the left eye is hypertropic in the opposite field of gaze. ''Paroxysmal skew deviation''[1] is an intermittent variety of skew deviation that may be part of an ocular tilt reaction.[6] The ocular tilt reaction is the normal coordination of agonist and antagonist muscle groups in response to utricular stimulation accompanying head tilt. Intermittent aperiodic alternating skew deviation[5] tends to be a more complex variety of the paroxysmal skew deviation with the hyperdeviation occurring at irregular intervals. Mitchell et al.[9] have reported a case of periodic alternating skew deviation. All patterns of skew deviation are associated with posterior fossa disease.

☐   **Foveal displacement syndrome.**[2] Some patients with subretinal neovascular membranes before or after photocoagulation therapy may develop binocular diplopia due to displacement of the foveomacular receptor elements, producing a rivalry between central and peripheral fusional mechanisms. Thus, if the eyes are not misaligned (the circumstance most of the time as peripheral fusional mechanisms are stronger than central mechanisms), the fovea of the involved eye is displaced (dragged) relative to the fovea of the normal eye, and the patient experiences diplopia. If the "diplopia" is neutralized by prisms, a small comitant deviation will be induced (measured); however, in spite of prescribing the neutralizing prism, diplopia recurs in a matter of minutes as the peripheral mechanisms realign the eyes. There is little that can be done to make these patients binocularly comfortable, but a few of them can tolerate a small central occluder in the visual axis of their spectacle correction in front of the involved eye.

REFERENCES

1. Allerand, CD: Paroxysmal skew deviation in association with brain stem glioma, Neurology 12:520, 1962.
2. Burgess, D, Roper-Hall, G, and Burde, RM: Binocular diplopia associated with subretinal neovascular membranes, Arch Ophthalmol 98:311, 1980.
3. Burian, HM, and von Noorden, GK: Binocular vision and ocular motility, St. Louis, 1974, The CV Mosby Co, p 395.
4. Cogan, DG: Neurology of the ocular muscles, ed. 2, Springfield, Ill, 1956, Charles C Thomas, Publisher, pp 133-134.
5. Corbett, JJ, Schatz, NJ, Shults, WT, Behrens, M, and Berry, RG: Slowly alternating skew deviation: description of a pretectal syndrome in three patients, Ann Neurol 10:540, 1981.
6. Hedges, TR, III, and Hoyt, WF: Ocular tilt reaction due to an upper brainstem lesion: paroxysmal skew deviation, torsion, and oscillation of the eyes with head tilt, Ann Neurol 11:537, 1982.
7. Keane, JR: Ocular skew deviation, Arch Neurol 32:185, 1975.
8. Kirkham, TH, Bird, AC, and Sanders, MD: Divergence paralysis and raised intracranial pressure, Br J Ophthalmol 56:776, 1972.
9. Mitchell, JM, Smith, JL, and Quencer, RM: Periodic alternating skew deviation, J Clin Neuro-ophthalmol 1:5, 1981.

PART III

Incomitant strabismus and associated diseases

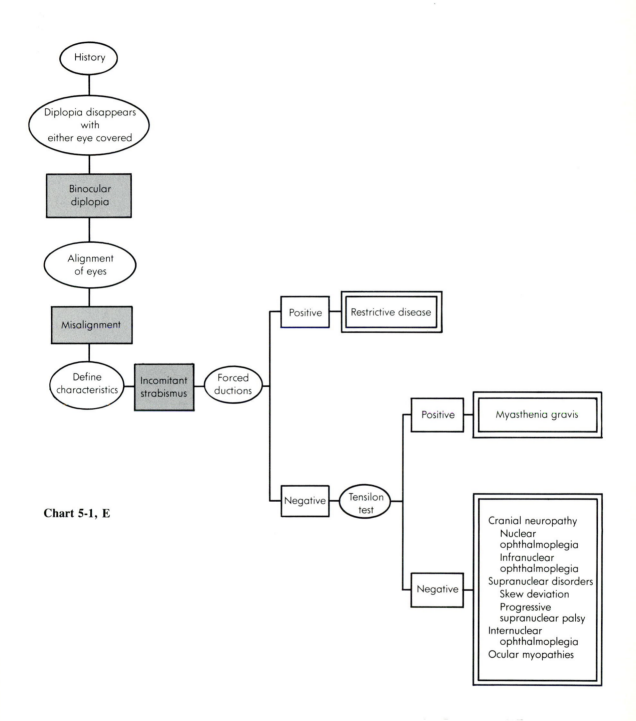

Chart 5-1, E

In all patients with incomitant deviations it is necessary to exclude two disease entities: restrictive ophthalmopathy and myasthenia gravis. The principal tests used to make this distinction are the forced duction and Tensilon (edrophonium chloride) tests.

○   **Forced duction test.** The presence of a mechanical restriction is most easily confirmed by the use of forced (passive) duction testing. Appropriate use of topical anesthetics makes the performance of forced duction testing comfortable for the patient, thus assuring the examiner of the best chance of detecting minimal restrictions of movements. Topical proparacaine solution should be instilled in the inferior cul-de-sac of each eye. Then a cotton-tipped applicator soaked in proparacaine is placed in the fornix over the insertion of the rectus muscles to be manipulated for approximately 15 to 20 seconds. If a restriction is marked, it can be demonstrated using the cotton-tipped applicator.

The patient is asked to look in the direction of the gaze limitation. The cotton-tipped applicator is placed over the presumed involved rectus muscle, and an attempt is made to move this eye in the direction of gaze restriction. Failure of movement or retraction of the globe into the orbit on passive movement signifies the presence of a restrictive process. This same sequence is then repeated on the other eye, comparing the ease and range of passive movement of the globe. If the globe is pushed back into the orbit inadvertently as pressure is applied, an otherwise positive test may be made equivocal. In pushing the eye back into the orbit the relative length of the tethered muscle is increased, allowing the eye to move more easily. This retrodisplacement of the globe produces a false sense of freedom of movement.

If the result obtained using the cotton-tipped applicator is equivocal, passive duction testing may be repeated by grasping the muscle insertion using a large blunt-toothed forceps. The use of the forceps allows the examiner to make the diagnosis of more subtle restrictions. Even at that, it may be impossible to determine if minimal ductional deficits are caused by restriction.

Some patients are unable to cooperate for either of these maneuvers. In these patients the intraocular pressure should be measured in the primary position and again with the eyes moved voluntarily into the direction of limited gaze. Although originally described using Goldmann applanation tonography, accurate results can be obtained more easily using a hand-held tonometer. A pressure rise of greater than 4 mm Hg in moving from one gaze position to another is diagnostic of a restrictive problem.[22,75] Patients with inferior rectus restriction often have elevated intraocular pressures in the primary position. Thus these patients may be identified mistakenly as glaucoma suspects or "ocular hypertensives." Unless there is evidence of progressive optic disc changes and visual field loss, no treatment is indicated.

☐ **Restrictive disease**

There are many disease processes that cause mechanical limitation of extraocular movements, that is, positive forced ductions, although dysthyroid orbitopathy is the most common (see Box). Brown's superior oblique tendon sheath syndrome, which mimics an isolated inferior oblique palsy, is an often overlooked syndrome. It can be either congenital or acquired. The acquired form often is associated with pain on attempted upgaze in the adducted position and tenderness in the region of the trochlea. The diagnosis is made by passive forced duction testing. Suggested treatment of the acquired form includes sub-Tenon injections of corticosteroids in the region of the trochlea in acute cases,

---

MECHANICAL (RESTRICTIVE) CAUSES
OF ACQUIRED DIPLOPIA

Dysthyroid orbitopathy
Orbital pseudotumor
Orbital myositis
Brown's superior oblique tendon sheath syndrome
Orbital mass lesions $\begin{cases} \text{Primary} \\ \text{Metastatic} \end{cases}$
Trauma

---

but spontaneous improvement often occurs with time. Surgery may be attempted in cases with a persistent deficit, but none of the suggested procedures is universally successful.

☐ Myasthenia gravis

If forced duction testing is negative, a Tensilon or neostigmine (Prostigmin) test should be performed to exclude the possibility of myasthenia gravis. Myasthenia gravis may mimic any single or combined extraocular muscle palsy, supranuclear or internuclear ophthalmoplegia (see Box).

Seventy-five percent of myasthenic patients[51] will present with ocular symptoms, and approximately 90% eventually will develop ocular involvement. It is believed that if no systemic signs develop within a period of 2 years, the disease is likely to remain localized to the extraocular muscles.[28] For the most part the diagnosis of myasthenia gravis depends on a positive Tensilon test. It is helpful to obtain photographs of the patient before and after the injection of Tensilon in order to document the results of the test procedure (see Box) and thus to avoid the need for repeated testing.

In performing the Tensilon test a measurable end point must be obtainable. One cannot rely on the subjective response of the patient or the qualitative judgment of the examiner. The only reliable indicator of a positive response is a quantitative change in the ptosis or measured ocular deviation. If ptosis is present, a change in the amount is certainly the easiest parameter to quantitate; however, Eaton has reported in his series of ocular myasthenics that 23% of patients who have diplopia do not have ptosis.[17]

OPHTHALMIC SIGNS OF MYASTHENIA GRAVIS

Ptosis	Pseudointernuclear ophthalmoplegia
Extraocular muscle palsies	Lid twitch[11]
Pseudogaze palsies	Orbicularis weakness[50]
Pseudoconvergence paresis	Nystagmus
Quiver movements	

Retzlaff et al.[55] demonstrate the necessity of measuring the effect of Tensilon in more than one position of gaze utilizing the Lancaster red-green test. They show that the response varies according to gaze position. These changes must occur within 30 to 60 seconds of injection and return to the pretest measurements within 4 to 5 minutes. The changes must be repeatable on subsequent testing. There are four possible responses to the Tensilon test, one negative and three positive. A negative response, that is, no change in the ocular alignment, generally means that the patient does not have myasthenia gravis but does not absolutely exclude the diagnosis. A small percentage (unquantitated) of patients with myasthenia will have a negative response to intravenous injection of Tensilon. They may show a positive response to more specialized tests, for example, electromyography with repetitive nerve stimulation or regional curare testing.

The three types of positive responses may occur in any myasthenic patient depending on the gaze position in which the deviation is measured:

Type 1: An improvement in alignment
   (Large tropia* → Small tropia → Fusion)
Type 2: A worsening of alignment
   (Small tropia* → Large tropia)
Type 3: A reversal in alignment
   (Right hypertropia → Left hypertropia)

*Vertical deviation: minimum change $\geqq 3^\Delta$. Horizontal deviation: minimum change $\geqq 5^\Delta$.

Paradoxical responses (types 2 and 3) to Tensilon include a worsening or a reversal of ocular misalignment; that is, a right hypertropia would increase by more than 3^Δ, or a right hypertropia would become a left hypertropia. A similar reversal can be seen in a patient with ptosis wherein the ptotic lid develops retraction, and the normal lid becomes ptotic. It is our impression and that of Liesegang and Glaser[42] that a type 1 response (improvement) is only seen in myasthenic patients, while a type 2 or 3 response may be seen in approximately 10% of nonmyasthenic ophthalmoplegias. The Tensilon test using small increments (0.2 ml) of Tensilon will often (but not always) produce a type 1 response in patients who have previously had type 2 or 3 responses to the sequence outlined above, as well as in patients with myasthenia who are not adequately treated with anticholinesterase agents.

The side effects of Tensilon are those of cholinergic hyperactivity and include tearing, salivation, gastric distress, and mild bradycardia as well as lid fasciculations. The safety of the Tensilon test has been well documented.[71]

For the most part, ocular myasthenia gravis is resistant to treatment with anticholinesterase agents such as pyridostigmine (Mestinon). Prednisone therapy has been effective and may be initiated with daily doses of 80 to 100 mg[65] and converted to an alternate-day regimen. Alternatively, treatment may be initiated with alternate-day prednisone, 25 to 100 mg.[19] Although systemic corticosteroids may cause an exacerbation of systemic signs in patients with generalized myasthenia, leading to extreme weakness and in some cases respiratory failure, this is less likely to occur in patients with ocular myasthenia.[19]

Once the desired response is achieved, the patient is slowly weaned to the lowest level of alternate-day prednisone that keeps the patient symptom free. The elimination of diplopia in response to alternate-day steroids in patients with ocular myasthenia is remarkable, approaching 90% to 100%.[19] In our experience patients with ocular myas-

TENSILON TEST

Tensilon (edrophonium hydrochloride) is supplied in single-dose, 10 mg/1 ml, break-neck vials; that is, there is 1 mg/0.1 ml.

A definite goal or end point must be selected. If ptosis is present, then a measured change in the amount of ptosis is satisfactory. (Polaroid pictures before and during the test are easily taken and are a good record. A copy given to the patient will save him from being "drowned in a veritable sea of Tensilon.") If no ptosis is present, it is necessary to quantitate a change in the deviation using a Hess or Lees screen. Some clinicians choose to pretreat all the patients with 0.4 mg of intramuscular atropine 15 minutes before performing the test. Others prefer to use 0.4 mg of intravenous atropine when needed.

Alternative A

1. Tensilon should be drawn up into a 1 cc tuberculin syringe.
2. 0.4 mg of injectable atropine sulfate should be drawn up into a 1 cc tuberculin syringe.
3. A 10 cc syringe should be filled with injectable saline.
4. A scalp-vein needle (21 or 23 gauge) should be placed into a dorsal hand vein.
5. A multiswitch stopcock may be used, or the syringes changed as necessary.
6. Inject 1 ml saline solution and observe for 1 minute.
7. a. Inject 0.2 ml Tensilon and flush tubing with 1 ml saline; observe for 1 minute. *If no response,* inject a bolus of 0.8 ml Tensilon and flush tubing with 1 ml saline; connect atropine syringe to tubing.

   or

   b. Inject 0.2 ml Tensilon and flush with saline. Continue slow injection of Tensilon by slowly flushing with saline after priming tube with remaining 0.8 ml.

   or

   c. Inject 0.2 ml Tensilon and flush with saline; observe for 1 minute. Inject 0.4 ml Tensilon and flush with saline; observe for 1 minute. Inject remaining 0.4 ml Tensilon and observe for 1 minute.

Alternative B

1. Draw Tensilon into 1 cc tuberculin syringe with a ⅝ inch, 27-gauge needle. Inject directly with tuberculin syringe and needle into dorsal hand vein. Make sure the syringe can be detached from the needle before inserting it into the vein.
2. Injections are made as in Alternative A.

Alternative C

Preferred in children, uncooperative adults, and in patients in whom a long duration of action is desired. Intramuscular atropine, 0.4 mg, is given 15 minutes prior to an intramuscular injection of neostigmine (Prostigmin). The dose of neostigmine is calculated

$$\frac{\text{Weight (kg)}}{70 \text{ (kg)}} \times 1.5 \text{ mg} = \text{Dose}$$

The patient should be reexamined 30 to 45 minutes after the injection.

thenia can be started on low doses of alternate-day steroids, that is, 10 mg of prednisone every other day. The dose is slowly increased until the desired effect is achieved. We estimate that about 80% of such patients will become free of diplopia over a wide range of gaze positions.

☐ Nuclear and infranuclear ophthalmoplegia

Once both restrictive disease and myasthenia gravis have been excluded (Chart 5-1, *E*), the vast majority of patients with incomitant strabismus will have processes affecting the ocular motor nuclei, their fascicles, or the cranial nerves themselves. The localization of the lesion causing ocular motor abnormalities is aided by the associated neurologic symptoms and signs.

Oculomotor nerve (third cranial nerve)

Anatomy. The third cranial nerve innervates five extraocular muscles: the levator palpebrae superioris; superior, inferior, and medial rectus; and the inferior oblique. It also supplies the presynaptic parasympathetic outflow to the ciliary ganglion controlling pupillary sphincter function and accommodation. The anatomy of the oculomotor nuclear complex in primates has been well worked out by Warwick (Fig. 5-14).[73] It is assumed that these findings are applicable in man, and clinically this appears to be true. The levator is bilaterally innervated by the central caudal nucleus. The medial rectus, inferior rectus, and inferior oblique muscles are ipsilaterally innervated. The superior rectus muscle is innervated contralaterally with the decussation of fibers occurring at the caudal end of the complex.[5]

The visceral nuclei extend from the rostral end of the complex caudally. The most rostral portion of the complex consists of paired central nuclei, the anterior median nuclei (one on each side of the midline). Dorsally and caudally the visceral complex divides into slender columns that subdivide again into a medial and lateral column. Caudally the lateral column subdivides again with the most lateral column extending around the central caudal nucleus. Between the masses of the somatic motor nuclei is found the nucleus of Perlia, which also makes up part of the visceral system. The visceral outflow is totally ipsilateral in projection.[8]

The oculomotor complex is cupped by the medial longitudinal fasciculus and lies ventral to the central gray matter. Fascicles arise along its entire length and sweep ventrally to exit the midbrain as multiple rootlets in the interpenduncular fossa. The nerve then turns rostrally, traveling in the subarachnoid space suspended under and over the anteriorsuperior cerebellar and posterior cerebral arteries to enter the lateral wall of the cavernous sinus. The pupillary fibers travel in the dorsomedial portion of the nerve. The nerve enters the orbit through the superior orbital fissure, and either at the anterior end of the cavernous sinus or the posterior aspect of the orbit it divides into a superior and inferior division (see Box). Because of this particular anatomic origin and projections, lesions at different levels tend to produce different signs.

• • •

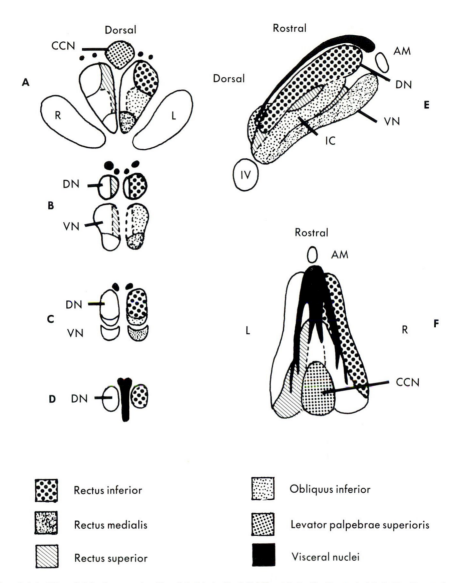

Rectus inferior

Rectus medialis

Rectus superior

Obliquus inferior

Levator palpebrae superioris

Visceral nuclei

Fig. 5-14. Warwick's figure. **A,** Caudal third. **B,** Middle third. **C,** Rostral third. **D,** Rostral end. **E,** Right lateral aspects. **F,** Dorsal aspect. *DN,* Dorsal nucleus; *VN,* ventral nucleus; *CCN,* caudal central nucleus; *IC,* intermediate column; *IV,* trochlear nucleus; *AM,* anterior median nucleus.

DIVISIONS OF THE THIRD CRANIAL (OCULOMOTOR) NERVE*

1. Superior division
    a. Superior rectus muscle
    b. Levator palpebrae superioris muscle
2. Inferior division
    a. Medial rectus muscle
    b. Inferior rectus muscle
    c. Inferior oblique muscle
    d. Parasympathetic innervation to sphincter pupillae muscle and ciliary muscles

*Divisions formed proximal to or at the superior orbital fissure.

Table 5-2. Comparison of causes of third cranial nerve palsy in adults

	Rucker[58] (335 cases)		Rucker[59] (274 cases)		Green et al.[26] (130 cases)		Goldstein and Cogan[25] (61 cases)		Rush and Younge[60] (290 cases)	
	No.	%	No.	%	No.	%	No.	%	No.	%
Aneurysm	64	19	50	18	38	30	11	18	40	14
Vascular disease*	63	19	47	17	25	19	28	47	60	21
Trauma	51	15	34	13	14	11	5	8	47	16
Syphilis	6	2	0	0	12	9	0	0	0	0
Neoplasm	35	11	50	18	5	4	6	10	34	12
Undetermined	95	28	55	20	33	23	7	11	67	23
Miscellaneous	21	6	38	12	5	4	4	6	42	14

*Including diabetes mellitus.

The causes of cranial nerve palsies in adults[25,26,58-60] and children[30,43] are different. Although the information available in the published series is not derived from a similar population base, the results are remarkably parallel within both the adult and children's series.

Third nerve palsies in adults. As just mentioned, the five major published series are not parallel in derivation (Table 5-2).[25,26,58-60] Some of these papers include patients with neurologic deficits other than third nerve palsies, excluding involvement of the fourth and sixth cranial nerves,[58-60] while others deal with truly isolated third nerve palsies.[26] The three series from the Mayo Clinic[58-60] include a variety of patients with acquired impairment of ocular motility; some were ambulatory and had only diplopia, and others were hospitalized with serious illness. Although these patients with oculomotor nerve paresis had no other ocular motor (trochlear and abducens) palsies, many did have other accompanying neurologic signs. This is in contrast to the patients reported by Green et al.[26] who had *isolated* oculomotor palsies, that is, no other neurologic signs.

The most common causes of third cranial nerve palsies in adults are aneurysms and vascular disease (hypertension, atherosclerosis, and diabetes mellitus), each accounting for approximately 20% of the total. Trauma and tumors each account for 10% to 15% of cases. These tumors include pituitary tumors with lateral extension, parapituitary mass lesions, meningiomas within the cavernous sinus, and metastatic or primary disease within the brain stem.[30,43,48,63] Parasellar mass lesions are reported to cause the acute onset of a third nerve palsy in association with a history of minimal trauma.[18]

A wide spectrum of miscellaneous neurologic and systemic diseases including sinusitis, Hodgkin's disease, herpes zoster, temporal arteritis, meningitis, encephalitis, collagen vascular disease, Paget's disease, as well as postoperative complications of neurosurgical procedures have been implicated as the cause of oculomotor paralysis. These entities, although rare, take on added importance when third cranial nerve palsies are evaluated on an age-related basis. It is important to emphasize that ocular motor palsies (third or sixth cranial nerve) may be the presenting sign in 12% of patients with giant cell arteritis.[34] Therefore patients over the age of 55 presenting with an ocular motor palsy should be questioned for a history of polymyalgia rheumatica, headache, or scalp tenderness and should have an immediate erythrocyte sedimentation rate performed. Appropriate therapy should be instituted as necessary.

Recognition of differential involvement of components of the oculomotor nerve in an adult is often helpful in terms of localization of the offending lesion.

Third nerve palsy involving all components. In a total isolated paralysis of the oculomotor nerve the globe is turned out and slightly down. The pupil is dilated and unreactive to direct or consensual stimuli. The eye may float toward the midline with attempted gaze toward the contralateral side (inhibition of the abducens nerve), and intorsion can be induced on attempted downgaze if the trochlear nerve is intact. Such findings usually indicate involvement between the base of the midbrain and the superior orbital fissure.

Patients with involvement of "all" the somatic components of the third nerve may demonstrate certain clinically apparent findings that are of diagnostic significance: pupillary sparing and aberrant regeneration.

Pupillary sparing and its importance. In adult patients presenting with retroorbital or periorbital pain and the acute onset of an isolated third nerve palsy, most either have an aneurysm in the distribution of the internal carotid artery compressing the third nerve, or they have suffered an infarction of the nerve substance itself. The decision facing the clinician is to determine which patients in this group are likely to have aneurysms and are therefore in need of arteriography with its inherent morbidity (mortality). In 1960 Goldstein and Cogan[25] demonstrated that pupillary sparing, that is, normal pupillary function, is the hallmark of third nerve palsies, presumably due to vascular occlusion (80%). On the other hand, pupillary sparing is rarely found (<10%) in patients with third nerve palsies due to aneurysms.[38] To further complicate matters, in aneurysmal third nerve palsies, pupillary function can remain normal for days and only later will become abnormal.[38,49] Temporary or initial pupillary sparing can be found in 8% to 15% of these cases.[38,49]

Pupillary findings must be related to the remainder of third nerve function. Pupillary sparing is a relative concept. For example, if a patient has a total paresis of the extraocular muscles, but the pupil on the involved side is only 1 to 2 mm larger than the other pupil and reacts fairly well to light stimuli (even though less briskly than its counterpart), we would consider this patient to have a "relative pupillary sparing third nerve" palsy.* However, if there is subtotal involvement of the extraocular muscles and the pupil is minimally, but definitely, involved, we would *not* consider the patient to have "relative pupillary sparing."

The explanation for pupillary sparing lies in the anatomy of the third nerve and its blood supply. Kerr and Hollowell[37] and Sunderland and Hughes[67] have shown that pupillary fibers travel superficially and superonasally in the third nerve and therefore are at risk early for involvement in compressive lesions, for example, aneurysm or midline shift prior to herniation of the isthmus through the tentorium cerebelli. Dreyfus et al.[16] and Asbury et al.[3] have demonstrated that pupillary sparing is produced by an occlusion of one of the vasa nervorum in the intracranial course of the third nerve. This produces an ischemic infarct of the core of the nerve while relatively sparing the superficial fibers including those destined for the pupil.

Vasculopathic—a definition. Although the so-called "pupillary sparing third cranial nerve palsy" has been classically associated with diabetes mellitus, it is most often found in patients who do not demonstrate abnormalities of glucose metabolism. The more general term of "vasculopathic paresis" has been applied, implying small-vessel infarction due to diabetes mellitus, atherosclerosis, hypertension, or other undefined vascular diseases. A vasculopathic etiology has also been postulated as a frequent cause of isolated fourth and sixth cranial nerve palsies. Such a palsy may be recurrent but almost always occurs as a mononeuropathy. Total recovery in weeks to months (up to 6) is the rule. These patients do not develop aberrant regeneration. If more than one ocular motor nerve is involved simultaneously,[40] the diagnosis of a vasculopathic paresis should be suspect.

Aberrant regeneration. Aberrant regeneration of the oculomotor nerve consists of a constellation of various clinical findings, the most common of which is lid retraction in downgaze (pseudo-von Graefe phenomenon[32]). Other findings include lid elevation or pupillary constriction on attempted adduction or unilateral globe retraction on upgaze or downgaze. Aberrant regeneration is presumed to be due to miswiring following a break in the axon cylinders within the third nerve with misdirection of sprouting axons.[33] Aberrant regeneration almost always occurs following an acute oculomotor palsy, but Schatz et al.[63] have noted aberrant regeneration without such a history. Their patients all had meningiomas of the cavernous sinus, and they believe that primary aberrant regeneration, that is, aberrant regeneration without a previous history of a third nerve palsy, indicates an indolent mass lesion in the sinus. Cox et al.[12] have reported similar findings in a patient with an intracavernous aneurysm.

Divisional involvement. Anatomically the oculomotor nerve lies above and medial to the trochlear nerve in the anterior part of the cavernous sinus. It separates into its two

*As far as we know, this concept of relative pupillary sparing is not discussed elsewhere in the literature. Based on our clinical experience, we believe that relative pupillary sparing and absolute pupillary sparing should be treated as one entity.

divisions either in the anterior cavernous sinus or in the region of the superior orbital fissure. Pathologic processes in this area therefore can involve either the superior or inferior branches separately.

Inferior divisional paresis is marked by internal ophthalmoplegia and paresis of the medial and inferior rectus muscles as well as paresis of the inferior oblique muscle. Inferior divisional palsies have been reported with trauma secondary to neoplasms and presumed viral insults. For the most part, in presumed viral cases the paresis tends to recover spontaneously.[68]

Superior divisional paresis is marked by ptosis and superior rectus muscle paresis. Isolated superior divisional paresis is rare. One case has been reported, presumably of a viral etiology in which spontaneous recovery occurred.[15] It has been noted that in patients with intracavernous aneurysms there tends to be a relative sparing of the inferior division of the oculomotor nerve. Additionally, these individuals, for the most part, had involvement of other cranial nerves (V and VI).[70]

Single muscle paresis. A series of cases of isolated inferior rectus muscle palsies presumed secondary to small-vessel occlusion in the brain stem have been reported.[57] These patients all recovered spontaneously. Warren et al.[72] have reported a series of cases with partial third nerve palsies involving one or two muscles and the pupil. These deficits were accompanied by other signs of intrinsic midbrain disease such as rubral tremor (involvement of the red nucleus) or cerebellar signs (involvement of the brachium conjunctivum). Using Warwick's model of the component parts subserving individual muscle function within the third nerve nucleus, they postulated specifically located lesions within the mesencephalon as being the cause of the neurologic deficits.

Isolated paresis of the inferior oblique muscle of unknown etiology has also been reported.[21,64] The finding of what appears to be an isolated inferior oblique palsy mandates excluding the so-called "Brown superior oblique tendon sheath syndrome."[7] The diagnosis is made by forced duction testing.

A dilated, unreactive pupil with no other signs of third nerve dysfunction is not a third nerve paresis. These patients should be evaluated for signs of possible ocular trauma, pharmacologic blockade, or Adie's syndrome.

Third nerve palsies in children. The causes of isolated third nerve palsies in children are different from those in an adult population[26,30,48] (Table 5-3). Between 43% and 47% of cases are congenital; between 13% and 23% are traumatic; neoplasms account for approximately 10% and aneurysms for 7% of cases. Both Miller[48] and Harley[30] point out that a high percentage of their cases of congenital oculomotor palsy had aberrant regeneration (61% and 93%, respectively). Since most of these patients have nonprogressive defects and negative radiographic studies, intrauterine or birth trauma is the most likely etiology.

Cyclic oculomotor paresis. Three of the patients in Miller's series[48] with congenital oculomotor paralysis developed cyclic oculomotor paralysis. Cyclic oculomotor paresis is a movement disorder usually present at birth. A child with a third nerve palsy will have spastic movements of the muscles innervated by the third cranial nerve resulting in lid elevation, adduction, miosis, and increased accommodation. These movements occur at regular intervals, lasting 10 to 30 seconds on the background of a total third nerve palsy.[43] Thus, cyclic oculomotor paresis is a misnomer, since the paralysis is present

Table 5-3. Comparison of causes of third cranial nerve palsy in children

	Miller[48] (30 cases)		Harley[30] (32 cases)		Green et al.[26] (6 cases)	
	No.	%	No.	%	No.	%
Congenital	13*	43	15	47		
Aneurysm	2	7				
Neoplasm	3	10	3	9		
Vascular disease			2†	6		
Trauma	6	20	4	13	4	X
Inflammation	4	13	3	9	2	X
Miscellaneous	2‡	7	5§	16		

*Includes birth trauma.
†Ophthalmoplegic migraine.
‡Limited information.
§Three cases of ophthalmoplegic migraine.

most of the time. A better term would be cyclic oculomotor spasm in association with oculomotor paralysis.

Ophthalmoplegic migraine. Ophthalmoplegic migraine is a rare syndrome that almost always has its onset in childhood. Patients with a migrainous ophthalmoplegia usually develop the third cranial nerve palsy as the headache phase abates, although it may occur at any time in relation to the pain phase. In fact the onset of the ptosis in many of these patients is the signal that the headache is about to disappear. The extraocular muscle weakness tends to last longer with each episode, and in a few individuals a permanent oculomotor paresis has developed.[14]

Management. Our recommendations for the evaluation of patients presenting with *isolated* third nerve palsies follow:

1. All patients under the age of 40 years who present with third nerve palsies should have a CT scan, cerebrospinal fluid (CSF) studies, and cerebral angiography, regardless of the state of the pupil.
2. All patients with symptoms or signs of subarachnoid hemorrhage should have a CT scan, CSF studies, and an angiogram.
3. The select group of patients who are in the vasculopathic age group (over age 40) and who present with pupillary-sparing third nerve palsies* should be observed daily for 5 to 7 days, then weekly for 1 month, and then monthly for 6 months.

   An appropriate diagnostic workup should include measurement of the systemic blood pressure and at least a 2-hour postprandial blood sugar. If the pupil becomes involved or signs and symptoms of subarachnoid hemorrhage develop, the patients should have immediate angiography.

*We believe this includes patients with relative pupillary sparing. Because there are no data to substantiate this clinical impression, we consider it to be reasonable to submit patients with such pupillary findings to immediate angiography.

4. All patients over the age of 40 presenting with nonpupillary-sparing third nerve palsies should have a CT scan, CSF examination, and a cerebral angiogram.

    Because 10% to 20% of patients with ischemic third nerve palsies will have pupillary dysfunction,[25,58] even using these guidlines there will be a certain number of negative angiograms.

    If the resolution of intravenous digital subtraction angiography (DSA) improves substantially, the risk-benefit ratio may be altered in favor of performing this test in all patients with third cranial nerve palsies regardless of the status of the pupil.

5. If aberrant regeneration is found, an appropriate evaluation for the presence of a mass lesion must be initiated, as aberrant regeneration is a sign of a compressive lesion except in cases of major head trauma.

6. Minor trauma should not be invoked as a cause of isolated third'nerve palsy. Another cause must be sought by appropriate diagnostic evaluation.

Trochlear nerve (fourth cranial nerve)

Anatomy. The trochlear nerves arise from a pair of motor neurons in the ventral mesencephalon under the inferior colliculi, contiguous to the caudal end of the third nerve complex. The fibers course dorsally to decussate completely in the anterior medullary velum, the roof of the fourth ventricle where the fibers are vulnerable to trauma. They emerge posterior to the inferior colliculi and travel rostrocaudally to enter the cavernous sinus just behind the posterior clinoid process. They lie inferior to the third nerves in the lateral walls of the cavernous sinuses and enter the orbits through the superior orbital fissures.

Trochlear nerve palsies in adults. The recent literature is replete with reports of varying entities causing isolated fourth cranial nerve palsies. This apparent increase of interest in isolated fourth nerve palsies is most likely secondary to the improved diagnostic acumen of both ophthalmologists and neurologists. This fact is reflected in the most recent series from the Mayo Clinic in which Rush and Younge[60] report 172 cases of fourth nerve palsies recognized among 1000 patients with ocular motor palsies seen between 1966 and 1978. This is almost twice as many as reported by Rucker in his previous series[58,59] surveying patients seen prior to 1966 in the same institution. The four largest series of fourth nerve palsies are listed in Table 5-4.[9,58-60] In spite of the availability of improved diagnostic techniques the number of cases remaining without a specific diagnosis is still approximately 30%. The most common cause of fourth cranial nerve palsies is trauma. Bilateral fourth nerve palsies are often seen following vertex blows to the head such as occur in motorcycle accidents. It is postulated that the mechanism is distension of the fourth ventricle causing a physiologic disruption of the crossing fibers in the anterior medullary velum (the anterior roof of the fourth ventricle).

    Vascular disease, including hypertension, atherosclerosis, and diabetes mellitus, accounts for approximately one fifth of the cases. Most isolated trochlear nerve palsies occurring in the fourth and fifth decades tend to improve spontaneously over a period of 2 to 6 months. Grimson and Glaser[27] have described six patients with fourth nerve palsies following herpes zoster ophthalmicus. The onset of the fourth nerve palsy occurred from

Table 5-4. Comparison of causes of fourth cranial nerve palsy

	Rucker[58] (67 cases)		Rucker[59] (84 cases)		Burger et al.[9] (33 cases)		Rush and Younge[60] (172 cases)	
	No.	%	No.	%	No.	%	No.	%
Aneurysm	0	0	0	0	1	3	3	2
Vascular disease	24	36	13	15	6	18	32	18
Trauma	24	36	22	27	13	39	55	32
Neoplasm	3	4	7	8	7	21	7	4
Undetermined	9	13	29	33	2	6	62	36
Miscellaneous	7	10	13	15	3	9	13	8

2 days to 4 weeks following the onset of the cutaneous eruption. Three patients were left with a permanent diplopia.

Rush and Younge[60] report three cases of isolated trochlear nerve palsy due to aneurysm, one in the cavernous sinus, one due to a large basilar artery aneurysm, and one associated with a subarachnoid hemorrhage. Miscellaneous causes include collagen vascular disease, neonatal hypoxia, hydrocephalus, complications of intracranial surgery and coronary angiography, and encephalitis.

Trochlear nerve palsies in children. In a review of 18 cases of trochlear nerve palsies, Harley[30] found a distribution of causes that was quite different from that in adults: 12 were considered to be congenital in origin (5 bilateral and 7 unilateral), 5 were secondary to head trauma, and 1 case followed encephalitis.

The sudden onset of vertical diplopia in late childhood to the middle to late forties in the absence of head trauma, which can be isolated to a single superior oblique muscle, should alert the clinician to the possibility of decompensation of a ''presumed'' congenital trochlear nerve palsy.[24,47] These patients tend to have large fusional amplitudes, often being able to fuse 10^Δ to 15^Δ from the neutral point. Old photographs demonstrating the presence of a head tilt, even in infancy, are extremely helpful. Vertical prisms often alleviate the patient's symptoms. If these patients are not made asymptomatic by the use of vertical prisms, a torsional problem is usually present. Under these circumstances a variety of extraocular muscle surgical procedures should be considered.[44]

Management. A child or adult who has a nontraumatic isolated fourth nerve palsy without large fusional amplitudes must be carefully examined for signs of tectal compression and should have a Tensilon test. Adult patients should have a general medical evaluation to exclude the presence of hypertension and diabetes mellitus. *Nonischemic causes of neurologically isolated trochlear nerve palsies are rare, and further investigation should only be undertaken if there is progression of the paresis or other neurologic signs develop.*

Our recommendations for the evaluation of patients presenting with isolated nontraumatic fourth nerve palsies follow:

1. Patients of all ages with large vertical fusional amplitudes need no further evaluation. They have decompensating congenital fourth nerve palsies.

Table 5-5. Comparison of causes of sixth cranial nerve palsy

	Rucker[58] (409 cases)		Rucker[59] (515 cases)		Shrader and Schlezinger[66] (104 cases)		Rush and Younge[60] (419 cases)	
	No.	%	No.	%	No.	%	No.	%
Aneurysm	16	4	15	3	0	0	15	3
Vascular disease	57	14	46	9	38	37	74	18
Trauma	57	14	55	11	3	3	70	17
Neoplasm	82	20	159	31	7	7	61	15
Multiple sclerosis	15	4	36	7	13	13	18	4
Syphilis	7	2	0	0	10	10	0	0
Undetermined	129	32	112	21	25	24	124	29
Miscellaneous	46	11	92	18	8	8	57	14

2. Patients of all ages without large vertical fusional amplitudes should have a Tensilon test performed to exclude myasthenia gravis.
3. Adult patients without large fusional amplitudes who have a negative Tensilon test should be evaluated for hypertension and diabetes mellitus.
4. Only those patients who demonstrate a progression of their fourth nerve palsy or who develop additional signs or symptoms of neurologic disease should be thoroughly evaluated both medically and neurologically, including high-resolution CT scanning and cerebral angiography.

Abducens nerve (sixth cranial nerve)

Anatomy. The sixth cranial nerves arise from a paired group of motor cells whose location is marked on the floor of the fourth ventricle (facial colliculi) by the passage of the fascicles of the seventh cranial nerves from their nuclei on the way to exit laterally in the brain stem. This group of motor cells consists of a central group that directly innervates the lateral rectus muscle and a surrounding group (paraabducens nuclei), which receives impulses from the paramedian pontine reticular formation and sends axons via the contralateral medial longitudinal fasciculus to the opposite medial rectus subnucleus of the third cranial nerve complex.

The motor cells lie dorsal and medial to the vestibular nuclei and lateral to the medial longitudinal bundles. The fascicles course ventrally through the pontine tegmentum, without crossing, to exit ventromedially at the pontomedullary junction. After emerging, they take a sharp turn rostrally, being anchored to the tips of the petrous pyramids by the petrosphenoidal ligaments (Dorello's canal, Gruber's ligament), to enter the substance of the cavernous sinuses and lie adjacent to the carotid arteries. They enter the orbits through the medial one third of the superior orbital fissures.

Sixth nerve palsies in adults. Sixth cranial nerve palsies are the most frequently reported ocular motor palsies. In the four largest series[58-60,66] (Table 5-5) approximately 25% of patients with sixth nerve involvement remained without a diagnosis. In these series the sixth nerve palsies were not truly isolated. Other neurologic signs were often

---

CAUSES OF SIXTH CRANIAL NERVE PALSIES

Vascular
   Intrinsic brain stem
   Intrinsic nerve (arteritis and occlusive)
   Compressive (aneurysm)
Trauma
Multiple sclerosis
Raised intracranial pressure of any cause, unilateral or bilateral
Wernicke's disease
Cervical manipulation
Meningitis
Sarcoidosis
Following spinal puncture
Following correction of spinal deformities
Tumor
   Intrinsic brain stem (glioma, metastasis early)
   Compression of nerve
Migraine
Sinusitis

---

present. There are no data on the etiologies of truly isolated unilateral sixth nerve palsy. It is our clinical impression that in patients over the age of 40 years the most common cause is, as in isolated pupil-sparing third nerve palsy and fourth nerve palsy, infarction of the nerve trunk. As in these other mononeuropathies, the function of the nerve typically returns completely within 3 to 6 months. A relatively complete list of causes of acquired sixth nerve palsies may be found in the Box on p. 188.

By contrast, bilateral sixth nerve palsy is never caused by infarction at any age. In Keane's inpatient series of 125 cases,[35] 28 (25%) were caused by tumor, 17 (13%) by multiple sclerosis, 16 (14%) by subarachnoid hemorrhage, 12 (10%) by meningeal or parameningeal infection, and 11 (8%) by head trauma. In the palsies caused by tumor about half were believed to be the result of local irritation or compression and half the result of the nonspecific effect of increased intracranial pressure or a shift of brain substance related to a remotely situated mass.

Bilateral sixth nerve palsies have been reported following lumbar myelography,[46] chiropractic manipulation of the neck, and lumbar puncture. Occasionally patients with Wernicke's encephalopathy may present with bilateral or asymmetric sixth nerve palsies. If such a patient is seen in the emergency room and appears dehydrated or semistuporous, the use of intravenous glucose solutions is contraindicated without thiamin supplementation because of the danger of inducing a hemorrhagic encephalopathy.

Sixth nerve palsies in children. In children the abducens nerve was the most commonly affected of the ocular motor nerves, accounting for approximately 95% of the cases surveyed in Harley's series of ocular motor palsies in children.[30] Trauma and neoplastic disease accounted for 40% and 33% of cases, respectively. Robertson et al.[56] reviewed 133 cases of isolated acquired sixth nerve palsies and found that 52 cases (38%) were due to primary brain stem gliomas. In 15 of 133 cases an isolated abducens palsy was the first sign of disease. Packer et al.[52] have emphasized the dismal course in children with brain stem gliomas. These tumors spread by infiltration, causing multiple cranial nerve deficits, pyramidal tract dysfunction, and cerebellar ataxia. One third of their patients (5 of 15) developed meningeal gliomatosis, and three of these patients presented with meningeal symptoms before other signs of posterior fossa involvement. Although CSF studies were universally abnormal, malignant cells were detected in only one patient. Most of these patients die of local recurrences following a course of radiation therapy with a median survival time of 12 to 15 months.[23]

Of the 10 cases originally diagnosed as having Gradenigo's syndrome (a sixth nerve palsy with ipsilateral ear and facial pain) in the series reported by Robertson et al.,[56] three subsequently proved to have mass lesions. With the exception of tumor cases the prognosis for spontaneous improvement in their series was excellent. Robertson and his co-workers found that any improvement in sixth nerve function was complete within 4 months of onset.

Knox et al.[39] have noted the occurrence of benign abducens nerve palsies in children. These pareses are always isolated and resolve within 10 weeks. The assumption is that these are postviral syndromes and benign, and thus invasive procedures should be avoided unless progression occurs. Robertson et al. reported three similar cases and cited two others within the text of their paper.[56] These palsies may be recurrent and eventually may leave the patient with a persistent abduction deficit.[54,74]

In an infant presenting with what appears to be bilateral abducens nerve palsies the diagnosis of congenital or infantile esotropia should be considered. Lifting the child up, holding him at arms' length, and spinning him around with you (the examiner) as the fulcrum should induce full ocular rotations if the problem is one of childhood esotropia rather than abducens paresis. In their series, Robertson et al.[56] found that about 20% (29 of 133) of sixth nerve palsies in children were bilateral. Ten children had primary brain stem gliomas, five were associated with trauma, and seven children had inflammatory disease.

Management. Our recommendations for the evaluation of patients presenting with *isolated,* unilateral, nontraumatic sixth nerve paresis follow.

1. In an individual younger than 14 years who presents with a unilateral sixth nerve palsy, we do not believe any investigation is warranted unless the child develops additional signs or symptoms of neurologic disease. The presumptive diagnosis is that of a benign sixth nerve palsy, and although a history of a recent viral illness[39] or immunization[74] is helpful, it is not necessary. Initially the child should be examined every 2 weeks to determine if there is any progression of the paresis or for the development of additional neurologic problems. If the process is an intramedullary neoplasm (glioma), little is to be gained even if it were possible to make the diagnosis at the time of presentation.

    If the sixth nerve paresis is complete, a patient often will develop contracture (? spasticity) of the ipsilateral medial rectus muscle, which will produce an increasing ductional deficit mimicking an increasing paresis. Forced duction testing is mandatory before making the diagnosis of a progressive ocular motor palsy.

These idiopathic sixth nerve palsies almost always clear completely by 10 to 16 weeks after onset. If there is *no* improvement over a 6-month period and the paresis remains isolated, a noninvasive investigation, that is, CT scan with and without contrast and magnetic resonance imaging (MRI), may be instituted, although in our experience such studies tend to be normal. These patients and those with only partial improvement of their sixth nerve paresis after 6 months should have surgery to maximize their fields of single binocular vision and thus assure binocularity.

2. The management of acute isolated sixth nerve paresis in a young adult (15 to 40 years) is controversial. Although in many of these patients the problem is benign and remitting, we recommend, at a minimum, a thorough medical and neurologic examination to exclude such entities as hypertension, collagen vascular disease, and multiple sclerosis.

   If the investigation is negative, the patient should be followed initially at biweekly intervals and then monthly. If the patient's recovery is incomplete, surgery should be considered 6 months after stabilization of the ocular misalignment. If other systemic or neurologic abnormalities develop, or if there is worsening of the paresis, that is, if there is increasing misalignment with absence of a positive forced duction test, an appropriate diagnostic evaluation including CT scan, magnetic resonance imaging, and metrizamide myelography should be instituted.

3. In the population over age 40 there will be an increasing incidence of microvascular infarction as an etiologic consideration. These patients often complain initially of periocular or retrobulbar pain for 5 to 7 days. The pain may precede the paresis. Since these vasculopathic palsies occur with greater frequency in patients with hypertension and diabetes mellitus, a general medical evaluation should be undertaken including a 2-hour postprandial blood sugar. If the patient is over age 55, an erythrocyte sedimentation rate should be obtained, since ocular motor palsies may be the presenting sign in 12% of cases with giant cell arteritis. A more aggressive evaluation, including neuroradiologic studies, may be in order in patients with a past history of carcinoma. Metastatic carcinomas of the breast and prostate are reported as causes of isolated sixth nerve palsies, and these cases may be amenable to radiotherapy or chemotherapeutic intervention.[62]

   If the paresis remains isolated and static for a period of at least 6 months, there is evidence that some of these patients will have basisphenoid tumors.[61,62] With the exception of one patient, all of those reported to have such tumors had relatively stable neurologic deficits, and surgical intervention was of little benefit. Although it is suggested that all patients with chronic and stable sixth nerve palsies should undergo aggressive neurologic investigations to exclude a petrous apex–cavernous sinus mass lesion,[13] we believe such investigations are not worthwhile since indolent lesions that might be uncovered are not treatable. An exception to this approach may be made if any other signs or symptoms of neurologic disease should become evident and mandate such a course.

4. The acute onset of a sixth nerve palsy associated with ipsilateral facial or retroauricular pain, at any age, mandates high-resolution CT scanning of the region of the petrous pyramid and mastoid bone. The combination of a sixth nerve paresis and ipsilateral facial pain implies either an inflammatory or neoplastic lesion involving the tip of the petrous pyramid.

5. In children as well as adults the presence of bilateral sixth nerve palsies should suggest the presence of raised intracranial pressure; therefore an intracranial mass lesion must be excluded. All patients presenting with bilateral sixth nerve palsies, including those associated with trauma, should have a thorough neuroradiologic investigation. The exception to this rule is the patient with a congenital sixth nerve paralysis accompanied by facial nerve weakness. This combination of findings suggests the diagnosis of Möbius syndrome (facial diplegia and horizontal pontine gaze deficits associated with clubfoot, pectoral muscle abnormalities, and branchial malformations).[31] In this case evaluation should be directed toward the extremity abnormalities, as the central nervous system deficits are stable.

In any infant or child presenting with a unilateral or bilateral ocular motor palsy, including a sixth nerve paresis, the diagnosis of battered child syndrome should be considered. Other stigmas of such maltreatment (bruises, basilar skull fracture, long bone fractures) should be sought.

Nonisolated ocular motor palsies

The topographic diagnosis of a lesion in a patient with a nonisolated ocular motor palsy depends upon the various combinations of associated neurologic deficits.

Intraaxial. The third nerve nucleus and fascicles are in close proximity to the medial longitudinal bundles, the red nucleus, the brachium conjunctivum, the substantia nigra, and pyramidal tracts. Involvement of the third nerve fascicles and the red nucleus produces Benedikt's syndrome (ipsilateral oculomotor paresis with an intention tremor of the contralateral foot, arm, and hand).[72] Involvement of the pyramidal tract produces Weber's syndrome (ipsilateral oculomotor paresis and contralateral hemiplegia). Cerebellar ataxia with either unilateral or bilateral involvement of the oculomotor nerve due to midline lesions is called Nothnagel's syndrome. Various combinations of vertical gaze paresis, with or without convergence retraction nystagmus, may be seen associated with brain stem involvement of the oculomotor complex.

The fourth nerve nucleus is contiguous with the end of the oculomotor nucleus, and thus processes involving the third nerve nucleus may also involve the trochlear nucleus. Since the trochlear nerve exits the brain stem dorsally, it is less frequently associated with intraparenchymal pathology than either the third or sixth cranial nerves. The abducens nucleus is located in an area in which there are a large number of structures associated with ocular movements including the paraabducens nuclei, medial longitudinal bundles, the paramedian pontine reticular formation, and the vestibular nuclei. In addition the fibers of the seventh nerve loop around the sixth nerve nucleus, and the first order neurons subserving the sympathetic innervation to the iris travel laterally adjacent to the descending sensory root of the trigeminal nerve in the tegmentum. The fascicles of the abducens nerve pass through the corticospinal tracts as they exit the brain stem ventrally.

Pathologic processes involving the pons in the region of the sixth nerve nuclei can produce a variety of distinctive syndromes: (1) Foville's syndrome (anterior inferior cerebellar artery syndrome), which includes ipsilateral paralysis of gaze, ipsilateral facial palsy, loss of taste from the anterior two thirds of the tongue, ipsilateral Horner's syndrome, ipsilateral facial analgesia, and ipsilateral deafness, and (2) Millard-Gubler syndrome, which includes ipsilateral sixth nerve paralysis with a contralateral hemiplegia. In addition, various combinations of sixth nerve paresis associated with horizontal gaze palsies and nystagmus should suggest pontine disease.

Extraaxial. Sixth nerve paresis associated wtih fifth (corneal sensation), seventh, and eighth (vestibular and auditory) nerve dysfunction can occur with cerebellopontine angle tumors. In children a sixth nerve paresis associated with ipsilateral facial pain and hearing loss indicates an osteitis of the tip of the petrous pyramid secondary to a chronic mastoiditis or middle ear infection (Gradenigo's syndrome). Involvement of the petrous pyramid by other processes such as cholesteatoma or metastatic carcinoma produces a similar syndrome, usually without hearing loss and with less pain. The diagnosis in all of these cases is made most accurately with CT scanning.

Unilateral ophthalmoplegia involving the third, fourth, and sixth cranial nerves can be evaluated with the following scheme in mind. Accompanying pain or altered sensation in the distribution of the first division of the trigeminal nerve with optic nerve involvement most likely implies orbital pathology. From the anterior cavernous sinus to the superior orbital fissure the involved nerves can be the first division of the fifth nerve and the third, fourth, and sixth nerves. In lesions of the region of the posterior to midcavernous sinus the involved nerves could include the first or second division of the fifth nerve and the third, fourth, and sixth nerves. In the retrocavernous space, all three divisions of the trigeminal nerve can be involved in addition to the optic chiasm or optic tract. The presence of other brain stem signs would, of course, suggest posterior fossa disease.

Bilateral ophthalmoplegia is indicative of more widespread involvement. Lesions at the base of the brain or involving midline structures must be excluded. In all of these cases the particular distribution of neurologic deficits will mandate the appropriate diagnostic tests including neuroradiologic, general medical, and CSF evaluation. The consecutive involvement of cranial nerves on both sides should suggest the possible diagnosis of a nasopharyngeal carcinoma. A diagnostic workup in these cases may include a blind biopsy in the area of Rosenmüller's fossa.

Two other entities should be considered in the differential diagnosis of patients with ocular motor paresis: botulism and acute infectious polyneuropathy. Botulism may present in one of two forms: (1) floppy baby syndrome[2,45,53] in the first year of life secondary to colonization of the gut with *Clostridium botulinum* or (2) an acute form at any age following the ingestion of contaminated food.[4,69] The clinical syndrome produced by this organism is due to the release of a species-specific exotoxin (A to E)[41] that interferes with cholinergic transmission. The exotoxins most often associated with ocular dysfunction are A and B.[10] The typical clinical picture of an alert patient with a dry mouth, swallowing difficulties, and flaccid paresis or weakness should alert the physician to the possibility of ingestion of botulinum toxin. The finding of dilated sluggish pupils with ptosis is an ominous sign, for in almost all individuals who develop respiratory distress these signs are present.[69] These patients are said to have accommodative paresis, but in most cases this is presumed on the basis of a complaint of blurred vision. The diagnosis is made by injecting graded dilutions of the patient's sera from suspected cases into laboratory animals and determining that dilution which causes death by respiratory paresis. Treatment includes the use of polyvalent antitoxin and supportive care in cases of acute poisoning and decontamination of the gut with antibiotics in floppy children.

Acute infectious polyneuropathy can occur in an ascending form of Guillain-Barré-Strohl syndrome[29,36] or a bulbar variant recognized by Fisher.[6,20] In the former state there is an ascending paresis with variable sensory loss that progresses to involve the bulbar musculature, producing some degree of facial diplegia and unilateral or bilateral ocular motor palsies. If the oculomotor nerves are involved, there is usually both an internal as well as an external ophthalmoplegia. In the Fisher variant the disease is characterized by areflexia, ataxia, and ocular motor palsies. In both syndromes involvement of the bulbar musculature may lead to respiratory and swallowing difficulties. These syndromes commonly follow a presumed "viral" illness.[29] Both variants are postulated to be due to a lymphocyte-mediated demyelination of the nerve roots, but this does not adequately explain all the clinical findings.

The diagnosis is confirmed by the finding of "albumino cytologic" dissociation on examination of the CSF, that is, elevated protein in the absence of a pleocytosis. Systemic corticosteroids are indicated in cases of involvement of the bulbar musculature, but their efficacy remains open to question.[1] For the most part therapy is supportive, including respiratory assistance in severe cases.

REFERENCES

1. Arnason, BGW: Inflammatory polyradiculoneuropathies. In Dyck, PJ, Thomas, PK, and Lambert, EH, editors: Peripheral neuropathy, vol 2, Philadelphia, 1975, WB Saunders Co, p 1110.
2. Arnon, SS, Midura, TF, Damus, K, Thompson, B, Wood, RM, and Chin, J: Honey and other environmental risk factors for infant botulism, J Pediatr. 94:331, 1979.
3. Asbury, AK, Aldredge, H, Hershberg, R, and Fisher, CM: Oculomotor palsy in diabetes mellitus: a clinicopathological study, Brain 93:955, 1970.
4. Barker, WH, Jr, Weissman, JB, Dowell, VR, Jr, Gutmann, L, and Kautter, DA: Type B botulism outbreak caused by a commercial food product. West Virginia and Pennsylvania, 1973, JAMA 237:456, 1977.
5. Bienfang, DC: Crossing axons in the third cranial nerve nucleus, Invest Ophthalmol 14:927, 1975.
6. Blau, I, Casson, I, Lieberman, A, and Weiss, E: The not-so-benign Miller Fisher syndrome. A variant of the Guillain-Barré syndrome, Arch Neurol 37:384, 1980.
7. Brown, HW: True and simulated superior oblique tendon sheath syndromes, Doc Ophthalmol 34:123, 1973.
8. Burde, RM, and Loewy, AD: Central origin of oculomotor parasympathetic neurons in the monkey, Brain Res 193:434, 1980.
9. Burger, L, Kalvin, N, and Smith, JL: Acquired lesions of the fourth cranial nerve, Brain 93:567, 1970.
10. Cherington, M: Botulism. Ten-year experience, Arch Neurol 30:432, 1974.
11. Cogan, DG: Myasthenia gravis: a review of the disease and a description of lid twitch as a characteristic sign, Arch Ophthalmol 74:217, 1965.
12. Cox, TA, Wurster, JB, and Godfrey, WA: Primary aberrant oculomotor degeneration due to intracranial aneurysm, Arch Neurol 36:570, 1979.
13. Currie, J, Lubin, JH, and Lessell, S: Chronic isolated abducens paresis from tumors at the base of the brain, Arch Neurol 40:226, 1983.
14. Dalessio, DJ, editor: Wolff's headache and other head pain, ed 4, New York, 1980, Oxford University Press, pp 111-113.
15. Derakhshan, I: Superior branch palsy of the oculomotor nerve with spontaneous recovery, Ann Neurol 4:478, 1978.
16. Dreyfus, P, Hakim, S, and Adams, R: Diabetic ophthalmoplegia, Arch Neurol 77:337, 1957.

17. Eaton, L: As quoted in Retzlaff, JA, Kearns, TP, Howard, FM, and Cronin, ML: Lancaster red-green test in evaluation of edrophonium effect in myasthenia gravis, Am J Ophthalmol 67:13-21, 1969.

18. Eyster, EF, Hoyt, WF, and Wilson, CB: Oculomotor palsy from minor head trauma. An initial sign of basal intracranial tumor, JAMA 220:1083, 1972.

19. Fischer, KC, and Schwartzman, RJ: Oral corticosteroids in the treatment of ocular myasthenia gravis, Neurology (Minneap) 24:795-798, 1974.

20. Fisher, M: Unusual variant of acute idiopathic polyneuritis (syndrome of ophthalmoplegia, ataxia and areflexia), N Engl J Med 255:57, 1956.

21. Frey, T: Isolated paresis of the inferior oblique, Ann Ophthalmol 13:936, 1982.

22. Gamblin, GT, Harper, DG, Galentine, P, Buck, DR, Chernow, B, and Eil, C: Prevalence of increased intraocular pressure in Graves' disease—evidence of frequent subclinical ophthalmopathy, N Engl J Med 308:420, 1983.

23. Gjerris, F: Clinical aspects and long-term prognosis of intracranial tumors in infancy and childhood, Dev Med Child Neurol 18:145, 1976.

24. Glaser, JS, editor: Neuro-ophthalmology, Hagerstown, Md, 1978, Harper & Row, Publishers, p 253.

25. Goldstein, J, and Cogan, D: Diabetic ophthalmoplegia with special reference to the pupil, Arch Ophthalmol 64:592, 1960.

26. Green, W, Hackett, E, and Schlezinger, N: Neuro-ophthalmologic evaluation of oculomotor nerve paralysis, Arch Ophthalmol 72:154, 1964.

27. Grimson, BS, and Glaser, JS: Isolated trochlear nerve palsies in herpes zoster ophthalmicus, Arch Ophthalmol 96:1233, 1978.

28. Grob, D: Course and management of myasthenia gravis, JAMA 153:529, 1953.

29. Guillain, G, Barré, J-A, and Strohl, A: Sur un syndrome de radiculo-névrite avec hyperalbuminase due liquide céphalo-rachidien sans réaction cellulaire: remarques sur les caractères cliniques et graphiques des réflexes tendineux, Bul Soc Med Hop Paris 40:1462, 1916.

30. Harley, RD: Paralytic strabismus in children. Etiologic incidence and management of the third, fourth, and sixth nerve palsies, Ophthalmology 87:24, 1980.

31. Henderson, JL: The congenital facial diplegia syndrome: clinical features, pathology, and aetiology. A review of sixty-one cases, Brain 62:381, 1939.

32. Hepler, RS, and Cantu, RC: Aneurysms, third nerve palsies: ocular status of survivors, Arch Ophthalmol 77:604, 1967.

33. Holland, G: Electromyographische Untersucheingen bei Fehileitung regenerierender Nerven faserer nach Okulomotorinsparese, Klin Monatsbl Augenheilkd 144:686, 1964.

34. Hollenhorst, RW, Brown, JR, Wagner, HV, and Shick, RM: Neurologic aspects of temporal arteritis, Neurology (Minneap) 10:490, 1960.

35. Keane, JR: Bilateral sixth nerve palsy. Analysis of 125 cases, Arch Neurol 33:681-683, 1976.

36. Kennedy, RH, Danielson, MA, Mulder, DW, and Kurland, LT: Guillain-Barré syndrome. A 42-year epidemiologic and clinical study, Mayo Clin Proc 53:93, 1978.

37. Kerr, F, and Hollowell, OW: Location of pupillomotor and accommodation fibres in the oculomotor nerve: experimental observations on paralytic mydriasis, J Neurol Neurosurg Psychiatry 27:473-481, 1964.

38. Kissel, JT, Burde, RM, Klingele, TG, and Zeiger, HE: Pupil-sparing oculomotor palsies with internal carotid–posterior communicating artery aneurysms, Ann Neurol 13:149, 1983.

39. Knox, D, Clark, D, and Schuster, F: Benign VI nerve palsies in children, Pediatrics 40:560, 1967.

40. Larson, D, and Auchincloss, JH: Multiple symmetrical bilateral cranial nerve palsies in patients with diabetes mellitus: report of 3 cases, Arch Intern Med 85:265, 1950.

41. Lewis, GE, Jr, and Metzger, JF: Botulism immune plasma (human), Lancet 2:634, 1978.

42. Liesegang, TD, and Glaser, JS: The edrophonium (Tensilon) test in normals, myasthenics and in non-myasthenic ophthalmoplegias, Arch Ophthalmol (in press).

43. Loewenfeld, IE, and Thompson, HS: Oculomotor paresis with cyclic spasms. A critical review of the literature and a new case, Surv Ophthalmol 20:81, 1975.

44. Metz, HS, and Lerner, H: The adjustable Harada-Ito procedure, Arch Ophthalmol 99:624, 1981.

45. Midura, TF, and Arnon, SS: Infant botulism: identification of *Clostridium botulinum* and its toxin in faeces, Lancet 2:934, 1976.

46. Miller, EA, Savino, PJ, and Schatz, NS: Bilateral sixth nerve palsy, Arch Ophthalmol 100:603-604, 1982.

47. Miller, MT, Urist, MJ, Folk, ER, and Chapman, LI: Superior oblique palsy presenting in late childhood, Am J Ophthalmol 70:212, 1970.

48. Miller, NR: Solitary oculomotor nerve palsy in childhood, Am J Ophthalmol 83:106, 1977.

49. O'Connor, PS, Tredici, TJ, and Green, RP: Pupil-sparing third nerve palsies caused by aneurysm, Am J Ophthalmol 95:395, 1983.

50. Osher, RH, and Griggs, RC: Orbicularis fatigue, Arch Ophthalmol 74:677, 1979.

51. Osserman, KE: Ocular myasthenia gravis, Invest Ophthalmol 6:277, 1967.

52. Packer, RJ, Allen, J, Nielsen, S, Petito, C, Deck, M, and Jereb, B: Brainstem glioma: clinical manifestations of meningeal gliomatosis, Ann Neurol 14:177, 1983.

53. Pickett, J, Berg, B, Chaplin, E, and Brunstetter-Shafer, M: Syndrome of botulism in infancy: clinical and electrophysiologic study, N Engl J Med 296:770, 1976.

54. Reinecke, RD, and Thompson, WE: Childhood recurrent idiopathic paralysis of the lateral rectus, Ann Ophthalmol 13:1037, 1981.

55. Retzlaff, JA, Kearns, TP, Howard, FM, and Cronin, ML: Lancaster red-green test in evaluation of edrophonium effect in myasthenia gravis, Am J Ophthalmol 67;13-21, 1969.

56. Robertson, DM, Hines, JD, and Rucker, CW: Acquired sixth nerve paresis in children, Arch Ophthalmol 83:574, 1970.

57. Roper-Hall, G, and Burde, RM: Inferior rectus palsies as a manifestation of atypical third cranial nerve disease, Am Orthopt J 25:122, 1975.

58. Rucker, CW: Paralysis of the third, fourth, and sixth cranial nerves, Am J Ophthalmol 46:787, 1958.

59. Rucker, CW: The causes of paralysis of the third, fourth, and sixth cranial nerves, Am J Ophthalmol 61:353, 1966.

60. Rush, JA, and Younge, BR: Paralysis of cranial nerves III, IV, and VI. Cause and prognosis in 1,000 cases, Arch Ophthalmol 99:76, 1981.

61. Sakalas, R, Harbison, JW, Vines, FS, and Becker, DP: Chronic sixth nerve palsy. An initial sign of basisphenoid tumors, Arch Ophthalmol 93:186, 1975.

62. Savino, PJ, Hilliker, JK, Cassell, GH, and Schatz, NJ: Chronic sixth nerve palsies, Arch Ophthalmol 100:1442-1444, 1982.

63. Schatz, NJ, Savino, PJ, and Corbett, JJ: Primary aberrant oculomotor regeneration. A sign of intracavernous meningioma, Arch Neurol 34:29, 1977.

64. Scott, WE, and Nankin, SJ: Isolated inferior oblique paresis, Arch Ophthalmol 95:1586, 1977.

65. Seybold, ME, and Drachman, DB: Gradually increasing prednisone in myasthenia gravis, N Engl J Med 290;81, 1974.

66. Shrader, EC, and Schlezinger, NS: Neuro-ophthalmologic evaluation of abducens nerve paralysis, Arch Ophthalmol 63:84, 1960.

67. Sunderland, S, and Hughes, ESR: The pupillo-constrictor pathway and the nerves to the ocular muscles in man, Brain 69:301-309, 1946.

68. Susac, JO, and Hoyt, WF: Inferior branch palsy of the oculomotor nerve, Ann Neurol 2:336, 1977.

69. Terranova, W, Palumbo, JN, and Breman, JG: Ocular findings in botulism type B, JAMA 241:475, 1979.

70. Trobe, JD, Glaser, JS, and Post, JD: Meningiomas, aneurysms of the cavernous sinus, Arch Ophthalmol 96:457, 1978.

71. Van Dyk, HJL, and Florence, L: The Tensilon test. A safe office procedure, Ophthalmology 87:210, 1980.

72. Warren, W, Burde, RM, Klingele, TG, and Roper-Hall, G: Atypical oculomotor paresis, J Clin Neuro-ophthalmol 2:13, 1982.

73. Warwick, RJ: Representation of the extraocular muscles in the oculomotor nuclei of the monkey, J Comp Neurol 98:449, 1953.

74. Werner, DB, Savino, PJ, and Schatz, NJ: Benign recurrent sixth nerve palsies in childhood. Secondary to immunization of viral illness, Arch Ophthalmol 101:607, 1983.

75. Zappia, RJ, Winkelman, JZ, and Gay, AJ: Intraocular pressure changes in normal subjects and the adhesive muscle syndrome, Am J Ophthalmol 71:880, 1971.

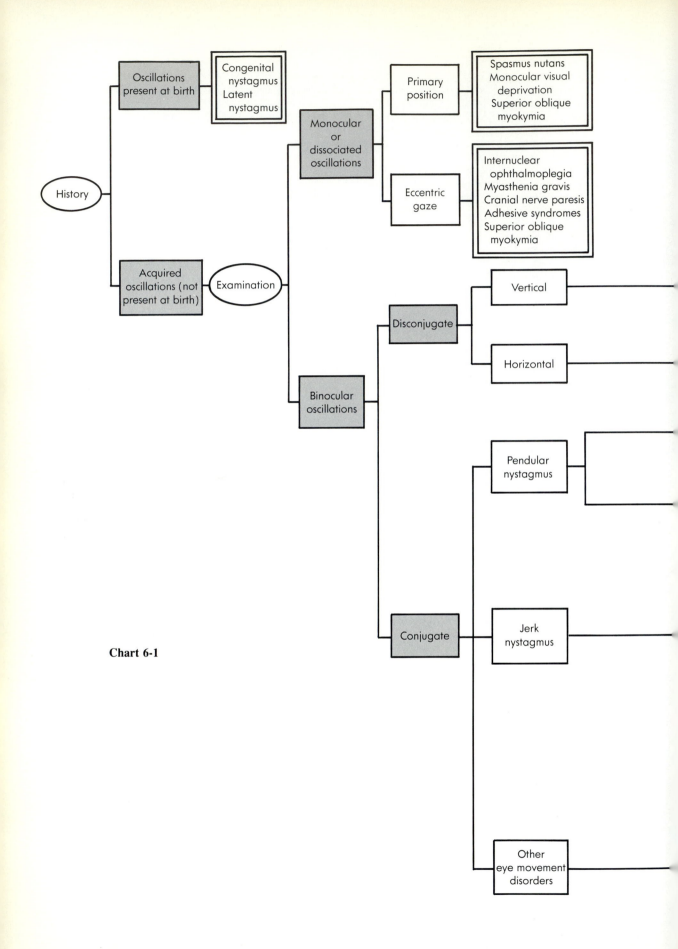

Chart 6-1

CHAPTER 6

Nystagmus and other periodic eye movement disorders

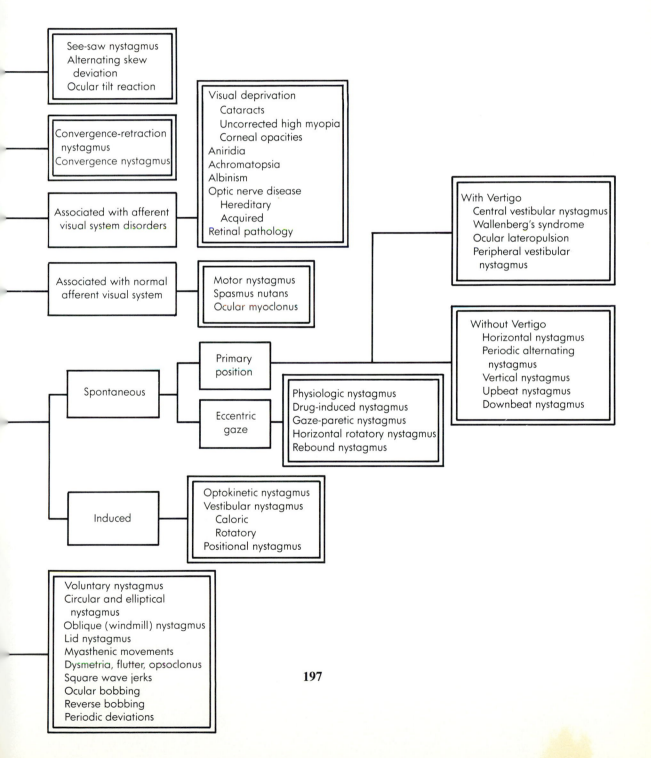

See-saw nystagmus
Alternating skew
  deviation
Ocular tilt reaction

Visual deprivation
  Cataracts
  Uncorrected high myopia
  Corneal opacities
Aniridia
Achromatopsia
Albinism
Optic nerve disease
  Hereditary
  Acquired
Retinal pathology

Convergence-retraction
nystagmus
Convergence nystagmus

Associated with afferent
visual system disorders

Associated with normal
afferent visual system

Motor nystagmus
Spasmus nutans
Ocular myoclonus

With Vertigo
  Central vestibular nystagmus
  Wallenberg's syndrome
  Ocular lateropulsion
  Peripheral vestibular
    nystagmus

Without Vertigo
  Horizontal nystagmus
  Periodic alternating
    nystagmus
  Vertical nystagmus
  Upbeat nystagmus
  Downbeat nystagmus

Spontaneous

Primary
position

Eccentric
gaze

Physiologic nystagmus
Drug-induced nystagmus
Gaze-paretic nystagmus
Horizontal rotatory nystagmus
Rebound nystagmus

Induced

Optokinetic nystagmus
Vestibular nystagmus
  Caloric
  Rotatory
Positional nystagmus

Voluntary nystagmus
Circular and elliptical
  nystagmus
Oblique (windmill) nystagmus
Lid nystagmus
Myasthenic movements
Dysmetria, flutter, opsoclonus
Square wave jerks
Ocular bobbing
Reverse bobbing
Periodic deviations

Nystagmus is a term used to describe oscillatory ocular movements that are "to a certain extent rhythmic."[14] Those ocular movements that are oscillatory, but not rhythmic, are called nystagmoid movements. In recent years elegant recording techniques have been used to study the waveforms, amplitudes, and velocities, as well as many other characteristics, of ocular oscillatory movement disorders. From these data rather structured and complex classification systems have been established. Some insight into the underlying pathology has been derived from mathematical modeling based on inferred neurophysiologic control centers and integrators. Despite this rapid proliferation of knowledge, little has been gained that is clinically applicable at this time.

Classically nystagmus has been divided into two broad categories depending upon the clinical appearance of the movements: (1) pendular nystagmus and (2) jerk nystagmus. Pendular nystagmus is characterized by bilateral ocular oscillations that are approximately equal in velocity in both directions.[15] These oscillations may vary in speed and amplitude, are almost always horizontal, and often have a jerk component in eccentric gaze with the fast phase in the direction of gaze. Jerk nystagmus is characterized by rhythmic oscillations in which the movement in one direction is recognizably faster than the movement in the other direction. The slow movement is the pathologic movement, and the fast movement is corrective. Even so, jerk nystagmus is named (defined) according to the direction of the fast phase or corrective movement. That position in which the intensity (amplitude and frequency) of the ocular oscillation is at a minimum (position of relative stability) is termed the *null point*.

The clinician must develop a method, usually diagrammatic (Figs. 6-1 and 6-2), to record the patterns of nystagmus or nystagmoid movements and how they are affected by movement into the various gaze positions. The patient must be observed at least for a period of minutes to determine if the observed movements change with time, for example, the reversal of direction of nystagmus in periodic alternating nystagmus or intermittent breaks in fixation of ocular flutter or square wave jerks. It may be necessary to place stress upon the ocular motor system in order to induce or unmask certain disorders (e.g., ocular dysmetria, superior oblique myokymia, or positional nystagmus). The discipline of diagramming is important for two reasons: (1) the mechanical completion of the diagramming assists the clinician in extracting all the available information from the observed movement, and (2) it serves as a permanent record enabling the clinician to determine the stability of the oscillation over prolonged periods of time.

Nystagmus and nystagmoid movements have been classified in various ways. The decision tree used in this chapter (Chart 6-1) does not attempt to formally classify ocular oscillations but rather suggests a series of pragmatic steps intended to help the physician recognize the particular movement disorder.

○ **History**

Certain historical data are helpful in keying the clinician to the presence and type of an oscillatory disturbance. The complaints may be vestibular or visual (oscillopsia). The symptoms of acute vestibular dysfunction are vertigo, tinnitus, and nausea.

Oscillopsia is best described as an illusory perception of environmental movement and may be gaze induced, position dependent, or affected by activity. Oscillopsia may assume three forms. The first form occurs with acquired jerk nystagmus. The patient reports that the environment is moving in one direction, opposite to the slow phase of

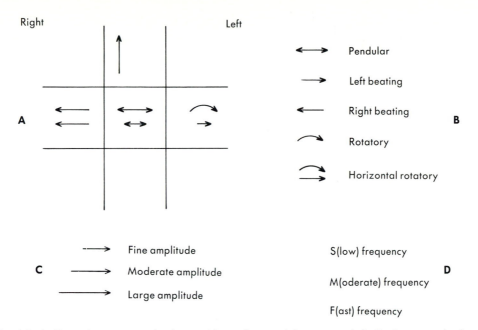

Fig. 6-1. A, Record movements in nine positions of gaze, right eye over left. B, Arrows point in direction of fast phase of nystagmus. C, Length of arrow reflects amplitude. D, *S, M,* and *F* designate frequency.

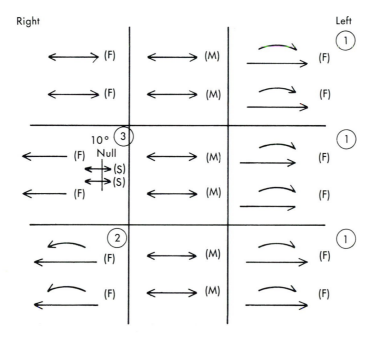

Fig. 6-2. Diagram of eye movements of patient with congenital nystagmus. *1,* Rotatory component in left gaze; *2,* rotatory component in right downgaze; *3,* null point 10° to right of primary position with small-amplitude, slow-frequency movement.

the nystagmus (i.e., in the direction of the fast phase). No movement is perceived during the fast phase as the visual threshold is elevated during fast eye movements. The second form of oscillopsia is associated with pendular oscillations. The patient perceives a to-and-fro movement of the environment. The third form of oscillopsia occurs with superior oblique myokymia. The patient experiences a pecular "jellylike" quivering of the environment during the rapid firing of the superior oblique muscle.

The patient's ability to function visually should be determined (Can the patient read? Is the patient independently mobile?). Attention should be directed toward investigating the broad topic of drug use and abuse (current and past) including medications, tranquilizers, antiepileptics, and antibiotics, as well as alcohol. Many drugs can induce ocular oscillations at therapeutic as well as toxic levels. A history of significant head or ocular trauma, or neurosurgical intervention, or of seizures is of value in suggesting the possibility of an underlying structural abnormality.

Oscillations present in perinatal period

The first relevant consideration is whether the nystagmus is present at birth or within the first few days after birth. If the oscillations are noted in this period, the diagnosis of congenital nystagmus can be made. Congenital nystagmus is traditionally divided into a motor and sensory type. The acquired oscillations associated with congenitally poor vision (deafferentation) usually do not develop until 2 to 3 months after birth, although they have been noted as early as 3 to 4 weeks postnatally in patients with Leber's congenital amaurosis. We consider this postnatal nystagmus an *acquired* oscillation and do not include it under the classification of congenital nystagmus. This type of sensory nystagmus is much more common than congenital (motor) nystagmus (10:1).[37] Similarly the oscillatory movements of spasmus nutans (usually a benign entity), which are often confused with congenital nystagmus, have their onset 4 to 6 months after birth. The presence of congenital nystagmus does not preclude concomitant diseases of the afferent visual system.

Congenital nystagmus. Congenital nystagmus includes all manifest nystagmus noted at birth or within the perinatal period. Clinically, congenital nystagmus may vary from an overt jerk nystagmus to what appears to be a purely pendular movement disorder (equal amplitude and velocity in each eye). The terms jerk and pendular do not really reflect the complexity of the underlying foveational strategies.[27] The nystagmus may be irregular but is almost always conjugate and horizontal. It is rarely purely vertical.

Congenital nystagmus is considered by some[27] to be a failure of the slow eye movement control subsystem. Others suggest a defect in the subcortical optokinetic system.[37] The result is fixation instability. The primary eye movement is a drift away from fixation, while the corrective movement is aimed at recovering fixation, which may or may not be achieved.[26] Attempted fixation tends to exaggerate the oscillations. Patients who have decreased vision for other reasons will also have a more severe nystagmus with attempted fixation. Even in the absence of a history of neonatal onset, the diagnosis of congenital nystagmus is relatively straightforward, as this movement disorder has characteristic findings. The nystagmus is bilateral and grossly symmetric in amplitude and frequency. The nystagmus remains horizontal in all gaze directions (even vertical), although a rotatory component may be superimposed in lateral gaze (Fig. 6-2). In spite of the almost continuous movement of the eyes, patients with congenital nystagmus are unaware of oscillopsia. The nystagmus disappears during sleep.

The patients almost always have a relative null point where the oscillatory movements are minimized. (The null point may be slightly different for each eye [Fig. 6-2].) They often assume a head turn to place the null point in the straight-ahead position, thereby maximizing their distance acuity. This is the basis for the Kestenbaum procedure in which the null point is placed in the primary position by recessing one pair of horizontal yoke muscles while simultaneously resecting the other pair. This often damps the nystagmus as well.

Patients with congenital nystagmus and *no* afferent visual system disease always have much better vision at near than at distance (e.g., 20/40 versus 20/80 to 20/200) as convergence damps the nystagmus. Dell'Osso[26] has suggested the use of prism glasses with two goals: (1) to optically place the null point in the straight-ahead position, obviating the need for a head turn, and (2) to induce convergence in order to improve distance acuity. In our experience this form of treatment is of doubtful efficacy.

Some patients with congenital nystagmus have head oscillations that appear to be compensatory for the eye movements. They become most apparent during attempted fixation. Inversion of the optokinetic reflex (i.e., an induced nystagmus in the opposite direction to that expected) is said to be present in 65% to 70% of patients with congenital nystagmus.[29] The need to search for an underlying sensory deficit cannot be over stressed because the visual handicap and genetic counseling differ, depending upon the concomitant afferent visual system deficits.

☐ **Latent nystagmus.** Latent nystagmus is a jerk nystagmus induced by monocular occlusion, usually of either eye, but may be induced by covering one eye only. The latent nystagmus may be made manifest with neutral density filters or high plus lenses placed in front of one eye. Although a congenital condition, generally it is not recognized until later in life. Under the artificial circumstances of attempting to determine monocular visual acuity during vision screening at school, children with latent nystagmus are found to have poor bilateral acuity. The jerk nystagmus is characterized by a slow-phase drift toward the covered side with a fast-phase corrective movement toward the side of the uncovered eye. The movements are bilateral, similar in amplitude and frequency, and symmetric.

Latent nystagmus has not been reported to be related to systemic or neurologic abnormalities. It has been reported to occur in association with congenital esotropia and dissociated vertical deviations. In patients with latent nystagmus who have amblyopia or strabismus and who are therefore fixing monocularly, the nystagmus may be present constantly and mimic congenital nystagmus.

Kestenbaum,[57] as well as Dell-Osso et al.,[28] have described manifest latent nystagmus, a binocular movement disorder in which the nystagmus fast phase beats in the direction of the fixating eye during alternating fixation in horizontal tropias. Accurate determination of the visual acuity in each eye in these patients is accomplished most easily by placing a central dot of tape on a plano lens in front of one eye, blocking central fixation (but allowing the eye to remain open), while refracting the other eye in order to determine the best corrected visual acuity. Similar results may be obtained by using a polarized acuity chart with polarizing lenses. Loss of vision in one eye in these patients often results in the induction of permanent nystagmus in the remaining eye,[70] causing a severe decrease in vision.

☐ Acquired nystagmus

If the nystagmus is not present within the first few weeks of life, we consider it to be a form of acquired nystagmus. Observation of the patient will reveal almost immediately whether the acquired oscillation primarily involves one or both eyes. If the oscillation is confined to one eye (monocular) or mainly involves one eye, that is, is bilateral but markedly asymmetric (dissociated), the disorders may be subdivided further by determining if movement is present in the primary position or whether it is evoked by eccentric gaze position (gaze-evoked).

☐ Monocular or dissociated oscillations in primary position (Chart 6-1, *A*)

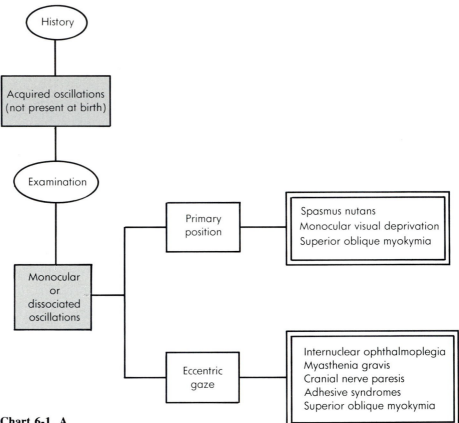

Chart 6-1, A

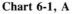 **Spasmus nutans.** Spasmus nutans is a rare, most often benign triad of torticollis, head nodding, and nystagmus, which appears monocular by gross inspection. It usually has its onset between the ages of 4 to 14 months but has been reported as late as 3½ years.[69] Cogan[16] has stated, ''Indeed it is the most common if not the only cause of unilateral horizontal nystagmus in infancy.'' Only two of the three characteristic findings of the triad need to be present to make the diagnosis. It often lasts less than 1 month but may last several months or years (average 12 to 24 months) and disappears by age 5. Classically the head nodding appears first, is rhythmic, and disappears with sleep and changes of head position. The pendular eye movement appears monocular, but on closer

inspection with a slit lamp or with a + 15 diopter lens dialed into a direct ophthalmoscope, it can be seen to be binocular with a fine conjugate shimmering movement apparent in the uninvolved eye. In our experience it may be horizontal, vertical, or rotatory in nature, and its amplitude and frequency tend to vary with gaze position.

Spasmus nutans has been reported to occur occasionally in association with developmental central nervous system disorders.[51] Acquired monocular nystagmus has been reported as the initial sign of chiasmal gliomas,[30,56,84] third ventricular tumors,[3,44] and degenerative disorders. The diagnosis of spasmus nutans is one of exclusion.[90] All children presenting with an acquired monocular or primarily monocular vertical oscillation(s) should have a high-resolution CT scan to exclude afferent visual system pathology. Since adequate sedation is a necessity for this procedure (may require general anesthesia), a concomitant fundus examination should be performed to evaluate the integrity of the optic discs and nerve fiber bundle layers of the retina.

☐ **Nystagmus of monocular visual deprivation.** It has been demonstrated that adults who sustain monocular visual loss may develop a fine, almost imperceptible, vertical oscillation of the damaged eye.[68,100] This oscillation may only be noted on slit lamp examination or during ophthalmoscopy. Uniocular adults may similarly develop nystagmus in their only eye associated with visual deprivation due to a cataract.[100]

Smith et al.[90] have reported strictly monocular, coarse (2° to 30°; 1 to 5 Hz) pendular, vertical oscillations occurring only in an amblyopic eye and developing years after uniocular visual loss (Heimann-Bielschowsky phenomenon). This visual loss can be due either to trauma or anisometropic or strabismic amblyopia.

☐ **Superior oblique myokymia.** Superior oblique myokymia is a monocular tremor caused by spontaneous firing of superior oblique muscle fibers. The patients complain of episodes of tilting of the image seen by one eye (episodic intorsion), oscillopsia, or of the awareness of ocular movement. The episodes are brief (seconds) but occur repeatedly. They may be induced by looking into the field of gaze of the involved superior oblique muscle or in moving the eye from that field back to the primary position. These patients are acutely aware of the onset and cessation of this microtremor.

Rosenberg and Glaser[77] emphasize that superior oblique myokymia can manifest itself as a slower, large-amplitude, intorsional movement causing vertical and torsional diplopia that can occur independently or be superimposed upon the monocular microtremor. In addition, other associated ocular movement disorders may be found including intermittent overaction of the superior oblique muscle, ipsilateral superior oblique paresis, and intermittent Brown's tendon sheath syndrome.

Hoyt and Keane[50] report rapid phasic activity in the involved superior oblique muscle and the absence of reciprocal phasic inhibition of the inferior oblique muscle. They postulate that this movement disorder is best explained by dysfunction in the brain stem fascicles of the fourth cranial nerve. Subsequent papers by Herzau et al.[47] and Kommerell and Schaubele[61] demonstrate single potentials of prolonged duration and high voltage utilizing electromyography. This finding is typical of neuronal damage with subsequent regeneration. This disorder always exists in isolation and requires no further workup.

The natural course of superior oblique myokymia includes recurrent spontaneous remissions and relapses. In those who are incapacitated a trial of carbamazepine is indicated.[94] Unfortunately, in our experience as well as that of others,[77] carbamazepine has not been uniformly successful in treating these patients. Intrasheath tenotomy of the superior oblique muscle also has been suggested to be effective in recalcitrant cases.[50,94]

Monocular or dissociated oscillations in eccentric gaze nystagmus (Chart 6-1, A)

In another group of primarily monocular oscillatory movement disorders the nystagmus is not present in primary position but only is noted when the eyes move to an eccentric gaze position.

☐ **Internuclear ophthalmoplegia.** Internuclear ophthalmoplegia (INO) has been discussed in detail elsewhere in this text. In its classic form INO is seen as a lag of the adducting eye, with nystagmus of the abducting eye occurring at the completion of a conjugate gaze movement. The decreased speed of movement of the adducting eye is caused by an interruption of the fibers to the agonist medial rectus muscle traveling in the medial longitudinal fasciculus (MLF). These fibers arise in the contralateral paraabducens nucleus and cross at the level of the sixth nerve nucleus to course rostrally in the MLF (see Fig. 4-1). The presence of an INO is indicative of intrinsic brain stem pathology. Numerous hypotheses have been offered to explain the presence of the nystagmus of the abducting eye, none of which has received universal acceptance.[59]

When the dissociation of movement is subtle, it may be made clinically more apparent by the use of an optokinetic stimulus.[89] The optokinetic target is moved toward the side of the lesion, thus activating the involved medial rectus muscle with each corrective saccade. Whether it is unilateral or bilateral, INO in a younger age group (<40 to 50) is most often due to multiple sclerosis, and in an older age group (>40 to 50) to stroke from atherosclerotic vertebrobasilar disease.

☐ **Myasthenia gravis.** In 1966 Glaser reported three cases of patients who had ptosis, adduction lag, and contralateral abducting nystagmus.[39] These patients all had myasthenia gravis, responding to the intravenous injection of Tensilon. Similar types of uniocular nystagmoid movements may be seen in the involved yoke muscle of any affected agonist; for example, if the right superior rectus muscle is weak, the left eye may demonstrate a nystagmoid movement in upgaze.

☐ **Cranial nerve paresis.** A patient who has a partial paresis of one of the extraocular muscles may or may not be able to fully complete an ocular movement into the field of action of the involved muscle. Once the eye has been moved as far as possible into the field of action of the paretic muscle, it will begin to drift back toward the primary position. This drift will be halted clinically by a fast corrective movement toward the eccentric gaze position. If the involved eye is used for fixation, one may see a dissociated nystagmus with larger amplitude movements in the contralateral eye.

☐ **Adhesive syndromes.** Dissociated eye movements may also be seen in adhesive syndromes in the field of action in which the tethering is occurring, that is, trapped inferior rectus muscle preventing the eye from moving upward. In certain cases of severe restrictive disease convergence-retraction movements can be mimicked. In bilateral dysthyroid orbitopathy with bilateral involvement of both the inferior rectus and medial rectus muscles, convergence movements with retraction can be produced in attempted saccadic upgaze (Fig. 6-3).

☐ **Superior oblique myokymia.** Superior oblique myokymia may be induced by moving the eyes into or away from the field of action of the involved superior oblique muscle.

Binocular oscillations

If the ocular oscillations involve both eyes to a relatively equal degree (see Chart 6-1), the first decision to be made is whether the movement is disconjugate (the eyes

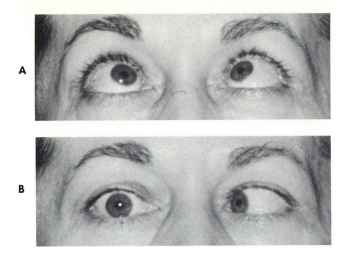

Fig. 6-3. A 56-year-old white woman who was admitted for a neurologic evaluation of convergence-retraction nystagmus. **A,** Marked bilateral medial deviation of eyes on attempted upgaze. **B,** Left esotropia in primary position with right eye fixing. This patient had dysthyroid ophthalmopathy with positive forced ductions.

moving in opposite directions) or conjugate (both eyes moving in the same direction). If the movement is disconjugate, it should be noted whether the movement is vertical or horizontal.

▧ Disconjugate vertical movements (Chart 6-1, *B*)

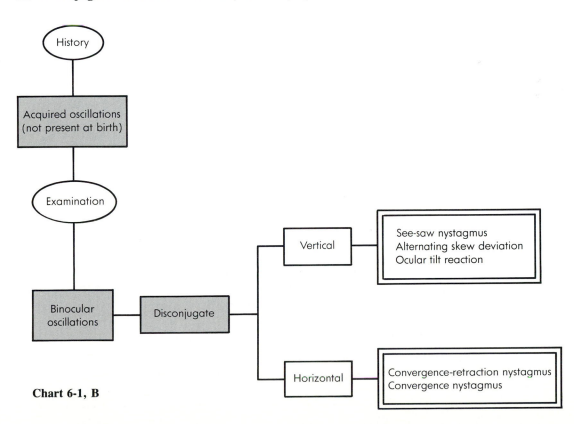

Chart 6-1, B

☐ **See-saw nystagmus.** This oscillatory movement is characterized by an alternate elevation and depression of one eye accompanied by a similar movement, but in the opposite direction, in the other eye (see-saw motion). The rising eye intorts, and the descending eye extorts. The torsional movements are present in all fields of gaze, whereas in general the see-saw effect is limited to the primary position.[19] The see-saw movement causes oscillopsia and a feeling of motion sickness in some patients. For the most part these patients have large parasellar tumors producing chiasmal and optic nerve compression. See-saw nystagmus has also been reported with septo-optic dysplasia.[19,25,64] Patients have decreased vision in one or both eyes with bitemporal visual field loss. Patching of the eye with poorer vision may damp the see-saw movement, improve visual acuity, and reduce the accompanying motion sickness feeling.[64] Vertebrobasilar disease and head trauma have also been implicated as causes of this peculiar movement complex.[83]

Hoyt and Gelbart[49] have reported five infants with oculocutaneous albinism, in all of whom see-saw nystagmus was the primary form of nystagmus noted during initial examination. Horizontal nystagmus subsequently supervened in all their patients, but brief periods of see-saw nystagmus are still seen in three of the patients, one of whom is 5 years old. There is an even rarer form of see-saw nystagmus, apparently congenital in nature, in which there is an inversion of the torting movement with intorsion in infraduction and extorsion in supraduction.[88]

☐ **Alternating skew deviation.** There are three types of alternating skew deviation: periodic alternating skew, aperiodic slowly alternating skew, and cyclic alternating skew. In each type, first one and then the other eye becomes hypertropic for a given period of time.

☐ **Ocular tilt reaction.** The ocular tilt reaction is an extremely rare intermittent movement disorder consisting of paroxysmal tonic skew deviation and torsion of the eyes coupled with ocular oscillations and head tilt due to a lesion in the region of the zona incerta of the diencephalon.[46] It can be produced experimentally in the monkey by stimulation near the interstitial nucleus of Cajal.[98]

▨ Disconjugate horizontal movements (Chart 6-1, *B*)

The horizontal gaze-evoked disorders are convergence-retraction nystagmus and convergence nystagmus.

☐ **Convergence-retraction nystagmus.** Convergence-retraction nystagmus (Parinaud's syndrome, sylvian aqueduct syndrome) is discussed elsewhere in this text. This movement disorder occurs with midbrain lesions. These lesions are most often extrinsic masses, but similar signs are seen with intrinsic lesions, usually infiltrative in nature. Initially most of these patients have a selective loss of the ability to voluntarily elevate their eyes; that is, upgaze saccades are replaced by a slow, undulating upward movement (side-to-side movement superimposed on the vertical movement). With time the patient loses the ability to make upward smooth pursuit movements, and eventually any attempt to produce upward saccades will induce a bilateral convergence movement with the eyes retracting into the orbits. This peculiar movement is demonstrated most easily by using an optokinetic stimulus moving downward to induce sequential corrective upward saccades.

Occasionally a patient with relatively symmetric bilateral dysthyroid orbitopathy, with an adhesive syndrome involving mainly the inferior and medial rectus muscles, will demonstrate similar convergence-retraction movements on attempted upgaze. All these patients have other signs of dysthyroid orbitopathy, including lid retraction (not to be confused with lid retraction caused by midbrain disease), stare, relative exophthalmos, and injection of the vessels over the insertions of the rectus muscles.

☐ **Convergence nystagmus.** Oscillations associated with convergence effort are rare.[86] In those few carefully documented cases the oscillations were variable in waveform, being either conjugate or disconjugate. Gresty et al.[42] have described a 28-year-old patient with a presumed cerebrovascular accident that left her with a comitant binocular convergent pendular nystagmus. Recordings of her eye movements demonstrated that the movements consisted of synchronized pendular movements of convergence and divergence at a frequency of 3 to 4 Hz.

Conjugate oscillations

The acquired binocular conjugate oscillations can be divided into three major categories: pendular nystagmus, jerk nystagmus, and distinctive or peculiar patterns (see Chart 6-1).

☐ **Pendular nystagmus** (Chart 6-1, *C*). In the majority of cases the finding of pendular nystagmus is indicative of poor visual acuity. If the afferent visual system does not mature as expected (i.e., an infant does not develop increasing visual acuity according to age norms), the child will develop wandering oscillations of both eyes. These oscillations tend to be pendular and at times are accompanied by synchronous contraversive head movements that attempt to compensate for the ocular movement.[14] The pendular movements are exaggerated by fixation effort and disappear with the eyes closed or during sleep.

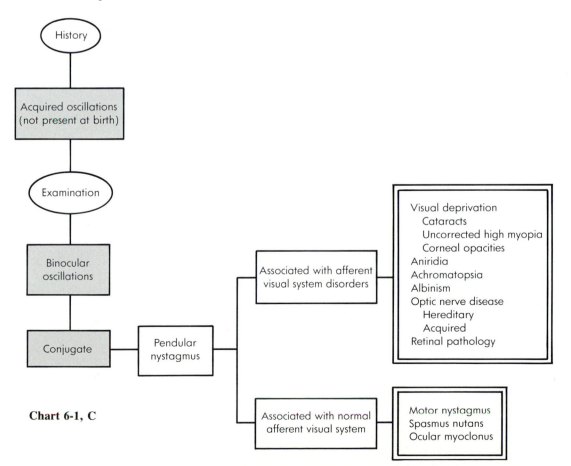

Chart 6-1, C

The acquired nystagmus associated with poor visual function cannot be distinguished from congenital nystagmus on the basis of eye movement recordings.[27] Both congenital nystagmus* and acquired sensory nystagmus seem to be initiated by a slow drift of the target off of the fovea[37] and have similar wave forms. Nystagmus caused by poor vision may coexist with congenital nystagmus, and these patients will have a history of ocular oscillations in the perinatal period. Gelbart et al.[37] have reported 132 patients with infantile nystagmus, 104 of whom had sensory defects. These defects included 41 patients with optic nerve hypoplasia, 9 of whom had paradoxical pupillary responses†; 33 patients with Leber's congenital amaurosis, 4 of whom had primarily vertical nystagmus at initial presentation but who subsequently became horizontal in all but one by the end of the first year of life, 24 of whom had a paradoxical pupillary response; 16 patients with oculocutaneous albinism, 5 of whom had transient see-saw nystagmus; 7 patients with cone dystrophies; and the remaining patients had such varied lesions as congenital stationary night blindness, CHARGE syndrome[71] and Aicardi's syndrome. Sixteen patients had anterior segment abnormalities. Adults who become blind at any age will develop pendular nystagmoid movements that may have superimposed convergence movements. A jerk component may be seen in lateral gaze as well.

☐   **Motor nystagmus.** Motor or efferent nystagmus is an acquired pendular nystagmus of low frequency and amplitude that is due to a defect in the ocular motor control systems. It may be monocular or binocular, conjugate or disconjugate, and have a nystagmus waveform that does not vary with gaze position.[4,42] This nystagmus is usually multivectoral rather than predominantly horizontal. It may be synchronous with other involuntary movements or be associated with head tremor. There is always other evidence of neurologic disease. These patients complain bitterly of oscillopsia. This nystagmus is believed to be due to a lesion either in the brain stem or cerebellum,[42] most often caused by demyelinating or vascular disease. Recent evidence suggests that the use of systemic scopolamine may damp the nystagmus and relieve the oscillopsia,[42] although we have found this not to be effective.

☐   **Ocular myoclonus.** Ocular myoclonus[12] is a continuous, rhythmic, to-and-fro pendular oscillation, usually vertical, occurring with similar synchronous movements of the face, palate, or extremities. The ocular movement is considered by some to be just a specific form of acquired pendular nystagmus.[42] This group of synchronous movements, oculopalatal myoclonus, indicates damage in the "myoclonic triangle" formed by the ipsilateral red nucleus and inferior olivary nucleus and the contralateral dentate nucleus of the cerebellum and their interconnecting fiber tracts. Histopathologically there is pseudohypertrophy of the inferior olivary nucleus. There is a latency period of weeks to months following the acute lesion (usually vascular infarction) before the development of myoclonic movements. These movements are present during sleep[95] and usually persist forever.

---

*Yee et al.[101] suggest that the nystagmus accompanying rod monochromacy may be separated from the large group of pendular movements by its low amplitude, directional asymmetry of optokinetic response, and smooth pursuit movements.

†Paradoxical pupillary responses may be demonstrated by decreasing the ambient illumination and finding pupillary constriction or by beginning in subdued illumination, switching the lights on, and noting pupillary dilatation.[8,36,41]

☐   **Jerk nystagmus** (Chart 6-1, *D*). Jerk nystagmus may be divided into that present spontaneously in primary position, that present only in eccentric gaze, and that induced by optokinetic or vestibular stimuli or upon assuming a particular head position.

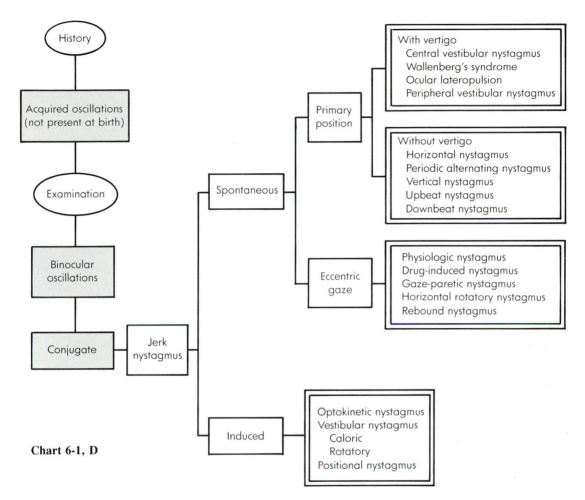

Chart 6-1, D

☐   **Primary-position jerk nystagmus.** Jerk nystagmus present in the primary position can be subdivided by the presence or absence of vertigo.

☐   **With vertigo.** The presence of vertigo indicates a lesion involving the labyrinth, the eighth cranial nerve, or the vestibular nuclear complex and its connections. Vestibular nystagmus is a rotatory (torsional), horizontal-rotatory, purely horizontal, or vertical jerk nystagmus present in the primary position that increases in intensity when the eyes are moved in the direction of the fast phase (Alexander's law).[1,31]

Lesions of the vestibular apparatus act as destructive lesions and mimic the effects of cold water irrigation. Thus a patient with a disease affecting the right vestibular apparatus will develop a left-beating nystagmus, and the environment will appear to move toward the left. The patient may experience the subjective sensation of spinning to the right, will past point to the right, and on standing, especially with his eyes closed, will tend to fall to the right. Peripheral and central vestibular dysfunction may be differentiated by the features listed in Table 6-1. Patients with nystagmus due to peripheral vestibular

Table 6-1. Peripheral vs central vestibular disease

	Peripheral	Central
Severity of vertigo	Marked	Mild
Duration of symptoms	Finite	May be chronic
Tinnitus/deafness	Common	Rare
Type of nystagmus	Usually mixed horizontal-rotatory	May be purely horizontal, rotatory, or vertical
	Visual fixation inhibits nystagmus	Visual fixation has no effect on nystagmus
Common causes	Infectious or inflammatory?	Acoustic neuroma
	Toxic	Ischemia
		Demyelinating disease

lesions have a fast phase that beats in the same direction independent of gaze position. Patients with central lesions have nystagmus that may reverse in direction as the gaze position changes. Patients with mixed signs (i.e., direction of the nystagmus and vertigo, pastpointing, and falling) will most likely have a central lesion.

Patients with Wallenberg's lateral medullary syndrome[96] have a distinct constellation of features including ipsilateral loss of pain and temperature sensation in the face and contralateral loss in the trunk and limbs, ipsilateral Horner's syndrome, dysarthria and dysphagia, ataxia of the ipsilateral limbs, vertigo, and a distinctive type of nystagmus. With the eyes open there is a horizontal rotatory jerk nystagmus beating away from the side of the lesion. With a disruption of fixation, for example, closing the eyes, the nystagmus either stops or reverses.[32] This syndrome is caused by an occlusion of the posterior inferior cerebellar artery. Depending on the amount of underlying cerebellar and brain stem damage, the physical findings will vary considerably.[32] In addition these patients may demonstrate ocular lateropulsion,[60,66] that is, a tendency for the eyes to deviate toward the side of the lesion. In fact, many of these patients will complain that their eyes are being pulled toward one side of their heads. Saccades are hypometric and pursuit is impaired away from the lesion, while saccades are hypermetric and pursuit is normal toward the side of the lesion. A veering of the eyes toward the side of the lesion is noted on vertical gaze movements.

☐ **Without vertigo.** Those patients having primary position jerk nystagmus without vertigo may be subdivided according to the plane of ocular movement. Horizontal jerk nystagmus without vertigo, occurring in the primary position, is limited to the entity of periodic alternating nystagmus. Periodic alternating nystagmus is a jerk nystagmus with a cyclically moving or wandering null point.[23] Thus, if the eyes are observed in one position of gaze, they will pass through a repetitive sequence consisting of a 10-second null period in which the eyes do not move or may beat downward. This is followed by a period of ascending and descending intensity (amplitude and frequency) of unidirectional nystagmus lasting approximately 90 seconds, followed by a null period and then a repeat of nystagmus cascade but with the fast phase in the opposite direction. Pathologic[53] and experimental[11] data suggest that the lesion is in the vestibular nucleus. Periodic alternating nystagmus may accompany other neurologic findings implicating structural posterior fossa disease, specifically the cervicomedullary junction.[23,54] High-resolution CT scanning supplemented by metrizamide opacification of the cerebrospinal fluid should provide all the information necessary to establish the presence or absence of a lesion. In our experience this disorder tends to occur without other evidence of neurologic disease but is visually disabling. Based on the report[43] that some patients have responded to treatment with baclofen with disappearance of their periodic alternating nystagmus, we advocate a trial of this agent in all patients.

Vertical nystagmus present in the primary position may be subdivided according to the direction of the fast phase into upbeat (fast phase up) and downbeat (down) varieties. Both upbeat and downbeat nystagmus may represent defects in the smooth pursuit mechanism in the direction of the fast phase.[24,102]

Upbeat nystagmus may assume various forms—large-amplitude upbeating that increases in upgaze, small-amplitude upbeating that decreases in upgaze but increases in downgaze, and an intermediate form. It has been suggested[22] that with one exception[38] the first type represents a cerebellar vermis lesion and the second type an intrinsic medullary lesion.

The finding of downbeat nystagmus in any position of gaze is usually indicative of cervicomedullary structural disease.[17] The most common causes of downbeat nystagmus are stroke, multiple sclerosis, Arnold-Chiari malformation, and platybasia. Downbeat nystagmus has also been reported in patients with communicating hydrocephalus,[73] magnesium deficiency,[81] and phenytoin[2] and carbamazepine[99] intoxication. Drug intoxication rarely produces this sign. Downbeat nystagmus may be exaggerated or induced by having the patient assume a lateral gaze position or look below the midline. We recommend that all patients with isolated downbeat nystagmus have a CT scan and metrizamide myelography.[52]

☐ **Eccentric gaze jerk nystagmus** (Chart 6-1, *D*). This is a jerk nystagmus present in eccentric but not primary gaze.

☐ **Physiologic nystagmus.** Physiologic or endpoint nystagmus is a low-amplitude jerk nystagmus of irregular frequency with the fast phase toward the field of gaze. It is poorly sustained. It usually does not occur until the eyes have been held eccentrically for a few seconds and is typically dissociated, being more prominent in one eye than it is in the other.

☐ **Drug-induced nystagmus.** The most common causes of pathologic bidirectional gaze-evoked nystagmus are drugs, including barbiturates, tranquilizers, phenothiazines, and anticonvulsants. The nystagmus may have a rotatory component. Drug-induced upbeat nystagmus is the most common form of vertical nystagmus. As mentioned previously, drug-induced downbeat nystagmus is rare. In the absence of drugs, gaze-evoked nystagmus reflects brain stem or cerebellar dysfunction.

☐ **Gaze-paretic nystagmus.** Gaze-paretic nystagmus represents a failure to maintain an eccentric gaze position. Patients recovering from a gaze palsy pass through a stage where they are able to make a conjugate gaze movement but are unable to maintain the eccentric position. Following an adequate saccadic movement the eyes drift back toward the primary position, at which time a corrective saccade is initiated. A similar movement can be seen in patients with cerebellar disease. Normal subjects in the dark have similar ocular oscillations on eccentric gaze.[9] These movements have been reproduced in cerebellectomized animals[11,97] and thus are considered to represent some deficit of cerebellar modulation of brain stem function.[75]

☐   **Horizontal rotatory nystagmus.** Patients with extrinsic lesions in the cerebello-pontine angle often have a distinctive gaze-evoked pattern of nystagmus. Patients with right-sided lesions would have slow, large-amplitude, right-beating nystagmus on gaze to the right, left-beating nystagmus of medium amplitude and frequency in primary position, and fine horizontal rotatory left-beating nystagmus in left gaze.[7,82] Most of these extrinsic lesions, usually acoustic neuromas, grow so slowly that the patients do not have vertigo because of the adaptive ability of the vestibular system.

☐   **Rebound nystagmus.** Rebound nystagmus, a horizontal jerk nystagmus, is divided into two types. Type 1 occurs when a patient with cerebellar hemispheric degeneration due to alcohol abuse is made to sustain an eccentric gaze position. At first a gaze-evoked nystagmus will be seen that will slowly fatigue and be followed by the development of a jerk nystagmus in the opposite direction, that is, fast phase toward the primary position.[48] Rebound nystagmus type 2 is a transient primary position nystagmus that occurs when the eyes are returned to the primary position following sustained eccentric gaze. The nystagmus has its fast phase in the direction opposite to the sustained deviation and represents cerebellar parenchymal disease[103] not limited to the effects of alcohol.

☐   **Induced jerk nystagmus.** Jerk nystagmus can be produced in all normal individuals by either optokinetic or vestibular stimulation. Some people will develop a transient jerk nystagmus when they move their heads into particular positions (positional nystagmus). Positional nystagmus always indicates an abnormality of the vestibular system.

☐   **Optokinetic nystagmus.** Optokinetic nystagmus (OKN) is a type of induced nystagmus easily elicited in all alert persons whose vision permits them to count fingers. It represents activation of fixation and pursuit (slow movement) mechanisms followed by a fast-phase movement either foveating or at least corrective in the opposite direction. It is usually induced clinically by the use of a striped tape or rotating drum. The eyes involuntarily follow a moving stripe (object) of interest until it passes beyond the range of fixation, at which time a fast movement is made in the opposite direction. Thus a jerk nystagmus is induced in which slow-phase velocity depends on the speed of the stimulus, and fast-phase velocity depends on the innate saccadic velocity of the individual. A sustained optokinetic response is more consistently evoked with targets moving in the horizontal plane than in the vertical plane. Although the underlying physiologic mechanisms are not yet known,[101] the response is involuntary and cannot be suppressed if the optokinetic stimulus fills the entire visual field. The optokinetic response can be used as a relative test of visual acuity in children, in linguistically deficient patients, and in malingerers.

OKN abnormalities are seen in patients with deep occipitoparietal lesions but not in patients with pure occipitocortical lesions. Abnormal nystagmus is seen when the tape is rotated toward the side of the lesion and may take the form of either a relative asymmetry of response or a tonic deviation of the eyes without a fast phase. The optokinetic response will be absent in brain stem disease involving the ocular motor mechanisms. Optokinetic stimuli are also useful in exaggerating the dissociated movements of subtle INO and to induce convergence-retraction nystagmus in midbrain syndromes.

☐   **Caloric and rotatory vestibular nystagmus.** The vestibular apparatus plays a major role in controlling and coordinating the tone of the body musculature, including the extraocular muscles. Maintained postural deviations are controlled by the otoliths in the utricles and saccules, while postural movements resulting from acceleration are controlled by the hair cells in the semicircular canals. Varying degrees of nystagmus and vertigo can be produced in a normal person by stimulating the peripheral apparatus either by rotational or caloric testing. Such tests are useful clinically to determine the integrity of the labyrinth and its central connections.

The interpretation of both rotational and caloric testing assumes that horizontal canal function reflects the functional capability of the vertical canals as well. Rotational testing requires that the so-called horizontal canals be placed in the true horizontal plane. Since the horizontal canals in an erect or seated patient normally lie at a 30° tilt to the horizon, the patient so situated must tilt his head 30° forward in order to be appropriately positioned for testing. The patient's eyes are closed in order to prevent the development of OKN. The patient is rotated rapidly for approximately 20 seconds, and the movement is abruptly halted. The patient opens his eyes, and the after-nystagmus (i.e., the nystagmus present after the rotation is stopped) is studied along with postural deviation and pastpointing. Normally the slow phase of the nystagmus, the ocular and postural deviations, and pastpointing *will be in the direction of the recently completed movement.* That is, if the patient was rotated to the right, the slow phase of the nystagmus would be to the right; the fast phase would be to the left, and the vertigo would be toward the left. Rotational testing stimulates both canals with a greater effect on the canal toward which the patient is rotated.

Caloric testing depends upon producing convection currents in the endolymph by the use of a caloric stimulus introduced into the external auditory canal. To isolate and maximize this effect on the horizontal canal, it is necessary to position the patient's head so that the horizontal canal lies in the vertical plane. This is accomplished in the seated patient by tilting the patient's head backward 60°, or in the supine position by tilting his head forward 30°. Thermal stimulation will produce a directional jerk nystagmus most easily remembered by the mnemonic COWS—Cold, Opposite; Warm, Same—with cold and warm referring to the type of stimulus and with opposite and same referring to the direction of the fast-phase response. The advantage of the caloric test is that the vestibular apparatus on each side can be tested separately, and no sophisticated equipment is required.

In comatose individuals or those with loss of voluntary supranuclear control mechanisms, for example, progressive supranuclear palsy, the integrity of the brain stem mechanisms may be determined by calorics or by moving the patient's head in a horizontal and then a vertical plane, producing contraversive eye movements, the so-called oculocephalic or doll's eyes maneuver. An alert individual will not produce such contraversive movements.

☐ **Positional nystagmus.** Positional nystagmus is a jerk nystagmus induced by altering the position of the body or the head. The patient complains about the acute onset of vertigo with changes in body orientation. There are two types of positional nystagmus: (1) central, involving the vestibular nerve, nuclei, or their connections, and (2) peripheral, involving the membranous labyrinth.[45]

In *central positional nystagmus* the nystagmus begins immediately upon changing to the inducing head position, does not fatigue nor habituate if the test is repeated, and is associated with mild vertigo.

Peripheral positional nystagmus has a measurable latency before onset after moving the head into the appropriate position, fatigues within a short period of time, habituates with repeat testing, and is associated with severe but limited-duration vertigo. This variety of positional nystagmus, although bothersome to the patient, is almost always a benign disorder; therefore in these patients no further evaluation is necessary.

☐   **Other eye movement disorders** (Chart 6-1, *E*). The remaining entities consist of a collection of distinctive movement disorders in which no unifying feature other than the conjugacy of the oscillation is apparent.

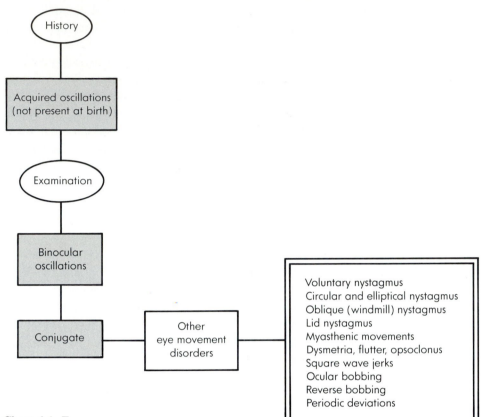

Chart 6-1, E

☐   **Voluntary nystagmus.** To the observer, voluntary nystagmus appears to be a low-amplitude, high-frequency pendular oscillation that occurs in bursts and cannot be maintained for more than a few seconds. By eye movement records, voluntary nystagmus has been established to be a series of sequential saccades.[87] The ability to produce this nystagmus is frequently a familial trait[5] and is often used as a parlor trick. The importance of recognizing this syndrome is the identification of patients feigning illness who present with the complaint of the sudden onset of oscillatory movements following an alleged injury. This movement will completely disappear if the patient is forced to keep his eyes open. In general this feature is enough evidence to establish the diagnosis of voluntary nystagmus.

☐   **Circular and elliptical nystagmus[4].** These are forms of nystagmus in which the globe oscillates continuously in a circular or elliptical pattern without torsion. They can be congenital in nature but also occur in an acquired form.[63]

☐   **Oblique nystagmus.** Oblique or diagonal nystagmus may be seen in patients with cerebellar disease associated with multiple sclerosis. An oblique nystagmus in which the directional vectors continuously change, producing so-called windmill nystagmus, also has been reported.[79]

☐ **Lid nystagmus.** Lid nystagmus is a rhythmic upward jerking of the upper eyelids that usually accompanies vertical ocular nystagmus. There are three types of lid nystagmus. The first is the exaggeration of the normal lid movement that accompanies vertical nystagmus; only the amplitude of the lid movement exceeds that of the ocular movement. The second type is evoked on lateral gaze, and the fast movements of the lids and horizontal nystagmus are synchronous.[21] The third type has been associated with convergence effort.[80]

☐ **Myasthenic (quiverlike) movements.** In patients with myasthenia gravis with marked involvement of all their muscles, a jellylike bilateral quiver movement may be clinically recognized at the initiation of a saccadic movement.[18] This quiver movement is considered to be specific of myasthenia gravis. In addition, myasthenic patients with ocular involvement may appear to have a gaze paresis including the development of a gaze-paretic type of nystagmus. This nystagmus[55] fatigues rapidly with the eyes assuming a position short of the target. These movement disorders are markedly improved by the injection of Tensilon.

☐ **Dysmetria, flutter, and opsoclonus.**[33] These constitute a group of ocular oscillations that, in listed order, occur with increasing degrees of cerebellar dysfunction.

Ocular dysmetria[13] occurs at the end of refixation saccades. It is often more apparent when the eyes move from the lateral gaze position to the primary position than in the opposite direction. It is manifested either as a binocular conjugate undershooting or overshooting followed by a to-and-fro saccadic oscillation around the fixation point before foveation is accomplished, or as a conjugate overshoot followed by a single corrective saccade in large-amplitude refixation movements.

Ocular flutter is a spontaneous binocular break in fixation followed by horizontal oscillations around fixation. It is almost never present in the absence of dysmetria, and its presence probably represents a further deterioration of cerebellar function.

When cerebellar input to the paramedian pontine reticular formation is entirely disrupted, rapid, involuntary, continuous, repetitive, conjugate saccadic eye movements in all directions are seen. This movement disorder is termed *opsoclonus* or *saccadomania*. These movements persist during sleep. Patients who recover go through a reverse sequence in which brief periods of opsoclonus interrupt stable periods of fixation, followed by a period in which flutter and dysmetria are present. The flutter then disappears, and finally with total recovery the dysmetria also disappears.

Opsoclonus in a child is indicative of occult neuroblastoma[91] until a CT scan of the adrenal region excludes this diagnosis. In children and adults opsoclonus can occur as part of a postinfectious syndrome with ataxia, extremity myoclonus, and tremulousness. This postinfectious syndrome is somewhat responsive to corticosteroid therapy. Opsoclonus in older adults has been reported as a remote effect of visceral carcinoma.

☐ **Square wave jerks.** Square wave jerks and macrosquare wave jerks[62] are relatively rare ocular movement disorders. Clinically there is a break in fixation followed by a rapid single movement of refoveation. To inspection, both square wave and macrosquare wave jerks may look like primary position horizontal nystagmus but are identified by their characteristic electronystagmographic pattern. Square wave jerks are subtle and may be easily missed clinically (amplitude, 0.5° to 3°; latency to refixation, 200 ms), whereas macrosquare wave jerks are quite easily seen (amplitude, 4° to 30°; latency to refixation, 50 to 150 ms) and are distinctive. Both types of disorder are in general associated with cerebellar disease.

☐   **Ocular bobbing.** Ocular bobbing is indicative of brain stem dysfunction and is not precisely localizable.[10] In ocular bobbing the eyes repeatedly move briskly downward from the primary position, remain eccentric for a few seconds, and then slowly drift back to the primary position.[35] The movement may be more apparent in one eye than the other.[67] Although ocular bobbing has been classically associated with intrinsic brain stem lesions including vascular accidents,[93] pontine glioma,[20] toxic,[72] hepatic,[74] and metabolic[93] encephalopathies, multiple sclerosis,[6] and encephalitis,[78] it has been reported with extraaxial lesions compressing the stem as well.[34,93] *Reverse bobbing*[58,76,93] consists of a rapid deviation of the eyes upward and a slow return to the horizontal. Ocular dipping or *inverse bobbing*[58,76] is an arrhythmic, slow downward movement followed by a fast upward component. This type of disorder has been reported with intracerebral hematomas and metabolic encephalopathy.[10] In patients with ocular bobbing, inverse or reverse bobbing, horizontal eye movements are usually absent.

☐   **Periodic deviations.** Periodic deviations are of two types—periodic alternating gaze deviation and periodic alternating ping-pong gaze.

Periodic alternating gaze deviation[40] is an involuntary, continuous cyclic disorder of eye movements that disappears during sleep. A cycle consists of a binocular horizontal slow deviation of the eyes to one eccentric gaze position; the eyes remain in lateral gaze for about 2 minutes, and then a slow conjugate movement of the eyes occurs to the opposite lateral gaze position, where the horizontal deviation is maintained for 2 minutes, and then the cycle begins again.

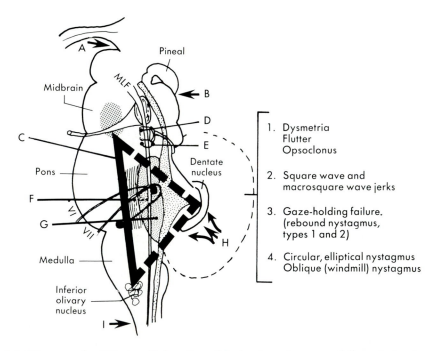

Fig. 6-4. Diagram of midline sagittal section of brain stem. Arrows and lines designate unique regions in which pathologic processes produce labeled eye movements. *A,* See-saw nystagmus; *B,* convergence-retraction nystagmus; *C,* ocular myoclonus; *D,* superior oblique myokymia; *E,* internuclear ophthalmoplegia; *F,* gaze-paretic ocular bobbing; *G,* periodic alternating nystagmus, vestibular; *H,* upbeat nystagmus; *I,* downbeat nystagmus.

Periodic alternating ping-pong gaze is a cyclic disorder of eye movements in which the eyes deviate briefly far to the right and then rapidly reverse direction to the left with a periodicity of a few seconds.[65,85,92] Both of these movements are seen in comatose patients, and the underlying pathology remains speculative.

PATHOANATOMIC APPROACH TO ACQUIRED OCULAR OSCILLATIONS

There is another approach[82] to patients with acquired ocular oscillations. It is anatomical, relating each of the oscillatory disorders to its presumed site of pathology in a rostrocaudal orientation. A modified, more inclusive diagram is included in this chapter (Fig. 6-4).

REFERENCES

1. Alexander, G: Die Ohrenkrankheiten im Kindesalter. In Pfaundler, M, and Schlossmann, A, editors: Handbuch der Kinderheilkunde, Leipzig, 1912, Vlg FCW Vogel, pp 84-96.
2. Alpert, JN: Downbeat nystagmus due to anticonvulsant toxicity, Ann Neurol 4:471, 1978.
3. Antony, JH, Ouvrier, RA, and Wise, G: Spasmus nutans. A mistaken identity, Arch Neurol 37:373, 1980.
4. Aschoff, JC, Conrad, B, and Kornhuber, HH: Acquired pendular nystagmus with oscillopsia in multiple sclerosis: a sign of cerebellar nuclei disease, J Neurol Neurosurg Psychiatry 37:570, 1974.
5. Aschoff, JC, Becker, W, and Rettelbach, R: Voluntary nystagmus in five generations, J Neurol Neurosurg Psychiatry 39:300, 1976.
6. Ash, PR, and Keltner, JL: Neuro-ophthalmic signs in pontine lesions, Medicine 58:304, 1979.
7. Baloh, RW, Konrad, HR, Dirks, D, and Honrubia, V: Cerebellar-pontine angle tumors. Results of quantitative vestibulo-ocular testing, Arch Neurol 33:507, 1976.
8. Barricks, ME, Flynn, JT, and Kushner, BJ: Paradoxical pupillary responses in congenital stationary night blindness. In Smith, JL, editor: Neuro-ophthalmology update, New York, 1977, Masson Publishing Co, pp 31-38.
9. Becker, W, and Klein, HM: Accuracy of saccadic eye movements and maintenance of eccentric eye positions in the dark, Vision Res 13:1021, 1973.
10. Bosch, EP, Kennedy, SS, and Aschenbrener, CA: Ocular bobbing: the myth of its localizing value, Neurology (Minneap) 25:949, 1975.
11. Burde, RM, Stroud, MH, Roper-Hall, G, Wirth, FP, and O'Leary, JL: Ocular motor dysfunction in total and hemicerebellectomized monkeys, Br J Ophthalmol 59:560, 1975.
12. Chokroverty, S, and Barron, KD: Palatal myoclonus and rhythmic ocular movements: a polygraphic study, Neurology (Minneap) 19:975, 1969.
13. Cogan, DG: Ocular dysmetria, flutter-like oscillations of the eyes and opsoclonus, Arch Ophthalmol 51:318, 1954.
14. Cogan, DG: Neurology of the ocular muscles, ed 2, Springfield, Ill, 1956, Charles C Thomas, Publisher, p 184.
15. Cogan, DC: Neurology of the ocular muscles, ed 2, Springfield, Ill, 1956, Charles C Thomas, Publisher, p 189.
16. Cogan, DG: Neurology of the ocular muscles, ed 2, Springfield Ill, 1956, Charles C Thomas, Publisher, p 192.
17. Cogan, DG: Downbeat nystagmus, Arch Ophthalmol 80:757, 1968.
18. Cogan, DG, Yee, RD, and Gittinger, J: Rapid eye movements in myasthenia gravis, Arch Ophthalmol 94:1083, 1976.
19. Daroff, RB: See-saw nystagmus, Neurology (Minneap) 15:874, 1965.
20. Daroff, RB, and Waldman, AL: Ocular bobbing, J Neurol Neurosurg Psychiatry 28:375, 1965.
21. Daroff, RB, Hoyt, WF, Sanders, MD, and Nelson, LR: Gaze-evoked eyelid and ocular nystagmus inhibited by the near reflex: unusual ocular motor phenomena in a lateral medullary syndrome, J Neurol Neurosurg Psychiatry 31:362, 1968.
22. Daroff, RB, and Troost, BT: Up-beat nystagmus, JAMA 225:312, 1973.
23. Daroff, RB, and Dell'Osso, LF: Periodic alternating nystagmus and the shifting null, Can J Otolaryngol 3:367, 1974.
24. Daroff, RB, Troost, BT, and Dell'Osso, LF: Nystagmus and related ocular oscillations. In Glaser, JS, editor: Neuro-ophthalmology, Hagerstown Md, 1978, Harper & Row, Publishers, pp 219-243.
25. Davis, GV, and Schock, JP: Septo-optic dysplasia associated with seesaw nystagmus, Arch Ophthalmol 93:137-139, 1975.

26. Dell'Osso, LF: Improving visual acuity in congenital nystagmus. In Smith, JL, and Glaser, JS, editors: Neuro-ophthalmology. Symposium of the University of Miami and the Bascom Palmer Eye Institute, vol 7, St Louis, 1973, The CV Mosby Co, pp 98-106.

27. Dell'Osso, LF, and Daroff, RB: Congenital nystagmus waveforms and foveation strategies, Doc Ophthalmol 39:155, 1975.

28. Dell'Osso, LF, Schmidt, D, and Daroff, RB: Latent, manifest, and congenital nystagmus, Arch Ophthalmol 97:1877, 1979.

29. Dichgans, J, and Jung, R: Oculomotor abnormalities due to cerebellar lesions. In Lennerstrand, G, and Bach-y-Rita, P, editors: Basic mechanisms of ocular motility and their clinical implications, Oxford, 1975, Pergamon Press, p 281.

30. Donin, JF: Acquired monocular nystagmus in children, Can J Ophthalmol 2:212, 1967.

31. Doslak, MJ, Dell'Osso, LF, and Daroff, RB: Alexander's law: a model and resulting study, Ann Otol Rhinol Laryngol 91:316, 1982.

32. Duncan, GW, Parker, SW, and Fisher, CM: Acute cerebellar infarction in the PICA territory, Arch Neurol 32:364, 1975.

33. Ellenberger, C, Keltner, JL, and Stroud, MH: Ocular dyskinesia in cerebellar disease, Brain 95:685, 1972.

34. Finelli, PF, and McEntee, WJ: Ocular bobbing with extraaxial hematoma of the posterior fossa, J Neurol Neurosurg Psychiatry 40:386, 1977.

35. Fisher, CM: Ocular bobbing, Arch Neurol 11:543, 1964.

36. Freeman, MI, Burde, RM, and Gay, AJ: A case of true paradoxical pupillary reaction, Arch Ophthalmol 75:740, 1966.

37. Gelbart, SS, Hoyt, CS, and Stone, RD: Congenital nystagmus: a clinical perspective in infancy, Arch Ophthalmol (in press).

38. Gilman, N, Baloh, RW, and Tomiyasu, U: Primary position up-beating nystagmus, Neurology (Minneap) 27:294, 1977.

39. Glaser, JS: Myasthenic pseudo-internuclear ophthalmoplegia, Arch Ophthalmol 75;363, 1966.

40. Goldberg, RR, Gonzalez, C, Breinin, GM, and Reuben, RN: Periodic alternating gaze deviation with dissociation of head movement, Arch Ophthalmol 73:324, 1965.

41. Goldhammer, Y: Paradoxical pupillary reaction. In Smith, JL, editor: Neuro-ophthalmology update, New York, 1977, Masson Publishing Co, pp 39-42.

42. Gresty, MA, Ell, JJ, and Findley, LJ: Acquired pendular nystagmus: its characteristics, localising value and pathophysiology, J Neurol Neurosurg Psychiatry 45:431, 1982.

43. Halmagyi, GM, Rudge, P, Gresty, MA, Leigh, RJ, and Zee, DS: Treatment of periodic alternating nystagmus, Ann Neurol 8:609, 1980.

44. Halpern, J: Spasmus nutans, Arch Neurol 37:737, 1980.

45. Harrison, MS, and Ozahinoglu, C: Positional vertigo: aetiology and clinical significance, Brain 95:364, 1972.

46. Hedges, TR, III, and Hoyt, WF: Ocular tilt reaction due to an upper brain stem lesion: paroxysmal skew deviation, torsion, and oscillation of the eyes with head tilt, Ann Neurol 11:537, 1982.

47. Herzau, V, Korner, F, Kommerell, G, and Friedel, B: In Kommerell, G, editor: Disorders of ocular motility. Neurophysiological and clinical aspects, Munich, 1978, Bergmann, pp 81-90.

48. Hood, JD, Kayan, A, and Leech, J: Rebound nystagmus, Brain 96:507, 1973.

49. Hoyt, CS, and Gelbart, SS: Vertical nsytagmus in infants with congenital ocular abnormalities, Arch Ophthalmol (in press).

50. Hoyt, WF, and Keane, JR: Superior oblique myokymia: report and discussion on five cases of benign intermittent uniocular microtremor, Arch Ophthalmol 84:461, 1970.

51. Jayalakshmi, P, Scott, TFN, Tucker, SH, and Schaffer, DB: Infantile nystagmus: a prospective study of spasmus nutans, congenital nystagmus, and unclassified nystagmus of infancy, J Pediatr 77:177, 1970.

52. Kapila, A, Elble, R, Ratcheson, RA, Burde, R, and Gado, MH: Radiologic demonstration of the dorsal medullocervical spur in adult Chiari malformation, J Clin Neuro-ophthalmol 2:235, 1982.

53. Karp, J, and Rorke, LB: Periodic alternating nystagmus, Arch Neurol 32:422, 1975.

54. Keane, JR: Periodic alternating nystagmus with downward beating nystagmus, Arch Neurol 30:399, 1974.

55. Keane, JR, and Hoyt, WF: Myasthenic (vertical) nystagmus. Verification by edrophonium tonography, JAMA 212:1209, 1970.

56. Kelly, TW: Optic glioma presenting as spasmus nutans, Pediatrics 45:295, 1970.

57. Kestenbaum, A: Clinical methods of neuro-ophthalmologic examination, ed 2, New York, 1961, Grune & Stratton.

58. Knobler, RL, Somasundaram, M, and Schutta, HS: Inverse ocular bobbing, Ann Neurol 9:194, 1981.

59. Kommerell, G: Unilateral internuclear ophthalmoplegia. The lack of inhibitory involvement in medial rectus muscle activity, Invest Ophthalmol Vis Sci 21:592, 1981.

60. Kommerell, G, and Hoyt, WF: Lateropulsion of saccadic eye movements, Arch Neurol 28:313, 1973.
61. Kommerell, G, and Schaubele, G: Superior oblique myokymia. An electromyographical analysis, Trans Ophthalmol Soc UK 100:504, 1980.
62. Leigh, RJ, and Zee, DS: The neurology of eye movements, Philadelphia, 1983, FA Davis Co, p 61.
63. Leigh, RJ, and Zee, DS: The neurology of eye movements, Philadelphia, 1983, FA Davis Co, p 204.
64. Lourie, H: Seesaw nystagmus. Case report elucidating the mechanism, Arch Neurol 9:531, 1963.
65. Masucci, EF, Fabara, JA, Saini, N, and Kurtzke, JF: Periodic alternating ping-pong gaze, Ann Ophthalmol 13:1123, 1981.
66. Meyer, KT, Baloh, RW, Krobel, GB, and Hepler, RS: Ocular lateropulsion, Arch Ophthalmol 98:1614, 1980.
67. Newman, N, Gay, AJ, and Heilbrun, MP: Disjugate ocular bobbing: its relation to midbrain, pontine, and medullary function in a surviving patient, Neurology (Minneap) 21:633, 1971.
68. Norton, EWD: Nystagmus. In Smith, JL, editor: Neuro-ophthalmology, Springfield, Ill, 1964, Charles C Thomas, Publisher, p 288.
69. Norton, EWD, and Cogan, DG: Spasmus nutans. A clinical study of twenty cases followed two years or more since onset, Arch Ophthalmol 52:442, 1954.
70. Ohm, J: Der latente Nystagmus nach Verlust eines Auges, Albrecht Von Graefes Arch Ophthalmol 144:617, 1942.
71. Pagon, RA, Graham, JM, Jr, Zonana, J, and Yong, S: Coloboma, congenital heart disease, and choanal atresia with multiple anomalies: CHARGE association, J Pediatr 99:223, 1981.
72. Paty, DW, and Sherr, H: Ocular bobbing in bromism. A case report, Neurology (Minneap) 22:525, 1972.
73. Phadke, JG, Hern, JEC, and Blaiklock, CT: Downbeat nystagmus—a false localising sign due to communicating hydrocephalus, J Neurol Neurosurg Psychiatry 44:459, 1981.
74. Rai, GS, Buston-Thomas, M, and Scanlon, M: Ocular bobbing in hepatic encephalopathy, Br J Clin Pract 30:302, 1976.
75. Robinson, DA: The effect of cerebellectomy on the cat's vestibulo-ocular integrator, Brain Res 74:195, 1974.
76. Ropper, AH: Ocular dipping in anoxic coma, Arch Neurol 38:297, 1981.
77. Rosenberg, ML, and Glaser, JS: Superior oblique myokymia, Ann Neurol 13:667, 1983.
78. Rudick, R, Satran, R, and Eskin, TA: Ocular bobbing in encephalitis, J Neurol Neurosurg Psychiatry 44:441, 1981.
79. Sanders, MD: Alternating windmill nystagmus. In Smith, JL, and Glaser, JS, editors: Neuro-ophthalmology Symposium of the University of Miami and the Bascom Palmer Eye Institute, vol 7, St. Louis, 1973, The CV Mosby Co, pp 133-136.
80. Sanders, MD, Hoyt, WF, and Daroff, RB: Lid nystagmus evoked by ocular convergence: an ocular electromyographic study, J Neurol Neurosurg Psychiatry 31:368, 1968.
81. Saul, RF, and Selhorst, JB: Downbeat nystagmus with magnesium depletion, Arch Neurol 38:650, 1981.
82. Schatz, NJ, and Savino, PJ: Nystagmus. In Symposium on neuro-ophthalmology. Transactions of the New Orleans Academy of Ophthalmology, St Louis, 1976, The CV Mosby Co, pp 84-89.
83. Schmidt, D, and Kommerell, G: Schaukel-Nystagmus (seesaw nystagmus) mit bitemporaler Hemianopie als Folge von Schadelhirnstraumen, Albrecht Von Graefes Arch Klin Exp Ophthalmol 178:349, 1969.
84. Schulman, JA, Shults, WT, and Jones, JR, Jr: Monocular vertical nystagmus as an initial sign of chiasmal glioma, Am J Ophthalmol 87:87, 1979.
85. Senelick, RC: "Ping-pong" gaze: periodic alternating gaze deviation, Neurology (Minneap) 26:532, 1976.
86. Sharpe, JA, Hoyt, WF, and Rosenberg, MA: Convergence-evoked nystagmus. Congenital and acquired forms, Arch Neurol 32:191, 1975.
87. Shults, WT, Stark, L, and Hoyt, WF: Normal saccadic structure of voluntary nystagmus, Arch Ophthalmol 95:1399, 1977.
88. Slatt, B, and Nykiel, F: See-saw nystagmus, Am J Ophthalmol 58:1016, 1964.
89. Smith, JL, and David, NJ: Internuclear ophthalmoplegia. Two new clinical signs, Neurology (Minneap) 14:307, 1964.
90. Smith, JL, Flynn, JT, and Spiro, HJ: Monocular vertical oscillations of amblyopia. The Heimann-Bielschowsky phenomenon, J Clin Neuro-ophthalmol 2:85, 1982.
91. Solomon, GE, and Chutorian, AM: Opsoclonus and occult neuroblastoma, N Engl J Med 279:475, 1968.
92. Stewart, JD, Kirkham, TH, and Mathieson, G: Periodic alternating gaze, Neurology (Minneap) 29:222, 1979.
93. Susac, JO, Hoyt, WF, Daroff, RB, and Lawrence, W: Clinical spectrum of ocular bobbing, J Neurol Neurosurg Psychiatry 38:771, 1970.
94. Susac, JO, Smith, JL, and Schatz, NJ: Superior oblique myokymia, Arch Neurol 29:432, 1973.
95. Tamoush, AJ, Brooks, JE, and Keltner, JL: Palatal myoclonus associated with abnormal ocular and extremity movements, Arch Neurol 27:431, 1972.

96. Wallenberg, A: Acute bulbaraffection (Embyolie derart: cerebellar post. inf. sinistr?) Arch Psychiatr Nervenkr 27:504, 1895.

97. Westheimer, G, and Blair, SM: Oculomotor defects in cerebellectomized monkeys, Invest Ophthalmol 12:618, 1973.

98. Westheimer, G, and Blair, SM: The ocular tilt reaction—a brain stem oculomotor routine, Invest Ophthalmol 14:833, 1975.

99. Wheeler, SD, Ramsay, RE, and Weiss, J: Drug-induced downbeat nystagmus, Ann Neurol 12:227, 1982.

100. Yee, RD, Jelks, GW, Baloh, RW, and Honrubia, V: Uniocular nystagmus in monocular visual loss, Ophthalmology 86:511, 1979.

101. Yee, RD, Baloh, RW, and Honrubia, V: Eye movement abnormalities in rod monochromacy, Ophthalmology 88:1010, 1981.

102. Zee, DS, Friendlich, AR, and Robinson, DA: The mechanism of downbeat nystagmus, Arch Neurol 30:227, 1974.

103. Zee, DS, Yee, RD, Robinson, DA, Cogan, DG, and Engel, WK: Ocular motor abnormalities in hereditary cerebellar ataxia, Brain 99:207, 1976.

CHAPTER 7

Anisocoria and abnormal pupillary light reactions

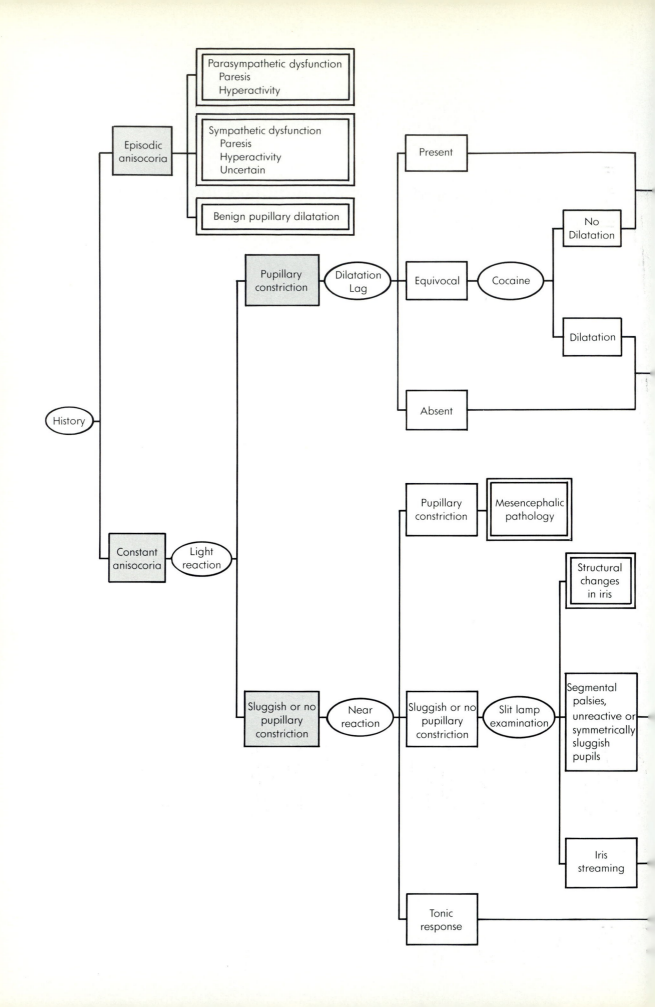

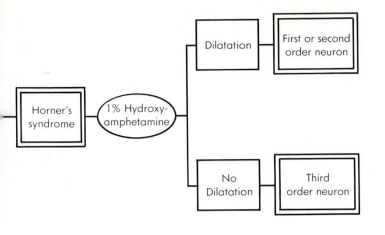

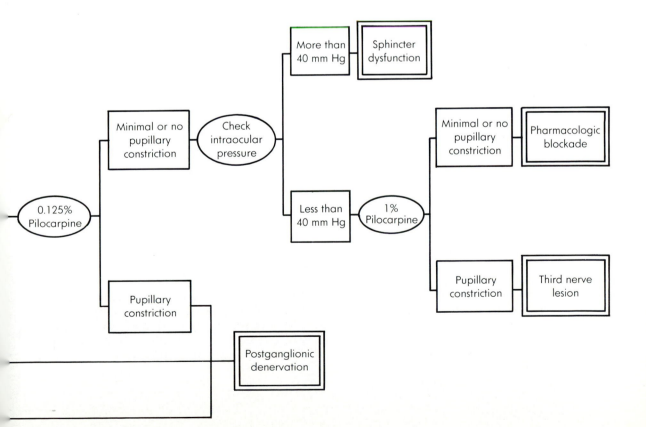

Anatomy and physiology

Analysis of pupillary abnormalities requires a basic understanding of the anatomic pathways and physiologic reactions underlying normal pupillary function. Although pupillary size and reactivity, as well as ciliary muscle tone, are basically controlled by the opposing limbs of the autonomic nervous system, the major role is played by the parasympathetic system due to the mechanical superiority of the sphincter muscle.

Parasympathetic control. The parasympathetic impulses arise in the Edinger-Westphal complex (EWC), a central paired subnucleus of the oculomotor nerve in the mesencephalon. The EWC consists of (1) the anterior median nucleus rostral to the oculomotor somatic complex, (2) visceral columns dorsally over the motor complex, and (3) Perlia's nucleus, which is in the midline between the paired motor groups (Fig. 7-1). The exact function that each of these nuclei control is not explicitly

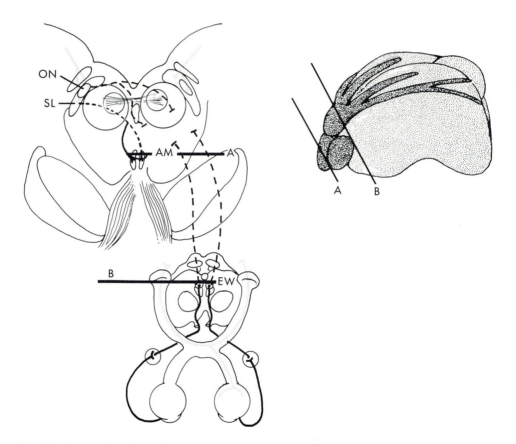

Fig. 7-1. *Upper right,* three-dimensional representation of oculomotor complex in primate. *Upper left,* coronal section of mesencephalon at level of anterior median *(AM)* nucleus *(ON,* pretectal olivary nucleus; *SL,* sublentiform nucleus). *Lower left,* coronal section of mesencephalon at level of Edinger-Westphal *(EW)* columns and somatic columns. Pupillary light reflex: lighter solid lines trace afferent pupillary fibers from retina, crossing in the chiasm to terminate in pretectal superior olivary and sublentiform nuclei. Broken lines trace pathway of intercalated neurons from pretectal nuclei to parasympathetic nuclei *(AM* and *EW)* of oculomotor nerve. Heavier solid lines trace efferent parasympathetic fibers via third cranial nerve, terminating in ciliary ganglion in orbit. Parasympathetic efferents arising in ciliary ganglion reach globe via short ciliary nerves.

known, but accommodation appears to be represented more rostrally than is pupillary function.[25]

When an individual is asleep, the pupils are miotic, reflecting unopposed parasympathetic tone. Upon awakening, this parasympathetic tone is modified by psychogenic factors (fear, alertness, stress, and noise), which inhibit the EWC directly, as well as by light stimuli relayed through the pretectal nuclei. Afferent input to the pretectal nuclei (sublentiform and olivary nuclei in the primate) originates in the retinal ganglion cells subserving, for the most part, macular function and sending divergent axon collaterals to the lateral geniculate body as well (Fig. 7-1).

Fiber projections from the pretectal nuclei decussate both dorsally and ventrally around the sylvian aqueduct and synapse in the EWC. Efferent pupillary fibers arise from the EWC and traverse the mesencephalon in the rostral fascicles of the third cranial nerve to enter the peripheral nerve in the interpeduncular fossa. Within the peripheral nerve they travel superficially in the superior nasal position, enter the orbit as part of the inferior division of the nerve, and arrive at the ciliary ganglion by means of the motor nerve to the inferior oblique muscle. Most of the pupillomotor fibers synapse in the main or accessory ciliary ganglia and reach the iris sphincter muscle via the short ciliary nerves. Interruption in this pathway from the EWC to the sphincter muscle will cause pupillary dilatation and decreased reactivity. Afferent visual system pathology does not produce a difference in pupillary size (anisocoria).

Pupillary constriction (miosis) is also a component of a number of synkinetic reactions involving parasympathetic activity: (1) near reflex—miosis, accommodation, and convergence; (2) Bell's phenomenon–levator inhibition, superior rectus muscle stimulation, and miosis; and (3) the Westphal-Piltz reaction—orbicularis spasm and pupillary miosis (unilateral or bilateral).

Sympathetic control. The oculosympathetic pathway is composed of three neurons (Fig. 7-2). The first order neuron arises in the hypothalamus and descends through the reticular substance, assuming a position contiguous to the vestibular nucleus, the mesencephalic root of the trigeminal nerve, and the paramedian pontine reticular formation at the pontomedullary junction. The first neuron synapses in the intermediolateral gray substance of the lower cervical and upper thoracic spinal cord (ciliospinal center of Budge-Waller, C_8-T_1). The second order neuron arises in the intermediolateral gray column, exiting by the ventral spinal roots and via the white rami communicans to ascend without synapse through the sympathetic paraspinal chain to the superior cervical ganglion. These two neurons make up the preganglionic portion of the three-neuron chain. From the superior cervical ganglion the postganglionic or third order neuron travels on the surface of the common carotid artery. At the bifurcation of the internal and external carotid arteries, fibers controlling facial sweating (with the exception in some cases of a small patch of skin over the superior orbital notch) follow the external carotid artery, while those destined for the eye and lid follow the internal carotid artery. In the cavernous sinus these eye and lid fibers join the fifth and sixth (?) cranial nerves and enter the orbit via the superior orbital fissure. Fibers destined for the dilator muscle enter the eye via the long posterior ciliary nerves or short posterior ciliary nerves (passing through the ciliary ganglion without synapse).

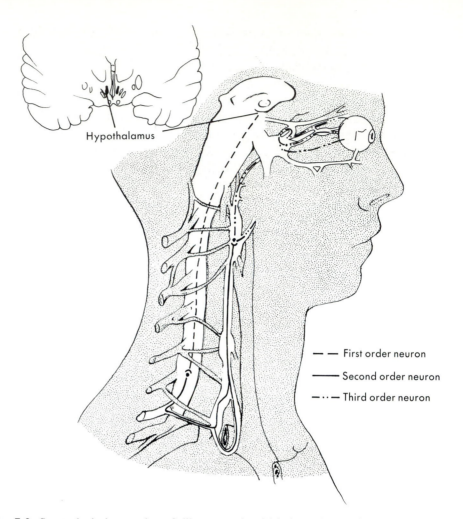

Hypothalamus

— — First order neuron

——— Second order neuron

—··— Third order neuron

Fig. 7-2. Sympathetic innervation of dilator muscle of iris is made up of a three-neuronal arc. First order neuron arises in hypothalamus and projects through brain stem to intermediolateral gray column of lower cervical and upper thoracic cords. Second order neuron arises in intermediolateral gray column, exits cord via white rami communicans, and travels rostrally with paravertebral sympathetic chain to synapse in superior cervical ganglion. Third order neuron originates in superior cervical ganglion and travels within pericarotid sympathetic plexus to cavernous sinus, where it joins first division of trigeminal nerve to enter the orbit and eventually enters globe and innervates dilator muscle of iris.

Light reaction

When determining pupillary size and reactivity to light stimuli it is necessary to control the testing situation to prevent pupillary constriction that accompanies various synkinetic reactions. The patient should fixate on a distant target, therefore preventing activation of the near reflex. The quality, that is, amplitude, latency, and speed, of the pupillary light reaction should somewhat parallel the patient's visual acuity except with decreased vision due to circumscribed foveal and bilateral occipital lobe disease. In patients with limited foveal disease visual acuity may be severely affected, but the majority of pupillary afferents from the macular region will be functioning normally, and the pupillary light reflex will be brisk and full. Similarly, since the pupil is driven by axon collaterals that branch before the visual fibers synapse in the lateral geniculate body, a patient with bilateral homonymous scotomas due to bilateral occipital lobe disease will have poor vision but clinically normal pupillary reactions.

In infants who are crying it is impossible to determine accurately the adequacy of the pupillary response because each time the baby squeezes his eyes closed, the pupils constrict (Westphal-Piltz phenomenon). The baby should be lifted with his neck supported and tilted with his head and body toward the examiner. Ordinarily the child will immediately stop crying and reflexly open his eyes. At this time a light may be projected into each pupil by an assistant and the status of the light reflex determined.*

Physiologic increase in sympathetic tone (anxiety pupils)

There are patients (usually children and young girls) who have normal visual function but relatively large, equally sized pupils that are bilaterally sluggishly reactive to light stimuli. The near reaction in these patients may be similarly sluggish, but usually less so. Under these circumstances the examination should be continued and the pupillary light reflexes rechecked later. On subsequent examination, invariably the light reflex will be brisk and symmetric. Pupils that are sluggishly reactive to light and that normalize during the examination are called Bumke's or anxiety pupils[8] and are postulated to be due to excess sympathetic tone. Similar reactions often are seen in patients with psychiatric disease.

Near reaction

The near reaction is a synkinesis consisting of convergence, accommodation, and pupillary miosis. The near reaction may be checked even in a blind person by using a proprioceptive target (one of the patient's own fingers). If a patient has a normal pupillary reaction to light with no specific complaints implicating a problem in the reading position, we believe it is superfluous to check the pupillary reaction to a near stimulus. If the patient has complaints involving proximal work, for example, diplopia or blurring of vision, then the components of the near reaction must be tested individually. The near reaction requires volitional effort on the part of the patient. Thus, only in the presence of pupillary miosis can the examiner be absolutely sure that the patient is trying to fixate on the near target. Unfortunately, in many pathologic states involving the mesencephalon all the components of the near reflex are affected concomitantly, and pupillary constriction does not occur. Under these circumstances, consistency in the measurements of range of accommodation and ocular misalignment at near is the only assurance that the patient is cooperating and has accommodative convergence paresis.

Decision tree

The decision tree (Chart 7-1) for the evaluation of anisocoria and abnormal light reactions is adapted from that proposed by Thompson and Pilley.[58] For the purposes of

---

*The integrity of the brain stem ocular motor connections can be tested at the same time, since the position in which the child has been placed is such that the horizontal canals of the labyrinthine apparatus are parallel to the floor. Thus the baby may be rotated to the right and left (the person holding the infant being the fulcrum), reflexly producing a tonic conjugate gaze movement opposite to the direction of the spin. Similarly the head can be moved passively up and down, inducing conjugate vertical excursions of the eyes.

this chapter we will exclude the pupillary abnormalities associated with afferent visual system dysfunction. The two major pupillary problems that concern the clinician are (1) anisocoria and (2) bilateral abnormal pupillary responses to light stimulation with or without light-near dissociation.

Patients may come to a physician because they, or their families and friends, have noted that one pupil is larger than the other, or anisocoria may be discovered incidentally during examination by a physician. The first critical piece of information to ascertain is whether the anisocoria has been intermittently or constantly present.

■ EPISODIC ANISOCORIA (Chart 7-1, *A*)

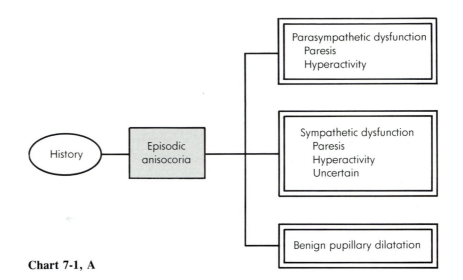

Chart 7-1, A

Either parasympathetic or sympathetic paresis or overactivity may produce intermittent anisocoria. In some cases the cause is not clearly evident.

□ **Parasympathetic paresis**

Uncal herniation. Patients with incipient uncal herniation with lateral brain stem compression due to a shift of midline structures[16] may pass through a phase in which there are intermittent mydriasis and sluggish pupillary reactions to light.[44] Other neurologic findings will contribute to the diagnosis, such as the patient's state of consciousness and motor function.

Seizure disorders. Unilateral pupillary dilatation is also an uncommon manifestation of seizure disorders.[64] The anisocoria may occur during the seizure or the postictal phase[41] and in some cases has been accompanied by conjugate deviation of the eyes. During these periods the pupil has been reported to be sluggishly reactive to light.

Migraine. Dalessio[12] and Edelson and Levy[14] have reported isolated pupillary mydriasis and loss of accommodation in patients with migraine headaches. The internal ophthalmoplegia tends to be transient.

□ **Parasympathetic hyperactivity**

Cyclic oculomotor paresis. Patients with congenital or acquired cyclic oculomotor palsy will demonstrate pupillary miosis during the spastic (shorter) phase and mydriasis during the longer (paralytic) phase.[30] This type of episodic phenomenon is recognized easily by the distinctive ocular motility disturbance.

   Parasympathetic spasm. Thompson and Corbett[59] have reported a single case of a young woman who suffered from the abrupt onset of intermittent spasm of the pupillary sphincter and ciliary muscles causing pupillary miosis and accommodative myopia. Both these muscles contracted several times a minute for 11 days and then stopped as suddenly as they started. The contractions were accompanied by a darkening of vision in the affected eye. No cause was found.

☐   **Sympathetic paresis.** Ipsilateral pupillary constriction and ptosis (Horner's syndrome), accompanied by conjunctival injection, lacrimation, and severe facial and periocular pain in the distribution of the external carotid system, are characteristic of cluster headache. The oculosympathetic paresis is initially transient (hours to days) but tends to persist for a longer period of time with each subsequent attack. These patients have involvement of the third order neuron.

☐   **Sympathetic hyperactivity.** Vijayan[61] has reported seven patients who sustained neck trauma with recurrent unilateral frontotemporal throbbing headaches associated with ipsilateral mydriasis and facial hyperhidrosis (Claude Bernard syndrome—mydriasis, lid retraction, and facial hyperhidrosis). Four of these patients had a transient (3 days) ptosis and miosis (Horner's syndrome) ipsilateral to the sympathetic hyperactivity following the headache. During the headache-free intervals pharmacologic testing suggested the existence of partial sympathetic denervation. Vijayan postulated that the probable site of the causative lesion was in the neck after the fibers had emerged from the T_1 segments.

☐   **Sympathetic dysfunction producing alternating anisocoria.** Patients with cervical cord lesions, such as from old trauma or syringomyelia, may have alternating anisocoria.[14,17,39] From one episode to the next, first one pupil is larger, then the other is larger. It is impossible to state categorically whether this anisocoria is due to an interruption of the sympathetic pathways, producing alternating Horner's syndrome (miosis, ptosis, and anhydrosis), or is secondary to irritative phenomena, producing an alternating Claude Bernard syndrome[9,28,39] (mydriasis, lid retraction, and excessive perspiration). The mechanism can only be determined by pharmacologic testing at the time of the anisocoria,[9,39] and the results of such testing are not universally available in the literature. These patients all have identifiable accompanying neurologic deficits such as limb weakness, paresthesias, or radicular pain. Occasionally a patient with thyroiditis or other inflammatory diseases in the neck contiguous to the second order sympathetic neurons may have an alternating anisocoria.

☐   **Benign pupillary dilatation.** If the anisocoria is unaccompanied by neurologic findings, then the diagnosis most likely is benign unilateral pupillary dilatation[14,20,63] (see Chart 7-1, *A*). This diagnosis should be limited to patients who maintain brisk light and near reflexes in the involved eye during the period of pupillary dilatation. Most of the cases purported to represent this entity have failed to satisfy this criterion,[14,20] as the affected pupil did not react briskly to light and near stimuli. Appropriate testing was not done to rule out pharmacologic blockade.[5,14,20] Most of the patients with benign pupillary dilatation complained of concomitant blurring of vision, and although the pupillary reactions are described as being brisk, the final pupillary diameter on the involved side always remained proportionately larger. Hypothetically, isolated sympathetic hyperactivity producing a transient Claude Bernard syndrome[28] could simulate benign pupillary dilatation, but in that case the pupillary light reaction should be sluggish. Patients with benign unilateral pupillary dilatation usually are young and often have associated headache. The springing pupil[4] has been described as an alternating pupillary dilatation of short duration with no other abnormality. We have not seen such a case. We believe that the terms *benign unilateral pupillary dilatation* and *springing pupil* should be used synonymously.[4]

Unilateral pupillary dilatation, episodic or not, always reflexly acts as a danger signal to the physician, raising the possibility of a posterior communicating or posterior cerebral artery aneurysm. Although Walsh and Hoyt[62] and Payne and Adamkiewicz[42] have each observed one case of isolated internal ophthalmoplegia as the presenting sign of posterior communicating artery aneurysm, they state that such cases are "exceptionally rare." We believe that any patient who presents with a dilated pupil without disturbances of extraocular muscle function, whether accompanied by a headache or not, should not be studied angiographically but rather should be observed at regular intervals.

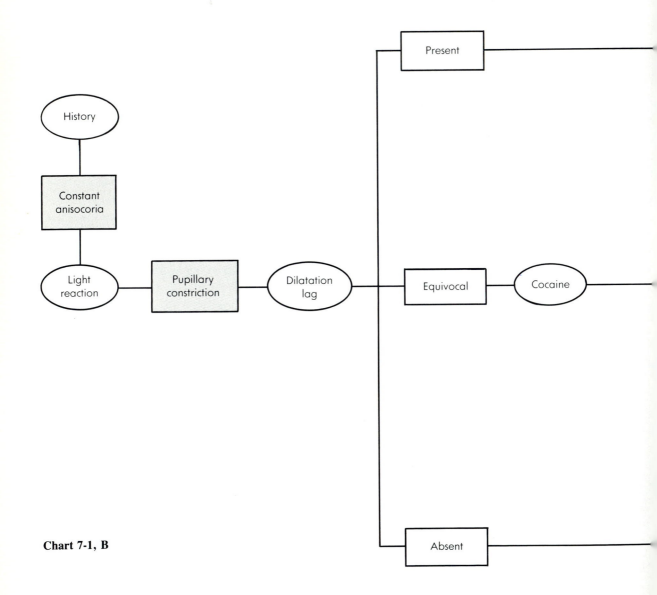

Chart 7-1, B

■ **CONSTANT ANISOCORIA** (see Chart 7-1)

   If there is a persistent inequality of pupillary size, the first step is to check the pupillary light reaction. If the pupillary response is normal, the anisocoria is either physiologic or the patient has Horner's syndrome. If one (or both) pupil reacts poorly (decreased speed and amplitude of response) to light, there is either a disturbance of the parasympathetic pathways to the sphincter muscle or damage to the sphincter muscle itself. Somewhat analogous conclusions can be reached by comparing the pupillary size in light and immediately after turning the lights off. In a patient without iris pathology, anisocoria that is exaggerated in the dark implies weakness of the dilator muscle on one side; anisocoria that is greater in the light implies weakness of the sphincter muscle.

■ **Normal light reaction: pupillary constriction** (Chart 7-1, *B*)

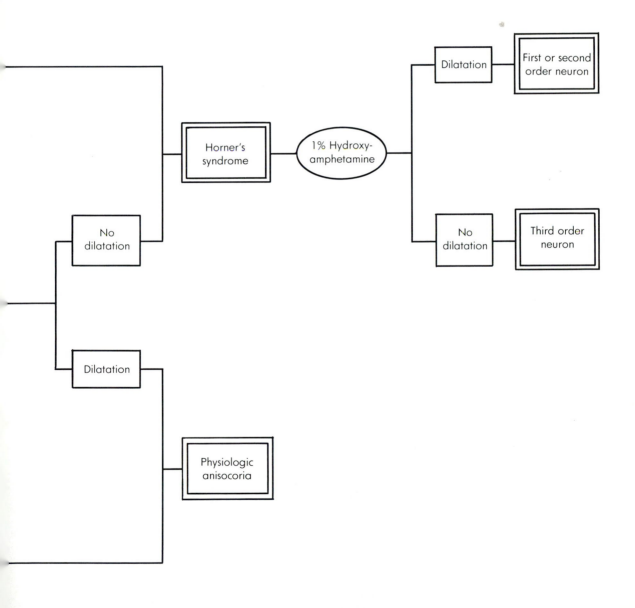

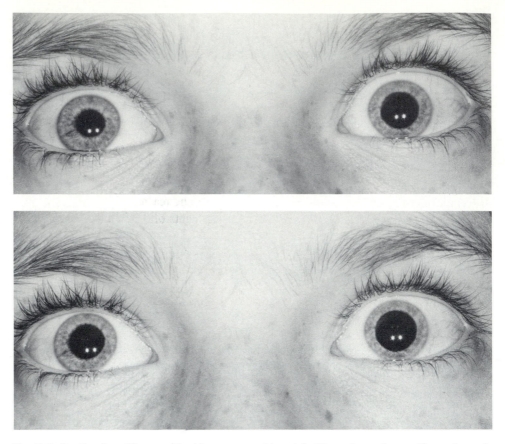

Fig. 7-3. Pupils of an 18-year-old white woman with a right Horner's syndrome. Upper frame is taken approximately 5 seconds after turning off room lights. Lower frame is taken after room lights have been off for 15 seconds. Note that anisocoria is maximal at 5 seconds versus 15 seconds (dilatation lag). (Courtesy H. Stanley Thompson, M.D.)

○ **Dilatation lag.** If the light reaction is normal in both eyes, the next step is to determine if there is a dilatation lag,[43] that is, if the anisocoria is exaggerated immediately following reduction of the background illumination. This is best demonstrated using flash Polaroid photography[11] (Fig. 7-3). If there is no dilatation lag, the diagnosis is physiologic anisocoria. Clinically, physiologic anisocoria is recognized when the difference in pupillary diameters exceeds 0.4 mm. The anisocoria may vary in degree over time, but rarely does the difference in pupillary size exceed 1 mm. Physiologic anisocoria[29] occurs in about 20% of the population under age 17 and in about 30% of the people over age 60. Four percent of the population will have a physiologic anisocoria that exceeds 1 mm.[34]

□ **Horner's syndrome.** Dilatation lag is due to a relative weakness of the dilator muscle and is diagnostic of oculosympathetic paresis. Therefore, if dilatation lag is found, other signs of oculosympathetic paralysis, Horner's syndrome[6] (ptosis and facial anhydrosis), should be sought. Enophthalmos has been mentioned as a feature of Horner's syndrome. The apparent enophthalmos of oculosympathetic paresis is produced by lower lid elevation secondary to denervation of the lower lid retractors.

Horner's syndrome is due to interruption of the sympathetic innervation to the eye.

A defect of the third order neuron proximal to the carotid bifurcation will produce ptosis, miosis, and ipsilateral facial anhydrosis. A lesion distal to the bifurcation tends to produce ptosis and miosis without anhydrosis. Patients with Horner's syndrome often have a transient increase in their amplitudes of accommodation. Psychosensory pupillary dilatation caused by startle or pain is reduced or absent on the involved side and can easily, although not reliably, be checked at the bedside by pinching the patient suddenly on the nape of the neck. Under normal conditions both pupils will dilate in response to both the pain and the unexpected manipulation (startle). The intraocular pressure on the involved side is lower initially than that in the uninvolved eye, but this normalizes with time. Whether the oculosympathetic pathways are partially or totally compromised, the pupillary light and near reactions are unimpaired.

Patients who have a disruption of sympathetic innervation to the eye early in life do not develop iris pigmentation on the involved side, that is, heterochromia iridis. This is due to the fact that the formation of pigment granules by stromal melanocytes is under sympathetic control. In addition to heterochromia, these patients have ipsilateral ptosis, miosis, and anhydrosis (congenital Horner's syndrome). This disruption of oculosympathetic tone is generally produced by natal or perinatal trauma, which usually also damages the brachial plexus.[23,24,30]

○   **Cocaine testing.** We recommend sequential pharmacologic testing to verify the diagnosis of Horner's syndrome.[19] Cocaine (5%) should be instilled in both eyes (2 drops at 5-minute intervals), and the patient's pupillary diameter should be measured under the same lighting conditions in approximately one-half hour. In patients with dark irides the response to cocaine may be extremely slow; it may take as long as 2 or 3 hours for the cocaine mydriasis to become established. If no mydriasis has occurred in either eye after one-half hour, an additional instillation of cocaine should be given and the patient observed for 1 to 2 hours.[56] Cocaine mydriasis results from blockade of the reuptake of tonically released norepinephrine by the postganglionic nerve fibers (third order neuron) innervating the iris dilator muscle. If there is an interruption of sympathetic tone anywhere from the hypothalamus to the iris dilator muscle, there will be a decrease in the amount of norepinephrine released, and the involved pupil will not dilate to the same extent as the uninvolved pupil.

If pupillary inequality increases after the topical use of cocaine, the presence of Horner's syndrome is confirmed. Minimal pupillary dilatation will occur frequently in patients with partial interruption of the sympathetic pathways.[18,56] A partial interruption is probably the explanation for the minimal pupillary dilatation seen in patients with first order neuron involvement.[18,56] The failure of the ipsilateral pupil to dilate provides no information about the site of the lesion and merely confirms the existence of oculosympathetic paresis. If both pupils dilate equally (no increase in the amount of anisocoria), the diagnosis is physiologic anisocoria.

○   **Hydroxyamphetamine 1%.** Hydroxyamphetamine 1% (Paredrine) is used to differentiate between preganglionic and postganglionic lesions causing Horner's syndrome. Hydroxyamphetamine acts by releasing norepinephrine from sympathetic granules at synaptic endings; thus the efficacy of hydroxyamphetamine in dilating the pupil depends upon the integrity of the third order neuron (superior cervical ganglion to the dilator pupillae muscle). If the suspect pupil fails to dilate 45 minutes after instillation of hydroxyamphetamine, or only partially dilates, then there is a sympathetic postganglionic third order neuron lesion. However, if the involved pupil dilates to the same extent as the normal pupil, the lesion is preganglionic, involving either the first or second order sympathetic neurons.

When using hydroxyamphetamine as a single drug screening test in patients presenting with Horner's syndrome, Maloney et al.[31] found a lack of pupillary dilatation in 89 patients, only 75 (84%) of whom later proved to have third order neuron lesions, whereas 14 (16%) had first or second order neuron sympathetic lesions that had been incorrectly localized. Thus hydroxyamphetamine had a diagnostic specificity of 84% for third order neuron lesions.

Hydroxyamphetamine had a diagnostic specificity of 97% for more proximal lesions. From another viewpoint the hydroxyamphetamine produced an appropriate response in 75 of 78 patients with third order neuron lesions, that is, a sensitivity of 96%, versus an appropriate response in 70 of 84 patients with proximal lesions, that is, a sensitivity of 84%. As mentioned previously, we recommend that pharmacologic confirmation of a diagnosis of Horner's syndrome be based on the sequential use of topical cocaine followed by hydroxyamphetamine testing.[56]

●　　●　　●

In children in the perinatal period the presence of Horner's syndrome without evidence of birth trauma mandates a CT scan to exclude the presence of cervical or mediastinal neuroblastoma.[23,24,50] Since iris coloration is only established after several months, heterochromia will not be a helpful feature,[23] especially during the perinatal period. In addition, in children who acquire Horner's syndrome the lesion most often affects the second order neuron.[24,46,48,50] Causative lesions include malignant tumors of neural crest origin,[24,46,50] occasionally benign tumors,[48] and trauma.[46,48] All children who develop Horner's syndrome must be carefully evaluated, including a CT scan of the mediastinum, for the presence of neck and mediastinal masses.

In adults Maloney et al.[31] found the following:

1. Malignant neoplasm is not as frequent a cause of Horner's syndrome as was previously believed (37 of 450 patients).[18]
2. Only 13 of 450 (3%) patients presenting with Horner's syndrome had a previously undetected malignancy. Of these 13 patients, 9 had concomitant complaints of arm pain, suggesting brachial plexus involvement and a diagnosis of Pancoast's tumor.[40]
3. Malignancies producing a Horner's syndrome[19,56] involved the first or second order neurons in 31 of 37 (84%) cases, typically the second order neuron.[31]

Since most third order neuron lesions are benign (idiopathic),[58] while first or second order neuron lesions are due to malignant neoplasms,[18,31,40] a patient who presents with an apparently isolated first or second order neuron lesion causing Horner's syndrome, at a minimum, should have a complete neurologic examination, palpation of the neck and thyroid gland, and a chest x-ray study with thoracic outlet views or body CT scan of the mediastinum and neck. In a patient who presents with an isolated Horner's syndrome localized to the third order neuron lesion, no investigation is necessary. The development of other neurologic complaints with time may alter this dictum and indicate the need for further evaluation.

Thompson et al.[51] have emphasized that the occurrence of ipsilateral ptosis and miosis does not make the diagnosis of Horner's syndrome. They reported 18 patients with ipsilateral ptosis and miosis referred for evaluation of Horner's syndrome who on pharmacologic testing were found not to have oculosympathetic paresis. They emphasize that miosis with a drooping lid ("pseudo-Horner's syndrome") can be produced by causes unrelated to oculosympathetic paresis. The majority of their patients had physiologic anisocoria with incidental ipsilateral lid dysfunction due to such diverse entities as levator dehiscence, dermatochalasis, and myasthenia gravis. The sequential use of cocaine and hydroxyamphetamine in these patients will lead to an appropriate diagnosis.

■ Abnormal light reaction: sluggish or no pupillary constriction (see Chart 7-1)

If one pupil does not react as well as the other to a light stimulus in a patient with anisocoria and a normal afferent visual system, there is either a structural or innervational defect in the iris sphincter. In anisocoria associated with an abnormal reaction to light the involved pupil will tend to be the larger of the two. The failure of the pupil to constrict may be limited to a sector, or it may involve the entire sphincter. The next step is to determine the pupillary reaction to a near target.

○   **Near reaction.** The near reaction can be (1) normal (light-near dissociation), (2) symmetric and sluggish, (3) asymmetric and sluggish (part of the pupil constricts while part does not), (4) absent, or (5) tonic (slow pupillary constriction to a near stimulus, which remains miotic with refixation on a distant target). A tonic response may be elicited on prolonged effort in patients who initially appear to have responses (2), (3), and (4). The presence of a tonic response is diagnostic of postganglionic parasympathetic denervation.[53]

If the pupillary near reaction is normal, the patient has a lesion affecting the pretectal mesencephalic regions of the brain stem, although having just one eye involved would be unusual. If the near response is sluggish, tonic, or absent (Chart 7-1, *C*), the next step is to determine the integrity of the iris by slit lamp examination.

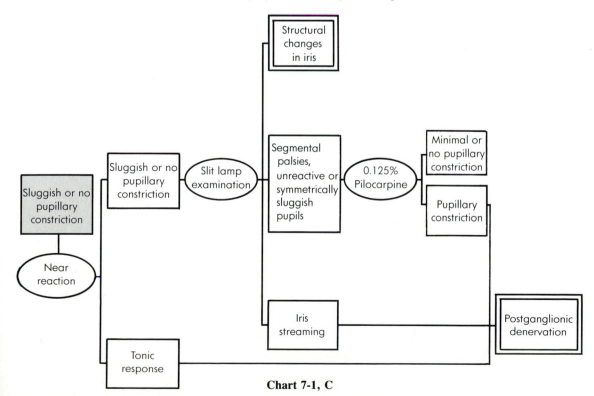

Chart 7-1, C

○   **Slit lamp examination.** Slit lamp examination will reveal immediately those patients with structural changes in the iris, such as sphincter rupture(s) and evidence of active or old inflammatory disease (keratitic precipitates, cells, flare, iris nodules, anterior or posterior synechiae), as well as the presence of mass lesions or rubeosis iridis with ectropion uveae. Transillumination of the iris may demonstrate subtle breaks in the iris sphincter or stroma.

If there are no structural defects of the iris, the entire sphincter may be partially or totally paretic, producing a pupil that is nonreactive or symmetrically sluggish, or there may be segmental paresis of the iris sphincter. There are two types of segmental palsy.[52] The first is characterized by a shifting of nonreactive iris stroma toward the area of the constricting sphincter, called *iris streaming,* and is diagnostic of postganglionic denervation. The second is much rarer and is marked by segmental constriction of the iris sphincter without iris streaming. This type of segmental palsy implies preganglionic third nerve palsy. Those patients who have nonreactive pupils or symmetrically sluggishly reactive pupils should be tested with weak parasympathomimetic agents for the presence of cholinergic supersensitivity, with rare exception a hallmark of postganglionic denervation.

☐   **Postganglionic denervation.** The most common cause of postganglionic denervation is Adie's syndrome.[53] Adie's syndrome is a disorder of pupillary sphincter function, usually associated with sector paresis and supersensitivity to weak cholinergic agents. In addition, patients with Adie's syndrome have regional corneal hypesthesia due to interruption of fibers of the ophthalmic division of the trigeminal nerve as they pass through the ciliary ganglion. These patients also have diminished or absent deep tendon reflexes throughout the body (90%).

Adie's syndrome is seen most often in young (second to fourth decades) women (70%). When first seen, these patients may have a dilated and fixed pupil that does not demonstrate cholinergic supersensitivity. In fact, in acute Adie's syndrome the pupil may not react to strong solutions of pilocarpine (1%), thus making it indistinguishable from pupils that are blockaded pharmacologically (anticholinergic drugs) and some cases of acute traumatic iridoplegia. With time and assumed resprouting of axons from a damaged ciliary ganglion, effective contractions of the pupillary sphincter become more evident, producing segmental palsies with iris streaming and pupillary and ciliary muscle tonicity. Concomitantly cholinergic supersensitivity develops as well.

Thompson[52] has pointed out the differences between the areas of innervated and denervated iris in Adie's syndrome. In the innervated areas (1) the sphincter reacts to light, contracts to near stimuli and to normal concentrations of instilled cholinergic drugs; (2) at the pupillary margin the stroma is bunched in folds with the radial lines of the iris stroma being taut to the periphery; and (3) in the pupillary zone and collarette the radial markings of the stroma tend to stream toward an active area. In denervated areas (1) the sphincter does not contract to light, often contracts to near, and is supersensitive to cholinergic agents; (2) at the pupillary margin the stroma seems spread out and thin, with the radial lines being lax; and (3) in the pupillary zone and collarette the radial markings of the stroma tend to stream toward the innervated area. Although Adie's syndrome is a unilateral condition initially (90%), it tends to become bilateral at a rate of about 4% per year.[53] The affected pupil will become more miotic with time and, in unilateral cases, may eventually be smaller than the unaffected pupil. In addition a small but definite further loss of sphincter function occurs progressively.[52]

Adler and Scheie[1] popularized the use of topical 2.5% methacholine for demonstrating the presence of pupillary cholinergic supersensitivity. Currently 0.125% pilocarpine is the agent of choice, although some prefer to use 0.0625% to 0.1% pilocarpine. Marked pupillary constriction in response to the topical application of these solutions is diagnostic of postganglionic denervation. About 80% (64%[45] to 100%[7]) of patients with Adie's syndrome will demonstrate supersensitivity to this solution.

The lack of pupillary response to light often causes glare problems outdoors or peculiar complaints of difficulty with fluorescent lamps. Accommodative difficulties due to ciliary muscle paresis often cause the patient to have problems with near tasks. If there is sector involvement of the ciliary muscles, lenticular astigmatism may cause visual distortion while reading. Some individuals are acutely aware of their inability to relax accommodation following prolonged close work. The use of weak solutions of pilocarpine in these patients will cause pupillary miosis due to cholinergic supersensitivity; however, this agent also induces marked myopia and brow ache in these patients and is not well accepted by them. Patients who have difficulty reading often are helped somewhat by the use of bilateral and equal bifocal or reading corrections.

Other causes of postganglionic denervation occur relatively infrequently and include (1) traumatic iridoplegia and (2) ciliary nerve damage produced by varicella,[13,37] orbital injury (including surgical), orbital or choroidal tumors, diffuse argon or xenon arc photocoagulation of the retina and choroid, extensive cryotherapy of the retina and choroid, and retrobulbar alcohol injections.

Bilateral segmental palsies may be seen in acute infectious polyneuritis (Fisher's syndrome),[26,38] as part of widespread peripheral neuropathies such as occur in patients with diabetes mellitus, or in the autonomic neuropathies including Riley-Day and Shy-Drager syndromes. In the Shy-Drager syndrome the patients will demonstrate sympathetic denervation as well, with failure to dilate to psychosensory stimuli, cocaine, or hydroxyamphetamine.

○   **Intraocular pressure** (Chart 7-1, *D*). If there is no evidence of iris pathology or postganglionic denervation, that is, absence of tonic response, iris streaming, or cholinergic supersensitivity, the next step is to measure the intraocular pressure. At pressure levels of 40 to 45 mm Hg a relative sphincter muscle paresis occurs, believed to be due to hypoxia of the iris muscles.[54] An occasional patient with acute angle-closure glaucoma or asymmetric, chronic angle-closure glaucoma occasionally may present without other symptoms. If the intraocular pressure is normal, it is necessary to exclude pharmacologic blockade.

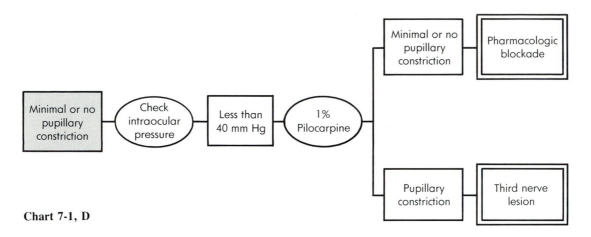

Chart 7-1, D

□   **Differentiating between pharmacologic blockade and third nerve lesion.** Patients with isolated anisocoria and subnormal or absent pupillary reactions and with no evidence of iris damage or postganglionic denervation are often suspected of having a partial third nerve palsy. However, in the absence of ptosis and an ocular motility defect, this diagnosis is untenable. Instead the physician should be alert to the possibility of pharmacologic blockade with atropinelike substances. Patients, their families, and medical personnel often contaminate their eyes unintentionally. People who picnic or work in areas where jimsonweed grows may inadvertently get the belladonna alkaloid from this plant in one or both eyes. In addition, individuals using retroauricular scopolamine patches (Transderm-Scop) to combat motion sickness may also have unilaterally or bilaterally dilated pupils.[10,33] Others may place these substances in their eyes in an attempt to feign illness. Such individuals have accommodative as well as pupillary paresis. These patients are usually seen in a hospital emergency room because of the dilated, nonreactive pupil(s) and accommodative paresis, often with additional complaints of blurred vision.

An additional cause of a unilaterally dilated, sluggishly reactive pupil is the topical ocular use of a strong sympathomimetic agent such as phenylephrine. These patients will always demonstrate pupillary constriction to strong light stimulus such as an indirect ophthalmoscope and will have a relatively normal range of accommodation. The diagnosis is often clinically apparent, as they also have ipsilateral lid retraction.

Fortunately it is possible to distinguish the pupillary dilatation of a third nerve palsy from the pharmacologic effect of parasympatholytic drugs on the pupil with the topical application of a 1% solution of pilocarpine.[57] In patients with third nerve palsies the pupil will constrict normally and become miotic, whereas in mydriasis due to pharmacologic blockade the pupillary response to 1% pilocarpine will be decreased. The amount of miosis will vary in relation to the strength of the mydriatic used and the time elapsed since its instillation.[57] A similar lack of miosis may be seen in traumatic iridoplegia and in rare cases of Adie's syndrome.

Cholinergic supersensitivity, as demonstrated by the use of weak solutions of pilocarpine (0.125%) to produce pupillary constriction, has been held as a diagnostic hallmark of postganglionic parasympathetic denervation of the intraocular muscles. Ponsford et al.[45] studied the pupillary responses to 2.5% methacholine in 14 patients with solely unilateral partial or complete third nerve palsies, 14 patients with Adie's syndrome, normal control subjects, and patients with neurologic disease not accompanied by third nerve dysfunction with normal pupils. They found that the involved pupils in both preganglionic third nerve palsies and Adie's syndrome respond to 2.5% methacholine by becoming miotic. They used the contralateral normal eye as an internal control. One difficulty with their study was the consistent finding of miosis following instillation of methacholine in the contralateral eye of patients with third nerve involvement.

After administration of the 2.5% methacholine to both eyes the response among patients with third nerve palsies and those with Adie's syndrome was quantitatively different if the response in the normal eye was subtracted from the response in the involved eye (third nerve:0.83 mm versus Adie's:1.69 mm difference between the two eyes), but in any event there was a clinically detectable response. A possible explanation for the development of supersensitivity in patients with third nerve palsies may be that a subset of fibers travels directly to the eye without synapsing in the ciliary ganglion.[22] Clinically a large difference in pupillary constriction between an involved eye and the contralateral eye to weak solutions of pilocarpine should be considered diagnostic of postganglionic denervation. If the response difference between the two eyes is small, other criteria should be used, such as the presence or absence of iris streaming, to make the diagnosis of postganglionic denervation.

☐ BILATERAL SLUGGISH OR NO PUPILLARY CONSTRICTION (Chart 7-2)

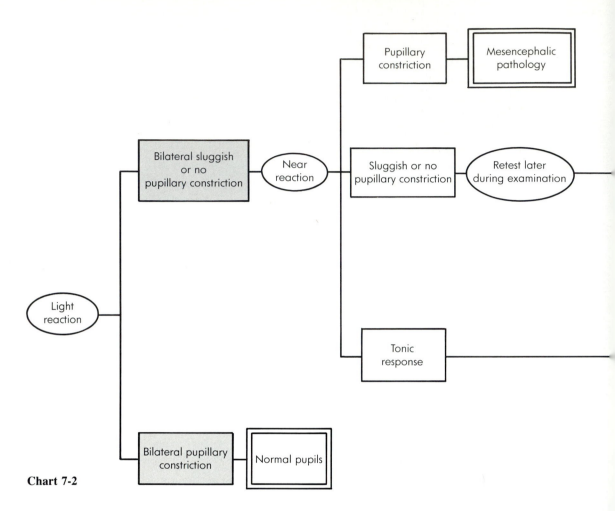

Chart 7-2

If a patient's visual function is normal or near normal and the pupillary light reflexes in both eyes are sluggish, the near reaction should be tested next. If the near reaction is normal, the lesion is presumed to be in the midbrain or pretectum. Such pupils are usually 4 to 5 mm in size, round, and regular and symmetrically react sluggishly to light and rapidly to near. Any disease affecting the intercalated fibers between the pretectal nucleus and the EWC can produce light-near dissociation. The best known cause of this type of light-near dissociation is Parinaud's syndrome produced by external pressure on the mesencephalon from a pineal mass lesion. Other causes of the sylvian aqueduct syndrome, such as infiltrating primary or metastatic tumors and infarction of the mesencephalon, also can produce light-near dissociation with middilated pupils.

Probably this type of light-near dissociation is most often seen in patients with diabetes mellitus, and it has been presumed to be due to vascular changes in the midbrain. On the other hand, Sigsbee et al.[49] have shown that about 75% of patients with diabetes will show cholinergic supersensitivity when tested with weak parasympathomimetic agents. This finding suggests the presence of a peripheral neuropathy, which may in fact

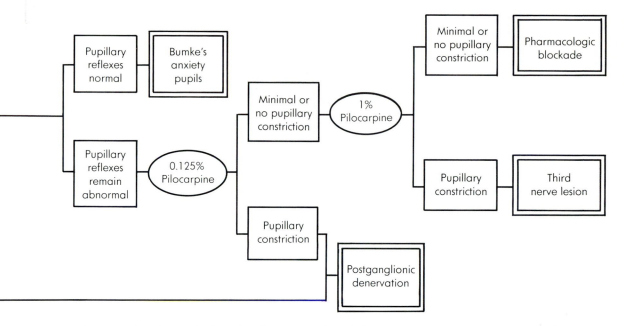

be causative in producing the light-near dissociation. A similar picture can be seen following panretinal photocoagulation or extensive peripheral cryotherapy.

The initial interest in light-near dissociation was due to the report of Argyll Robertson, who noted this finding in patients with central nervous system syphilis, most often tabes dorsalis.[3] The criteria used by Argyll Robertson[3] to describe these pupils included (1) miotic irregular pupils, (2) total absence of light response in the face of a retina sensitive to light (good vision), (3) brisk pupillary constriction to near stimuli, and (4) further pupillary constriction with physostigmine and poor dilatation to belladonna alkaloids. Apter demonstrated unilateral Argyll Robertson pupils in 12 of 46 patients with neurosyphilis.[2] Hooshmand et al.[21] have noted light-near dissociation in 86 of 241 (44%) patients with neurosyphilis. In our opinion patients with unilateral or bilateral miotic irregular pupils, normal vision, and light-near dissociation should have a VDRL and FTA-ABS (Fluorescent Treponemal Antibody Absorption) test. Although the location of the causative lesion has not been indisputably settled, it would appear that the most likely site of the pathology is in the mesencephalon just anterior to the anterior median nuclei (Fig. 7-1).

☐ **Bumke's anxiety pupils.** If the near reaction is sluggish and symmetric and the patient is young and otherwise healthy, or there is a history of psychiatric problems, the diagnosis of Bumke's anxiety pupils[8] must be considered. Under these circumstances the examination should be continued and the pupillary light reflexes checked again later, at which time they will almost invariably be normal. A similar lack of pupillary reactivity may be seen in patients taking systemic drugs with anticholinergic actions, such as those used to treat diarrhea, Parkinson's disease, or depression.

☐ **Postganglionic denervation.** If the patient does not fall into one of these categories and the near reaction is bilaterally sluggish, absent, or tonic, the most likely diagnosis is Adie's syndrome. Slit lamp examination at this time will exclude the unlikely possibility of bilateral structural iris abnormalities; for example, synechiae, sphincter rupture, and the presence of iris streaming will confirm the diagnosis of postganglionic denervation. Even in the absence of visible sector palsies we recommend the topical instillation of 0.125% pilocarpine to exclude the presence of cholinergic supersensitivity, which may be present prior to sphincter reinnervation.

Patients with the peroneal muscular atrophy of Charcot-Marie-Tooth disease (CMTD) are known to have bilateral pupillary abnormalities that resemble those of Adie's tonic pupil syndrome. Keltner et al.[27] have reported a kindred of 15 patients with CMTD, 13 of whom had pupillary abnormalities. These patients go through a sequence of changes reflecting progressive parasympathetic denervation. They often receive symptomatic relief from glare and reading problems with the use of topical 0.125% pilocarpine four times daily.

☐ **Pharmacologic blockade.** If pupillary constriction does not occur following the use of topical 0.125% pilocarpine, 1% pilocarpine should be instilled to exclude the presence of pharmacologic blockade, either due to the use of topical mydriatic agents or to the effect of various bacterial toxins (botulinum, diphtheria).

☐ **Third nerve lesion.** If both pupils fail to constrict to 0.125% pilocarpine but do constrict to 1% pilocarpine, then one must infer a lesion in the midbrain affecting the EWC, producing pupillary paralysis to both light and near stimuli.

OTHER PUPILLARY CONDITIONS

It should be noted that with increasing age an individual's pupils tend to become progressively more miotic. Morone,[35] as well as Thompson et al.,[55] demonstrated that patients with myotonic dystrophy tend to have pupils that are smaller in diameter than age-matched controls and are sluggishly reactive (amplitude and velocity) to light and near stimuli. These pupils dilate well in response to psychosensory stimuli. There is no evidence of cholinergic supersensitivity, since these pupils do not become more miotic in response to the topical application of 2.5% methacholine.

Extreme bilateral miosis (pinpoint pupils) may be produced by topical parasympathomimetic agents, narcotics, or pontine hemorrhage. Awareness of this differential diagnosis is important, especially when faced with a comatose patient with such pupils in an emergency room setting. If it could be established that the patient was using topical cholinesterase inhibitors and he required surgery, then the use of succinylcholine or a similarly acting agent should be avoided. A history of narcotic abuse would suggest that the use of a narcotic antagonist might be of value. In the face of a lack of brain stem reflexes the finding of pinpoint pupils may help to make the diagnosis. (When it is unilateral, extreme miosis suggests the use of topical parasympathomimetic agents, usually one of the cholinesterase inhibitors.)

There are some rare and curious pupillary abnormalities that defy classification. For example, Selhorst et al.[47] have noted intermittent corectopia (eccentric or oval pupils) in a patient with bilateral rostral midbrain infarction who subsequently died. In our experience midbrain corectopia is seen most frequently following severe head trauma. It represents selective central inhibition of sphincter tone.[44] The iris sphincter appears to consist of 70 to 80 separate motor units, which in a normal individual can be seen to fire somewhat asynchronously in low background illumination.[36] In patients with midbrain pathology this asynchrony can be carried to an extreme. A similar mechanism can be invoked to explain the oval pupils seen in patients with midbrain disease.[15]

Marshall et al.[32] suggest that midbrain corectopia represents a transitional stage in the development of third nerve compression during transtentorial herniation. On the other hand, Fisher[16] believes that third nerve involvement in such patients is secondary to a shift of midline structures, and the transtentorial herniation is a late and irreversible epiphenomenon. Marshall et al.[32] have reported the finding of oval pupils in 15 patients on a neurosurgical service, 14 of whom had raised intracranial pressure. Eleven of these patients had suffered closed head injuries. In 9 of the 14 patients with intracranial hypertension the oval pupil disappeared with relative normalization of the intracranial pressure. In our opinion the finding of oval pupils in the setting of neurologic disaster can represent either intrinsic midbrain dysfunction or shift of midline supratentorial structures.

Thompson et al.[60] have reported 26 patients with asymmetric pupillary dilatation. This is an intermittent pupillary abnormality in which the pupil can be seen to be distorted in one segment for a minute or more and then returns to normal. The episodes recur frequently throughout the day and usually continue for several days or a week and disappear spontaneously. Infrequently there may be a recurrence of a cluster of these episodes. Almost all the patients reported by Thompson et al.[60] experienced some unusual sensation in the affected eye, drawing attention to the pupil. Of the 29 patients, 17 complained of concomitant blurring of vision. Of these patients, 11 had Horner's syndrome, 4 had Adie's tonic pupils, and 8 had definite or probable migraine. Thompson et al. postulate that the underlying pathophysiology is a segmental spasm of the iris dilator muscle, and they call this distortion "tadpole-shaped pupils."

REFERENCES

1. Adler, FH, and Scheie, HG: The site of the disturbance in tonic pupils, Trans Am Ophthalmol Soc 38:183, 1940.
2. Apter, JT: The significance of the unilateral Argyll Robertson pupil. I. A report of 13 cases, Am J Ophthalmol 38:34, 1954.
3. Argyll Robertson, D: On an interesting series of eye symptoms in a case of spinal disease, with remarks on the action of belladonna on the iris, Edinburgh Med J 14:496, 1869.
4. Bach, L: Pupillenlehre, Berlin, 1908, S Karger, pp 153-157.
5. Boghen, D: Transient benign unilateral pupillary dilation, Arch Neurol 32:68, 1975.
6. Bonnet, P: L'historique due syndrome due sympathetic cervical, Arch Ophtal (Paris) 17:121, 1957.
7. Bourgon, P, Pilley, SFJ, and Thompson, HS: Cholinergic supersensitivity of the iris sphincter in Adie's tonic pupil, Am J Ophthalmol 85:373, 1978.
8. Bumke, O: Beiträge zur Kenntnis der Irisbewegungen, Zentralbl Nervenheilk Psychiatrie 27:89, 1904.
9. Burde, RM: Alternating Horner's syndrome or Bernard's sympathetic irritation, J Neurosurg 53:866, 1980.
10. Carlstan, JA: Unilateral dilated pupil, JAMA 248:31, 1982.
11. Czarnecki, JSC, Pilley, SFJ, and Thompson, HS: The analysis of anisocoria. The use of photography in the clinical evaluation of unequal pupils, Can J Ophthalmol 14:297, 1979.
12. Dalessio, DJ, editor: Wolff's headache and other head pain, ed 4, New York, 1980, Oxford University Press, p 111.
13. Dubois, HF, and van Bijsterveld, OP: Internal ophthalmoparesis: an uncommon complication of varicella, a common disease, Ophthalmologica 175:263, 1977.
14. Edelson, RN, and Levy, DE: Transient benign unilateral pupillary dilation in young adults, Arch Neurol 31:12, 1974.
15. Fisher, CM: Oval pupils, Arch Neurol 37:502, 1980.
16. Fisher, CM: Observations concerning brain herniation. Presented to the 108th Annual Meeting of the American Neurological Association, New Orleans, Louisiana, October 2-5, 1983. Abstract published in Ann Neurol 14:110, 1983.

17. Furukawa, T, and Toyokura, Y: Alternating Horner syndrome, Arch Neurol 30:311, 1974.
18. Giles, CL, and Henderson, JW: Horner's syndrome: an analysis of 216 cases, Am J Ophthalmol 46:289, 1958.
19. Grimson, BS, and Thompson, HS: Drug testing in Horner's syndrome. In Smith, JL, and Glaser, JS, editors: Neuro-ophthalmology, Symposium of the University of Miami and the Bascom Palmer Eye Institute, vol 8, St Louis, 1975, The CV Mosby Co, pp 265-270.
20. Hallett, M, and Cogan, DG: Episodic unilateral mydriasis in otherwise normal patient, Arch Ophthalmol 84:130, 1970.
21. Hooshmand, H, Escobar, MR, and Kopf, SW: Neurosyphilis. A study of 241 patients, JAMA 219:726, 1972.
22. Jaeger, RJ, and Benevento, LA: A horseradish peroxidase study of the internal structures of the eye, Invest Ophthalmol Vis Sci 19:575, 1980.
23. Jaffe, N: Reply to letter-to-the editor by Spigelblatt et al, J Pediatr 88:1068, 1976.
24. Jaffe, N, Cassady, R, Filler, RM, Petersen, R, and Traggis, D: Heterochromia and Horner syndrome associated with cervical and mediastinal neuroblastoma, J Pediatr 87:75, 1975.
25. Jampel, RS, and Mindel, J: The nucleus for accommodation in the midbrain of the macaque. The effect of accommodation, pupillary constriction, and extraocular muscle contraction produced by stimulation of the oculomotor nucleus on the intraocular pressure, Invest Ophthalmol 6:40, 1967.
26. Keane, J: Tonic pupils with acute ophthalmoplegic polyneuritis, Ann Neurol 2:393, 1977.
27. Keltner, JL, Swisher, CN, Gay, AJ, and Hepler, RS: Myotonic pupils in Charcot-Marie-Tooth disease. Successful relief of symptoms with 0.025% pilocarpine, Arch Ophthalmol 93:1141, 1975.
28. Kestenbaum, A: Clinical methods of neuro-ophthalmologic examination, ed 2, New York, 1961, Grune & Stratton, p 467.
29. Loewenfeld, IE: Simple, "central" anisocoria: a common condition, seldom recognized, Trans Am Acad Ophthalmol Otolaryngol 83:832, 1977.
30. Loewenfeld, IE, and Thompson, HS: Oculomotor paresis with cyclic spasms. A critical review of the literature and a new case, Surv Ophthalmol 20:81, 1975.
31. Maloney, WF, Younge, BR, and Mayer, NJ: Evaluation of the causes and accuracy of pharmacologic localization in Horner's syndrome, Am J Ophthalmol 90;394, 1980.
32. Marshall, LF, Barba, D, Toole, BM, and Bowers, SA: The oval pupil: clinical significance and relationship to intracranial hypertension, J Neurosurg 58:466, 1983.
33. McCrary, JA, and Webb, NR: Anisocoria from scopolamine patches, JAMA 248:353, 1982.
34. Meyer, BC: Incidence of anisocoria and difference in size of palpebral fissures in five hundred normal subjects, Arch Neurol Psychiatry 57:464, 1947.
35. Morone, G: Ricerche pupillografiche nella distrofia miotonica, Boll d'oculist 2:481, 1948.
36. Münch, K: Zur Frage der wurmförmigen Zuckungen am Sphinkter pupillae, Klin Monatsbl Augenheilkd 50:745, 1912.
37. Noel, L-P, and Watson, AG: Internal ophthalmoplegia following chickenpox, Can J Ophthalmol 11(3):267, 1976.
38. Okajima, T, Imamura, S, Kawasaki, S, Ideta, T, and Tokuomi, H: Fisher's syndrome: a pharmacological study of the pupils, Ann Neurol 2:63, 1977.
39. Ottomo, M, and Heimburger, RF: Alternating Horner's syndrome and hyperhidrosis due to dural adhesions following cervical spinal cord injury. Case report, J Neurosurg 53:97, 1980.
40. Pancoast, HK: Superior pulmonary sulcus tumor. Tumor characterized by pain, Horner's syndrome, destruction of bone and atrophy of hand muscles, JAMA 99:1391, 1932.
41. Pant, SS, Benton, JW, and Dodge, PR: Unilateral pupillary dilatation during and immediately following seizures, Neurology 16:837, 1966.
42. Payne, J, and Adamkiewicz, J, Jr: Unilateral internal ophthalmoplegia with intracranial aneurysm, Am J Ophthalmol 68:349, 1969.
43. Pilley, SFJ, and Thompson, HS: "Dilation lag" in Horner's syndrome, Br J Ophthalmol 59:731, 1975.
44. Plum, F, and Posner, JB: The diagnosis of stupor and coma, ed 2, Philadelphia, 1972, FA Davis Co, p 87.
45. Ponsford, JR, Bannister, R, and Pael, EA: Methacholine pupillary responses in third nerve palsy and Adie's syndrome, Brain 105:583, 1982.
46. Sauer, C, and Levine, HNMW: Horner's syndrome in childhood, Neurology 26:216, 1976.
47. Selhorst, JB, Hoyt, WF, Feinsod, M, and Hosobuchi, Y: Midbrain corectopia, Arch Neurol 33:193, 1976.
48. Shewmoon, DA: Unilateral straight hair in congenital Horner's syndrome due to stellate ganglion tumor, Ann Neurol 13:345, 1983.
49. Sigsbee, B, Torkelson, R, Kadis, G, Wright, JW, and Reeves, AG: Parasympathetic denervation of the iris in diabetes mellitus, J Neurol Neurosurg Psychiatry 37:1031, 1974.

50. Spigelblatt, L, Benoit, P, and Jacob, JL: Neuroblastoma with heterochromia and Horner syndrome (letter-to-the-editor), J Pediatr 88:1067, 1976.
51. Thompson, BM, Corbett, JJ, Lines, LB, and Thompson, HS: Pseudo-Horner's syndrome, Arch Neurol 39:108, 1982.
52. Thompson, HS: Segmental palsy of the iris sphincter in Adie's syndrome, Arch Ophthalmol 96:1615, 1978.
53. Thompson, HS: A classification of "tonic pupils," In Thompson, HS, editor: Topics in neuro-ophthalmology, Baltimore, 1979, The Williams & Wilkins Co, pp 95-96.
54. Thompson, HS: The pupil. In Moses, RA, editor: Adler's physiology of the eye, ed 7, St Louis, 1981, The CV Mosby Co, p 343.
55. Thompson, HS, Van Allen, MW, and von Noorden, GK: The pupil in myotonic dystrophy, Invest Ophthalmol 3:325, 1964.
56. Thompson, HS, and Mensher, JH: Adrenergic mydriasis in Horner's syndrome. Hydroxyamphetamine test for diagnosis of postganglionic defects, Am J Ophthalmol 72:472, 1971.
57. Thompson, HS, Newsome, DA, and Loewenfeld, IE: The fixed dilated pupil: sudden iridoplegia or mydriatic drops? A simple diagnostic test, Arch Ophthalmol 86:21, 1971.
58. Thompson, HS, and Pilley, SFJ: Unequal pupils. A flow chart for sorting out the anisocorias, Surv Ophthalmol 21:45, 1976.
59. Thompson, HS, and Corbett, JJ: Spasms of the iris sphincter, Ann Neurol 8:547, 1980.
60. Thompson, HS, Zackon, DH, and Czarnecki, JSC: Tadpole-shaped pupils caused by segmental spasm of the iris dilator muscle, Am J Ophthalmol 96:467, 1983.
61. Vijayan, N: A new post-traumatic headache syndrome; clinical and therapeutic observations, Headache 17:19, 1977.
62. Walsh, FB, and Hoyt, WF: Clinical neuro-ophthalmology, Baltimore, 1969, The Williams & Wilkins Co, vol 1, p 252.
63. Walsh, FB, and Hoyt, WF: Clinical neuro-ophthalmology, Baltimore, 1969, The Williams & Wilkins Co, vol 1, p 253.
64. Zee, DS, Griffin, J, and Price, DL: Unilateral pupillary dilatation during adversive seizures, Arch Neurol 30:403, 1974.

CHAPTER 8

Eyelid disturbances

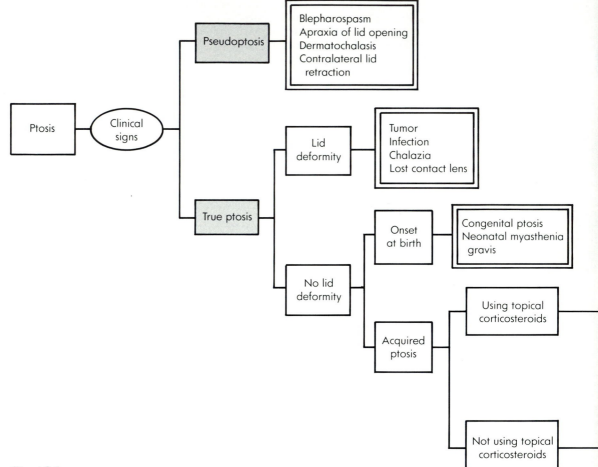

Chart 8-1

PART I

Ptosis

Blepharoptosis (ptosis) is the downward displacement of the upper lid caused by a dysfunction of the lid elevators. True ptosis must be distinguished from other conditions that produce true or apparent narrowing of the interpalpebral fissure unassociated with a myopathy, neuropathy, or myoneural dysfunction involving the upper lid elevators (pseudoptosis) (Chart 8-1).

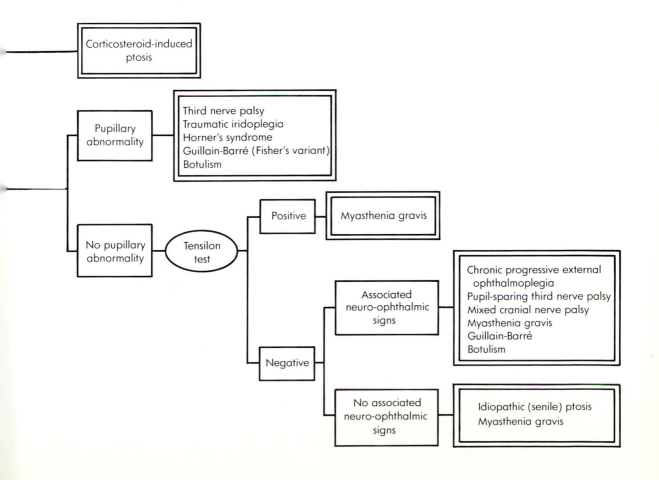

■ **Pseudoptosis** (Chart 8-1, *A*)

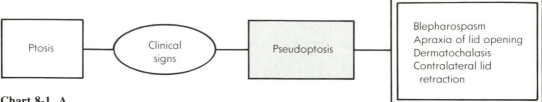

Chart 8-1, A

☐   **Blepharospasm.** Blepharospasm is a voluntary or involuntary lowering of the upper lid caused by orbicularis contraction, which is always associated with elevation of the lower lid and lowering of the brow. The inferior corneal limbus is covered by the lower lid. This does not occur in true ptosis except with Horner's syndrome. Blepharospasm frequently will be accompanied by visible twitching movements of the orbicularis muscle (Fig. 8-1, *A*).

☐   **Apraxia of lid opening.** Apraxia of lid opening is the inability to open the eyes despite normal functioning of muscles and nerves subserving lid opening. This condition is encountered in Parkinson's disease as well as with frontal lobe disease. The lids are closed and cannot be voluntarily opened by the patient, who must often lift the lid with a finger in order to see. At times a head-thrusting movement may result in lid opening.[10]

☐   **Dermatochalasis.** The presence of redundant skin on the upper lid causing narrowing of the interpalpebral fissure is termed dermatochalasis. This condition is usually seen in older patients and will often be accompanied by external signs of protrusion of orbital fat through an incompetent orbital septum (Fig. 8-1, *B*).

☐   **Contralateral lid retraction.** Subtle lid retraction of one upper lid may make the other lid appear ptotic even though it is in its normal position. Normally the upper lid covers the superior corneoscleral limbus when the eyes are in the primary position. Visibility of sclera above the superior limbus indicates upper lid traction and suggests that the suspected "ptotic" lid is in a normal position (Fig. 8-1, *C*).

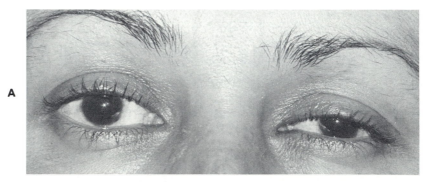

Fig. 8-1. Pseudoptosis. **A,** Blepharospasm: narrower lid fissure on left is due to lower upper lid but also to elevation of lower lid. Note flattening of left brow.

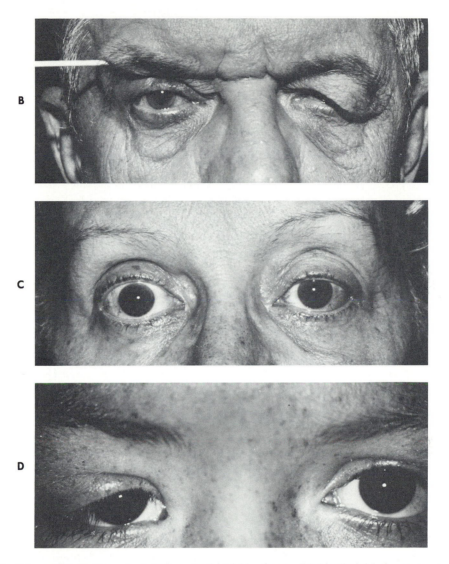

Fig. 8-1, cont'd. B, Dermatochalasis: redundant folds of upper lid skin diminish the apparent width of interpalpebral fissure. Elevation of right fold shows upper lid in its normal position. **C,** Contralateral lid retraction: right upper lid retracted, exposing sclera above superior corneoscleral limbus. Left upper lid is in normal position. **D,** Lid deformity: the thickened, S-shaped right upper lid is due to a neurofibroma in this patient with neurofibromatosis.

■ **True ptosis**
☐ **Lid deformity present** (Chart 8-1, *B*)

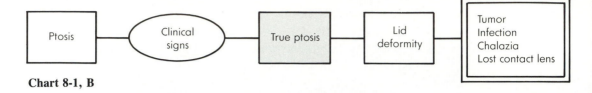

Chart 8-1, B

Once it has been determined that the patient has true ptosis and not pseudoptosis, local lid abnormalities that may weigh down the upper lid should be eliminated as causes. Any extra mass added to the upper lid will, by the force of gravity and thickening of the lid itself, result in its drooping. Tumors of the upper lid (Fig. 8-1, *D*) or infectious processes, which may be acute (preseptal cellulitis) or chronic (chalazion), may produce ptosis. Patients who are contact lens wearers should be asked about previously "lost" lenses. A contact lens may become trapped under the upper lid, and a granulomatous reaction around this retained foreign body can cause ptosis.[17] Double eversion of the upper lid will reveal the true nature of this ptosis.

☐ **No lid deformity** (Chart 8-1, *C*)

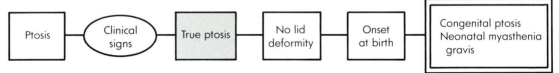

Chart 8-1, C

If no lid deformity or mass is apparent, the next critical distinction is to determine if the onset of the ptosis was at birth or was acquired later in life.

☐ **Onset at birth**

☐   **Congenital ptosis.** Congenital ptosis is present from birth. It may be isolated or associated with difficulty in elevation of the ipsilateral eye. At times ptosis may be part of a more complex syndrome of multiple congenital anomalies (Turner's syndrome, Smith-Lemli-Opitz syndrome, etc.)[9]. If there is doubt as to the presence of ptosis from birth, old photographs should be reviewed. Often a previously undetected congenital ptosis may be documented in this manner, thus avoiding the necessity for further evaluation.

☐   **Neonatal myasthenia gravis.** Children born of myasthenic mothers may show evidence of ptosis or other signs of myasthenia beginning within 24 hours of birth. The syndrome of neonatal myasthenia may last for weeks and may require supportive treatment with anticholinesterase agents. This transient form of myasthenia is produced by the passage across the placenta of antibodies against acetylcholine receptors.[6]

Congenital myasthenia gravis. Congenital myasthenia is a rare form of myasthenia; it is present from birth but, unlike neonatal myasthenia, is permanent. While the congenital form may be familial, the mother need not be a myasthenic.[14]

Infants may manifest intermittent retraction of a ptotic lid during chewing, jaw movement, or sucking. This movement (Marcus Gunn jaw-winking phenomenon) results from a presumed miswiring between the oculomotor and trigeminal motor pathways. At times tearing may be associated with jaw winking (crocodile tears). Jaw winking may become less marked as the patient grows older. These patients do not require a neurologic evaluation.

☐ **Acquired ptosis** (Chart 8-1, *D*)

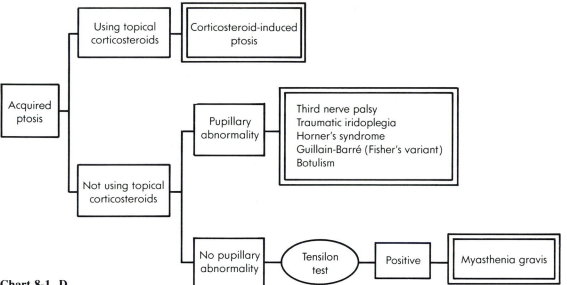

Chart 8-1, D

☐ **Topical corticosteroid–induced ptosis.** When it has been determined that the ptosis is acquired, the patient should be questioned about the use of topical corticosteroids, which have been implicated in the production of ptosis.[8] The true incidence of cortico-steroid-induced ptosis must be small, given the amount of topical corticosteroid dispensed without apparent difficulty. If no medication can be implicated as the cause of the ptosis, close inspection of pupillary size and reactivity should be performed.

☐ **Pupillary abnormalities present**

Several forms of pupillary abnormality may be associated with ptosis. The presence of a dilated, poorly reactive pupil ipsilateral to the ptotic lid suggests a third cranial nerve palsy (see chapter 5). Trauma may result in ptosis and a large pupil, but iris sphincter ruptures or tears will be detected on slit lamp examination. The association of ptosis and ipsilateral miosis suggests an oculosympathetic paresis (Horner's syndrome). (See Chapter 7). Rarely Fisher's variant of the Guillain-Barré syndrome and botulism may present with ptosis and pupillary dilation early in the course of their evolution.

☐ **Pupillary abnormalities absent**
◯ **Tensilon test positive**

☐ **Myasthenia gravis.** Acquired ptosis in the presence of normal pupils must be considered to be caused by myasthenia gravis until proven otherwise. Myasthenia is a

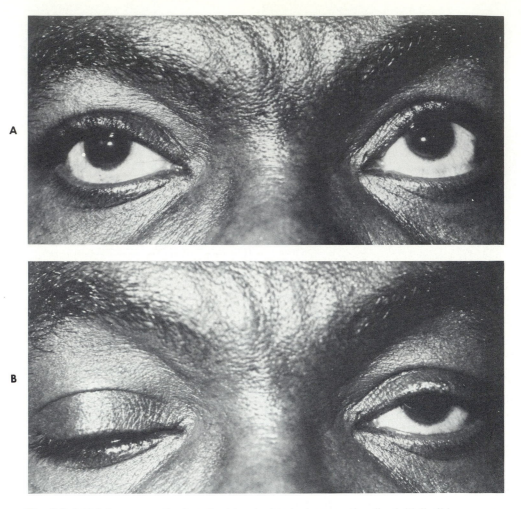

Fig. 8-2. Lid fatigue: myasthenic patient is asked to look up continually. Initially lids are open, **A;** however, after sustaining upgaze, lids droop, producing an almost complete right ptosis and a marked left ptosis, **B.**

disorder involving skeletal and not visceral musculature; therefore the pupils and accommodation are normal. The intravenous administration of edrophonium chloride (Tensilon test) should be carried out in all patients with acquired ptosis and normal pupils.

Myasthenia gravis is characterized by impaired transmission of impulses across the myoneural junction. The impaired transmission is due to the presence of antibodies to acetylcholine receptors in the motor end-plate of striate muscle. These antibodies block the receptor, while some also cause accelerated receptor degradation.[7] Ocular signs, particularly ptosis, may be the initial manifestation of myasthenia in up to 75% of patients.[15] If these ocular signs remain the only indications of myasthenia for longer than 2 years, it is unlikely that systemic myasthenia will develop. The ocular form of myasthenia is said to occur in approximately 20% of myasthenic patients.[4,15]

Variability of clinical signs and fatigability of specific muscle groups upon repeated

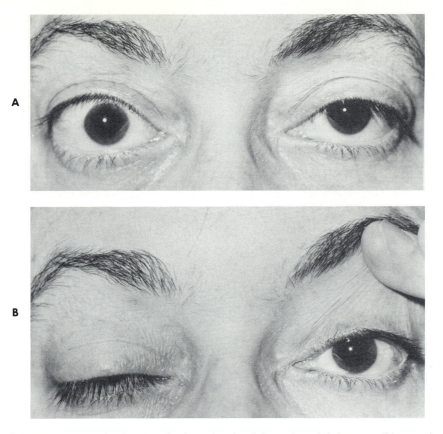

Fig. 8-3. Enhanced ptosis. **A,** Myasthenic patient has left ptosis and right upper lid retraction. **B,** Left lid is elevated manually, which produces a complete ptosis of previously retracted right upper lid.

function are the hallmarks of myasthenia. Ptosis will be improved or absent upon awakening but will become pronounced as the day progresses. Marked ptosis may be produced by having the patient sustain upgaze (Fig. 8-2). This curtain effect of the lids to sustained upward gaze is a useful office test in detecting myasthenic ptosis. Because ptosis from any cause may worsen during the day, fatigability is suggestive of but not specific for myasthenia.

When the ptosis is asymmetric, the patient may use the frontalis muscle to elevate both lids, producing what appears to be lid retraction on one side. If the examiner manually elevates the more ptotic lid, the previously retracted lid will fall (Fig. 8-3). This fall of the apparently retracted upper lid has been termed *enhanced ptosis*[11] and probably is explained by invoking Hering's law of equal innervation as applied to the levator palpebrae superioris. Lid retraction of dysthyroid orbitopathy is not affected by manually elevating the contralateral lid.

Cogan has described the lid-twitch sign as being characteristic of myasthenic ptosis.[3] The patient looks down for 10 to 15 seconds and is then asked to make a rapid refixational eye movement to the primary position. A positive lid-twitch sign consists of an upward overshoot of the lid, which then will slowly drop to its previous ptotic position. We have seen this sign with nonmyasthenic ptosis.

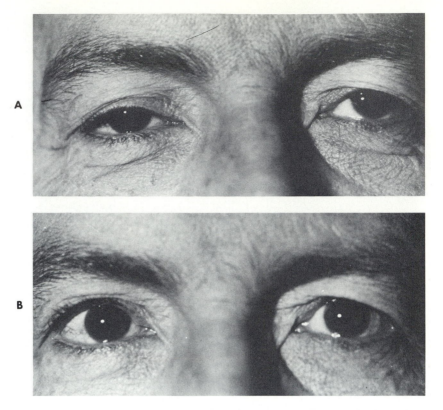

Fig. 8-4. Positive Tensilon test. **A,** Pre-Tensilon bilateral ptosis. **B,** Postinjection, widened inter-palpebral fissures with resolution of bilateral ptosis.

Myasthenic ptosis is frequently associated with orbicularis weakness. While the patient attempts forced lid closure, the examiner manually separates the lids. In myasthenia the lids may often be opened with little effort.

Ocular motility disturbances often accompany myasthenic ptosis. The ocular motility defects may resemble an isolated extraocular muscle weakness, cranial nerve palsy, or supranuclear motility disturbance (see Chapter 5).

Myasthenia and dysthyroidism, both immunologically mediated disorders, are often associated. Circulating antithyroid antibodies have been found in 30% to 40% of myasthenic patients.[12] When these disorders occur together, the ptosis of myasthenia may be masked by the lid retraction of Graves' disease. Connective tissue diseases also are found more frequently in myasthenia than in the general population.

When a variable or fatigable ptosis suggests myasthenia, the intravenous administration of edrophonium chloride (Tensilon) is the next test to perform. One positive Tensilon test establishes the diagnosis of myasthenia gravis (Fig. 8-4). However, myasthenia may exist even in the face of a negative Tensilon test, and one negative test does not exclude myasthenia as the cause of ptosis.

Electromyographic demonstration of neuromuscular fatigue may be present when pharmacologic testing is equivocal or negative.[6] It has been shown that in patients with purely ocular myasthenia the presence of an abnormal repetitive stimulation test in clinically uninvolved muscles does not predict that the disease will become clinically generalized.[1]

Once the diagnosis of myasthenia has been established, the patient should be referred to a neurologist to determine the extent of disease and for treatment. Even if ocular signs appear to be the only manifestation of myasthenia, treatment by a nonneurologist should be discouraged unless the treating physician is comfortable managing the bulbar aspects of myasthenia and the side effects of myasthenic treatment regimens.

Many treatment options are now available to the myasthenic patient. The time-honored initial treatment usually consists of oral pyridostigmine bromide (Mestinon). Systemic corticosteroids may be administered in conjunction with anticholinesterase medications if remission does not occur. Azathioprine[16] and plasmapheresis have also proved effective in the treatment of myasthenia. Myasthenic patients should have polytomography or CT of the chest to detect the presence of an enlarged thymus gland due to hyperplasia or a thymoma. Surgical removal of thymic masses often results in the remission of myasthenia. It has been suggested that all young generalized myasthenics, irrespective of the chest radiographic findings, should undergo thymectomy.[6] We do not advise thoracotomy in patients with purely ocular myasthenia unless a thymic mass is detected radiographically. Even in patients with severe bilateral ptosis, but without thymic enlargement, we would advise eyelid surgery rather than thymic extirpation.

Certain pharmaceuticals that may further compromise nerve conduction should be avoided in myasthenic patients. Curarelike drugs (e.g., succinylcholine chloride) are contraindicated during the induction of anesthesia. Of more practical impact is the contraindication of certain antibiotics in myasthenia. The aminoglycosides (gentamicin, colistin, polymyxin, neomycin, kanamycin, tobramycin) have a curarelike effect on the neuromuscular junction and must be used in myasthenic patients with caution and only when other antibacterial agents are not efficacious.

A myasthenic-like syndrome may be produced by penicillamine, although the exact mechanism remains unknown. Since this drug is used frequently in the treatment of rheumatoid arthritis, an arthritic patient who develops myasthenic symptoms should be asked about ingestion of penicillamine.[2] Myasthenic patients treated for cardiac arrhythmias with quinidine or procainamide may experience worsening of their myasthenia.[14]

○ **Tensilon test negative** (Chart 8-1, *E*)
☐ **Associated neuro-ophthalmic signs present**

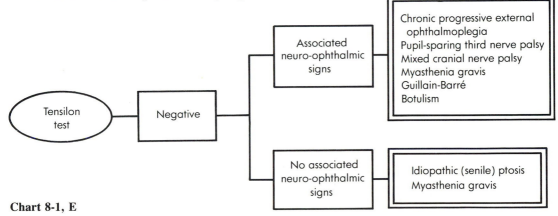

Chart 8-1, E

When the Tensilon test is negative, the examiner must determine if other neuro-ophthalmic signs are present or if the ptosis is truly isolated. Ocular motility disturbances associated with acquired ptosis and normal pupils may indicate a pupil-sparing third cranial nerve palsy, the syndrome of multiple cranial nerve involvement, chronic progressive external ophthalmoplegia, myotonic dystrophy,[13] Fisher's variant of the Guillain-Barré syndrome, or botulism.

☐ Associated neuro-ophthalmic signs absent

☐ **Idiopathic "senile" ptosis.** An isolated ptosis in the nonmyasthenic older patient may be classified as "senile" ptosis. This noninherited form of ptosis is believed to be due to disinsertions or dehiscences of the levator aponeurosis.[5] When the ptosis becomes a functional or cosmetic disturbance, surgical correction may be considered.

Finally, it should be recalled that ptosis with or without accompanying ocular motility disturbance may still be myasthenic despite repeatedly negative Tensilon tests.

REFERENCES

1. Bever, CT, Aquino, AV, Penn, AS, et al: Prognosis of ocular myasthenia, Neurology (Minneap) 30:387, 1980.
2. Bocanegra, T, Espinoza, LR, Vasey, FB, et al: Myasthenia gravis and penicillamine therapy of rheumatoid arthritis, JAMA 244:1822, 1980.
3. Cogan, DG: Myasthenia gravis: a review of the disease and a description of lid twitch as a characteristic sign, Arch Ophthalmol 74:217, 1965.
4. Daroff, RB: Ocular myasthenia: diagnosis and therapy. In Glaser, JS, editor: Neuro-ophthalmology Symposium of the University of Miami and the Bascom Palmer Eye Institute, vol 10, St Louis, 1980, The CV Mosby Co, p 62.
5. Dortzbach, RK, and Sutula, FC: Involutional blepharoptosis. A histopathological study, Arch Ophthalmol 98:2045, 1980.
6. Drachman, DB: Myasthenia gravis, N Engl J Med 298:136, 1978.
7. Drachman, DB, Adams, RN, Josifek, LF, and Self, SG: Functional activities of autoantibodies to acetylcholine receptors and the clinical severity of myasthenia gravis, N Engl J Med 307:769, 1982.
8. Fraunfelder, FT: Drug-induced ocular side effects and drug interactions, Philadelphia, 1976, Lea & Febiger.
9. Gellis, SS, and Feingold, M: Atlas of mental retardation syndromes, Washington, DC, 1968, US Department of Health, Education and Welfare, US Government Printing Office.
10. Goldstein, JE, and Cogan, DG: Apraxia of lid opening, Arch Ophthalmol 73;155, 1965.
11. Gorelick, PB, Rosenberg, M, and Pagano, RJ: Enhanced ptosis in myasthenia gravis, Arch Neurol 38:531, 1981.
12. Kiessling, WR, Pflughaupt, KW, Ricker, K, et al: Thyroid function and circulating antithyroid antibodies in myasthenia gravis, Neurology (Minneap) 31:771, 1981.
13. Lesell, S, Coppeto, J, and Samet, S: Ophthalmoplegia in myotonic dystrophy, Am J Ophthalmol 71:1231, 1971.
14. Lisak, RP, and Barchi, RL: Myasthenia gravis. Major problems in neurology, vol 11, Philadelphia, 1982, WB Saunders Co, p 6.
15. Osserman, KE: Ocular myasthenia gravis, Invest Ophthalmol 6:277, 1967.
16. Witte, AS, Cornblath, DR, Parry, GJ, et al: Azathioprine in the treatment of myasthenia gravis, Ann Neurol 14:112, 1983.
17. Yassin, JG, White, RH, and Shannon, GM: Blepharoptosis as a complication of contact lens migration, Am J Ophthalmol 72:536, 1971.

PART II

Lid retraction

In the absence of primary position ocular misalignment the upper lid covers the superior limbus by 1 to 2 mm. If sclera is visible between the superior limbus and the upper lid, the upper lid is considered to be retracted. While marked proptosis due to an orbital mass lesion may produce a widened interpalpebral fissure, lid retraction is most often caused either by cicatricial or innervational contraction of the lid elevators.

Dysthyroid orbitopathy. Lid retraction is caused most frequently by dysthyroid orbitopathy. The patient may have a typical "stare" appearance, and the widened palpebral fissure may produce the appearance of proptosis even if none is present. The upper lid may be delayed in following the eyes as they move into downward gaze. This momentary "hang-up" of the upper lids is termed *lid lag*.

The retracted upper lid remains elevated in downgaze in the dysthyroid patient (Fig. 8-5). This differentiates dysthyroid lid retraction from midbrain lid retraction (see Collier's sign), where the lids also are retracted in the primary position but are normal in downgaze.

The cause of dysthyroid lid retraction remains unknown. It is believed that initially the retraction is innervational but in the chronic state becomes cicatricial. Lid retraction is not related to the state of thyroid function. Retraction may remit when the hyperthyroid state is treated successfully, but it may remain unchanged or even worsen. No particular form of thyroid therapy appears to predictably influence its persistence or resolution.

Dysthyroid lid retraction should be treated when it results in corneal exposure or a severe cosmetic blemish. Many surgical approaches are available, and the type of lid surgery required will differ from patient to patient. Lateral tarsorrhaphy is a useful temporizing procedure to protect the cornea. Definitive lid surgery should be delayed until the dysthyroid orbitopathy is quiescent and stable for at least 6 months and until other surgery (orbital or extraocular muscle) has been completed. Topically applied guanethidine and thymoxamine will alleviate the lid retraction of dysthryoidism early in the course of the disease. However, these drugs cause a chemical keratitis, are poorly tolerated, and are not approved by the FDA for topical ocular use.[1]

Nondysthyroid cicatricial retraction. Upper lid retraction may result from alteration of the lid tissues themselves. Following trauma, scar formation may produce retraction of the upper lid. Scarring following lid inflammation may cause retraction, as after an attack of herpes zoster. This form of lid retraction is almost invariably accompanied by visible deformities of the lid itself.

Midbrain lid retraction (Collier's sign). A variety of lesions in the region of the upper dorsal midbrain may produce lid retraction. Masses in the periaqueductal gray region, especially pinealoma, are the most frequent causes in young adults, while hydrocephalus from any cause may produce this sign in young children. The combination of lid retraction and downward displacement of the eye gives infants the typical setting-sun sign.

Midbrain lid retraction is bilateral and symmetric but is occasionally unilateral.[4] It is frequently associated with upgaze paresis and light-near dissociation of the pupils (Parinaud's syndrome). There is no lid retraction in downward gaze as in dysthyroid orbitopathy. A patient with Collier's sign requires CT scanning with visualization of the third ventricular region.

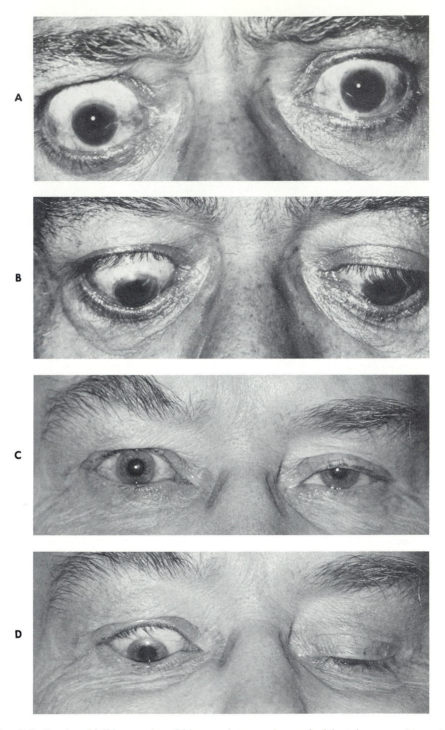

Fig. 8-5. Dysthyroid lid retraction. Lid retraction may be marked in primary position, **A,** and persist on downward gaze, **B.** The retraction also may be mild in primary position, **C,** but become evident by the appearance of severe retraction in downward gaze, **D.**

Sympathetic irritation (Claude Bernard's syndrome). This relatively rare phenomenon, the opposite of Horner's syndrome, consists of lid retraction and an enlarged ipsilateral pupil. It is said to be due to irritation of the sympathetic chain.[2] In our experience this is a very uncommon finding (see Chapter 7).

Metabolic lid retraction. Lid retraction without evidence of thyroid disease has been reported in 13 patients with hepatic cirrhosis.[3] Although thyroid studies were "normal," the more modern stimulation or suppression tests were not performed. Lid retraction due exclusively to cirrhosis must truly be a rare phenomenon.

Volitional lid retraction. Lid retraction may be produced as a volitional act by the patient. This is usually seen in anxious patients who are striving to be attentive. This form of bilateral lid retraction is accompanied by furrowing of the brow, indicating contribution by the frontalis musculature.

REFERENCES

1. Dixon, RS, Anderson, RL, and Hatt, MU. The use of thymoxamine in eyelid retraction, Arch Ophthalmol 97:2147, 1979.
2. Kestenbaum, A: Clinical methods of neuro-ophthalmologic examination, New York, 1961, Grune & Stratton, p 449.
3. Summerskill, WHJ, and Molnar, GD: Eye signs in hepatic cirrhosis, N Engl J Med 266:1244-1248, 1962.
4. Walsh, FB, and Hoyt, WF: Clinical neuro-ophthalmology, ed 3, Baltimore, 1969, The Williams & Wilkins Co, p 305.

PART III

Blepharospasm

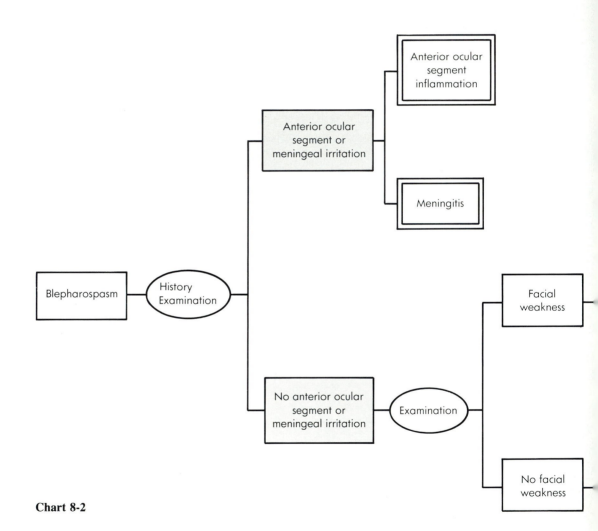

Chart 8-2

Blepharospasm is the term applied to intermittent or constant narrowing of the palpebral fissure caused by contraction of the orbicularis oculi. This should not be confused (but too often is) with narrowing of the fissure by a ptotic upper lid. The clue to this differentiation is that in orbicularis contraction the brow will often be lower and the lower lid higher than normal. By contrast, upper lid ptosis does not affect the position of the brow or lower lid (Chart 8-2).

Having established that the narrowing of the lid fissure is due to orbicularis spasm, the first consideration is trigeminal irritation.

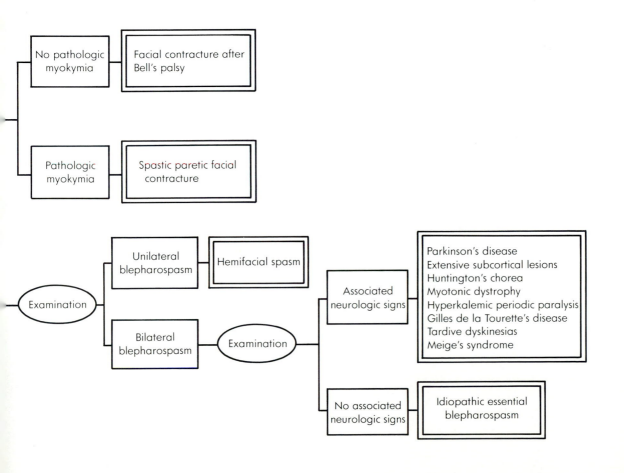

■ **Anterior ocular segment or meningeal irritation** (Chart 8-2, *A*)

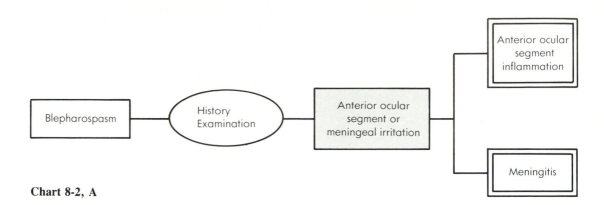

Chart 8-2, A

Trigeminal irritation is a frequent cause of blepharospasm, but rarely of a sustained type. The ophthalmic (first) division of the trigeminal nerve may be irritated by anterior ocular segment inflammation (keratitis, scleritis, uveitis, acutely elevated intraocular pressure) or by meningeal inflammation (meningitis, subarachnoid hemorrhage). The blepharospasm that results consists of squinting and painful aversion to bright lights (photophobia) (Fig. 8-6). Patients can always open their eyes to command, at least briefly. Ocular or meningeal inflammatory signs and symptoms are always evident, and there are no accompanying involuntary, stereotyped facial movements or tics. Patients with this type of blepharospasm are generally more troubled by the primary inflammatory symptoms than the resulting eyelid closure.

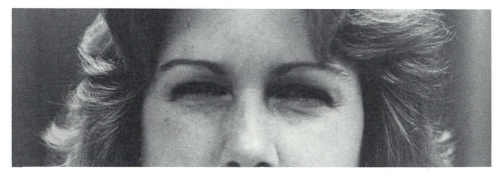

Fig. 8-6. Blepharospasm resulting from aversion to light (photophobia) secondary to keratitis. Note that palpebral fissure is not oblitered.

☐ **Facial weakness** (Chart 8-2, *B*)

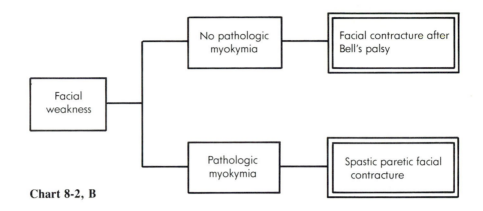

Chart 8-2, B

If ocular or meningeal inflammatory signs are absent, the examiner should look for the presence of facial weakness. Unilateral facial weakness suggests paretic facial contracture.

☐ **Facial contracture after Bell's palsy.** In the recovery phase of a lower motor neuron facial (Bell's) palsy the facial muscles on the involved side may be slightly contracted as compared to those on the normal side (Fig. 8-7). Upon attempted voluntary facial movements a residual paresis of the contracted side will be evident, as well as some synkinesis of facial muscles. Generally the electromyogram of the relaxed facial muscles on the involved side reveals a low frequency of motor unit potentials.

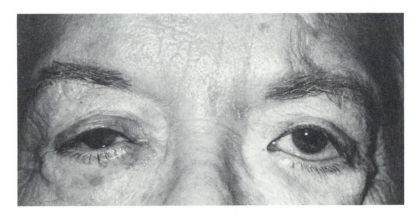

Fig. 8-7. Blepharospasm as part of facial contracture *(right)* following partially recovered Bell's palsy.

☐ **Spastic paretic facial contracture.** In other cases there is no history of previous facial palsy, and the contracture and paresis develop slowly. Superimposed on these signs are vermiform (wormlike) undulating contractions of the orbicularis oculi and other facial muscles known as *pathologic myokymia*. When these signs are found together, the diagnosis is spastic paretic facial contracture. Although usually caused by an intrinsic pontine neoplasm or multiple sclerosis, extramedullary compression by tumor has also been reported.[3,36] Pathologic studies have revealed lesions slightly rostral to, and sparing the seventh nerve nucleus. The pathogenesis of the combination of contracture, weakness, and myokymia is believed to be supranuclear "deafferentation" of the seventh nerve nucleus, rendering it hyperexcitable.[36]

Pathologic myokymia may also be caused by a variety of diseases affecting peripheral nerves. It must be distinguished from the occasional but persistent and bothersome fasciculations that often occur in the eyelids of otherwise healthy individuals, known as *benign myokymia*. Benign myokymia is believed to reflect transient peripheral hyperexcitability of a small group of seventh nerve axons.

☐ **Facial weakness absent** (Chart 8-2, *C*)

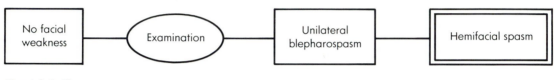

Chart 8-2, C

If facial weakness is not present, the clinician should observe if the blepharospasm is unilateral or bilateral. If unilateral, he must consider the diagnosis of hemifacial spasm.

☐ **Unilateral blepharospasm**

Hemifacial spasm. Hemifacial spasm is characterized by unilateral, involuntary bursts of tonic or clonic activity in the muscles of facial expression that last seconds to minutes.[9] These episodes have no clear-cut precipitants and may occur during sleep. Although some patients have a past history of an ipsilateral lower motor neuron facial paralysis (postparalytic), a majority have not (cryptogenic). Electromyography in hemifacial spasm has revealed synkinesis (simultaneous contraction) of orbicularis oculi and oris[1] but is otherwise indistinguishable from that of voluntary facial muscle contraction.[1] Patients with this disorder typically have no signs of facial palsy or pathologic myokymia.

The favored explanation for hemifacial spasm is that of Gardner and Sava,[13] who postulate that compression or other injury to the seventh nerve in its extraaxial course produces increased irritability with spontaneous firing. The synkinesis has been explained as spread of the impulse between axons of the nerve (ephaptic transmission), so that fibers directed toward one muscle group excite adjacent nerve fibers directed to another muscle group. Ferguson marshals experimental evidence to support his theory that proximal axonal damage results in deafferentation of the facial nucleus and unmasking of "automatic, associated and reflexive movements already present in the facial neuronal network."[9] Although extraaxial (cerebellopontine angle) tumors and intraaxial (brain stem) lesions have been described in association with hemifacial spasm, they are rare.[1] In most cases the seventh nerve is believed to be compressed by a stiff and tortuous cerebral vessel, the anterior or posterior inferior cerebellar artery.[1,13,20]

Patients with hemifacial spasm have had impressive relief of their disorder by a suboccipital craniectomy and placement of a nonabsorbable sponge between the seventh nerve at its exit from the lower pons and the indenting vessel.[20] Up to 15% of patients will have to forfeit hearing in the ipsilateral ear. Some authors question the Gardner-Sava hypothesis since good results may occur from sponge placement even where no compression of the seventh nerve is apparent.[7] Surgical therapy may not be necessary in some patients: carbamazepine often causes total remission or attenuation of spasm to acceptable levels. Dosages must be carefully titrated to avoid bone marrow suppression, hepatotoxicity, nausea, and disequilibrium. Some cases remit spontaneously.

Hemifacial spasm, especially in its initial stage, may be confused with focal epilepsy limited to the face. If there is no jacksonian march present, then the diagnosis of focal epilepsy rests upon finding an abnormal electroencephalograph (EEG).

☐ **Bilateral blepharospasm** (Chart 8-2, *D*)

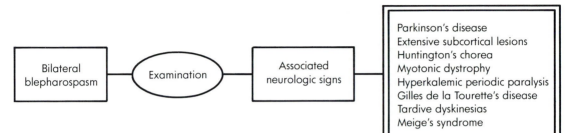

Chart 8-2, D

If involuntary lid closure is bilateral, the examiner must look for the associated signs of Parkinson's disease, Huntington's chorea, extensive subcortical strokes, myotonic dystrophy, Gilles de la Tourette's disease, tardive dyskinesias, and Meige's syndrome.

☐ **Parkinson's disease.** Blepharospasm was reported as a common feature of the dystonic facial grimacing found in patients with von Economo's encephalitis, which appeared in the decade following the 1919 influenza epidemic. Many of these patients went on to develop the postencephalitic form of parkinsonism. Blepharospasm is a documented feature of both the postencephalitic and idiopathic forms of parkinsonism. These patients may manifest reflex eyelid spasms when their lids or brows are touched. They may also have delayed lifting of the eyelids after normal or reflex closure (''apraxia of lid opening''[15]) without orbicularis spasm. Such patients may have to resort to head thrusts to facilitate eye opening. In most cases they must simply wait for the lids to open, because manipulation only results in further spasm (Fig. 8-8).

• • •

The reflex blepharospasm and ''apraxia of lid opening'' have also been reported in patients with Huntington's chorea and extensive subcortical destructive lesions.[10,15]

Myotonic dystrophy is an autosomal dominant disorder producing muscular weakness and wasting, frontal bladness, testicular atrophy, and cataracts. Generally the disease becomes apparent in early adult years, as the afflicted complain of distal weakness of myotonia. Facial muscles are typically quite weak and wasted; ptosis is often present, but patients also manifest delayed eyelid opening after forced eyelid closure (tonic blepharospasm), a phenomenon akin to the slow relaxation of a tight hand grip. A similar phenomenon is also observed in patients suffering from hyperkalemic periodic paralysis, a disorder of muscle membranes.[35]

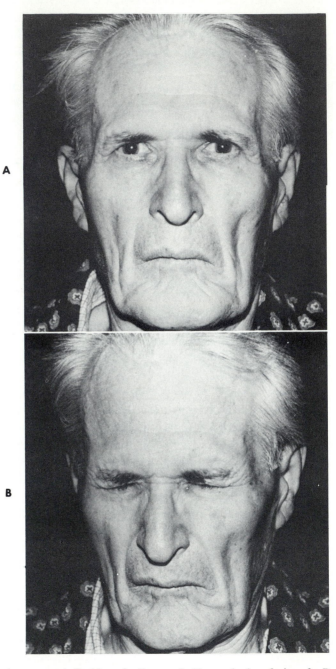

Fig. 8-8. Blepharospasm in Parkinson's disease. **A,** Expressionless facies of a Parkinson's disease patient. **B,** Blepharospasm after light tap on forehead.

☐   **Gilles de la Tourette's disease.** When facial tics, including blepharospasm, occur in childhood, they may be an initial manifestation of Gilles de la Tourette's disease.[29] Having its onset in the first decade, mainly in males, Tourette's disease consists of spasmodic contractions of facial, neck, or arm muscles, sometimes accompanied by vocal utterances (grunts, whistles), often including obscenities (coprolalia). No other consistent neurologic or psychopathologic abnormalities have been described. Signs of Tourette's disease can be dramatically reversed with haloperidol, a dopaminergic antagonist, especially if treated early in the course of the disease.

☐   **Tardive dyskinesias.** Blepharospasm has also been described as a rare manifestation of tardive dyskinesias, a movement disorder characterized by facial grimacing, intermittent jaw opening, lip smacking, and tongue protrusion.[6] Considered a manifestation of dopamine receptor supersensitivity, tardive dyskinesias are seen either spontaneously in the elderly, after levodopa treatment in Parkinson's disease, or, more commonly, after prolonged treatment of schizophrenics with neuroleptic medications, especially phenothiazines and butyrophenones. Discontinuation of the medication generally results in remission of the dyskinesias, but occasionally dopaminergic receptor blocking agents (such as reserpine) may have to be administered.

☐   **Meige's syndrome.** Patients who manifest prolonged bilateral (sometimes unilateral) contraction of mid and lower facial muscles along with their lid closure are said to have the syndrome of blepharospasm-orofacial dystonia, first described by Meige in 1910.[24] The term *dystonia* implies a more sustained contraction than a spasm. Such sustained contractions lead to abnormal postures that change as different muscle groups become involved. Blepharospasm is typically the initial sign, with progression to include tonic and clonic contractions of muscle groups variously involving the eyelids, eyebrows, lips, tongue, jaw, larynx and pharynx, neck, and rarely, the limbs.[26,33] Marsden[23] reported that of 30 cases of blepharospasm, 13 were isolated while 17 showed dystonic features involving other facial and neck muscles. Significantly, none of the 13 isolated cases developed dystonia elsewhere. No patients with this syndrome show neurologic deficits beyond the abnormal posturing. Meige's syndrome remains idiopathic; a single pathologic examination revealed no abnormalities.[12]

The pharmacotherapy of Meige's syndrome has included virtually every drug known to influence neurotransmitters. Based on the impression that blepharospasm was often linked to Parkinson's disease, there was great hope that the success of levodopa in treating that disease might apply to blepharospasm. Unfortunately it has not helped.

Meige's syndrome has also been likened to a hyperkinetic disorder such as Huntington's chorea, which responds to dopaminergic antagonists such as haloperidol, reserpine, and tetrabenazine. Beneficial results have thus far been sparse or transient.[6,23,34] Since an antagonism between dopamine and acetylcholine has been recognized in Parkinson's and Huntington's diseases, several investigators have attempted to manipulate the cholinergic system. But the use of cholinomimetic agents such as physostigmine, choline chloride, and lecithin has met with only limited success.[4,34]

There is some preliminary evidence that centrally acting anticholinergic agents may be more fruitful.[31] These favorable results are consistent with those observed recently in anticholinergic treatment of other dystonic diseases such as dystonia musculorum deformans[8] and spasmodic torticollis.[32]

Several investigators have reported some success in treating Meige's syndrome patients with baclofen, a gamma aminobutyric acid (GABA) agonist.[16] GABA is a central neurotransmitter with inhibitory effects. Baclofen relieves spasticity and helps in some cases of tardive dyskinesia, but its value in the dystonias is yet unproven.

Likening blepharospasm to a myoclonic (sudden, lightninglike muscle contraction) rather than a tonic (more sustained contraction) disorder has led to the use of anticonvulsants. These have not generally helped, although two patients with Meige's syndrome are reported to have responded to clonazepam (Clonopin), which contains sedative properties.[25] Valproic acid and carbamazepine have been used successfully in treating myoclonus but not blepharospasm.

If the characteristic features of a dystonia involving more than eyelid muscles are present in patients with blepharospasm, we make a presumptive diagnosis of Meige's syndrome and favor a trial of neurotransmitter agonists and antagonists and anticonvulsants, acknowledging that they may not be effective.

☐   **Idiopathic (essential) blepharospasm** (Chart 8-2, *E*). There remains a large group of blepharospastic patients between 50 and 70 years of age who may manifest some associated facial grimacing but who have no other neurologic abnormalities. Such patients do not qualify for a diagnosis of Meige's syndrome and should be considered to have idiopathic (essential) blepharospasm.[2,5,18-19] In these patients, excessive blinking is often the first symptom and is passed off as a habit spasm or sensitivity to light. The blinking leads to uncontrolled eyelid spasms that interrupt more and more waking activities, especially driving, reading, watching television, and social intercourse. The symptoms are frequently unilateral at first, leading to the misdiagnosis of hemifacial spasm. The distinction is made by the fact that the spasms spread to involve the eyelids on the other side rather than the mid and lower facial muscles on the same side. Whistling or humming or facial grimaces may at first reverse the blepharospastic attacks, but eventually nothing seems to help. The examiner may be struck by the fact that the eyelid closure disappears when the patient is distracted during the interview, only to recur with force when emotionally threatening topics are broached! No signs of cerebrovascular or Parkinson's disease are evident in this group of patients.

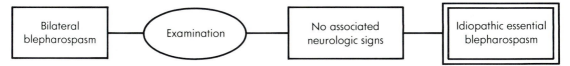

Chart 8-2, E

There is great controversy as to whether essential blepharospasm represents fundamentally a psychopathologic or neuropathologic disturbance. The psychopathologic theory holds that it is a conversion reaction.[21,22] In support of the psychopathologic etiology is the frequent documentation of altered affect,[5,23] especially depression, and the fact that blepharospasm resembles a facial tic—a brief, patterned, predictable, episodic movement usually involving the face. Although tics typically begin in childhood, their onset may be later in life. They are worsened by emotional tension and improved by distraction.

To buttress further the psychodynamic theory of blepharospasm are the frequent reports of relief with placebos, tranquilizing medications, psychotherapy,[21,27] behavior modification,[17,30] and hypnosis.[37] However, there have been no comprehensive reports of the psychic disturbances in these patients, and results of successful psychotherapy are limited to isolated case reports. In fact the frustratingly low success rate of psychotherapy has reinforced the neuropathologic theory of the origin of blepharospasm, which considers it a manifestation of an involuntary movement disorder. Blepharospasm may be the initial sign, with other muscles involved only years later.[19,23] Therefore it may be difficult to tell at the outset whether the blepharospasm is to remain limited or not. As long as it remains limited, we believe that neurotransmitter agonists or antagonists are not indicated.

We consider this limited form of blepharospasm to be psychogenic and advise sedatives, antidepressants, placebos, counseling, and behavior modification. If symptoms are disabling, selective seventh nerve section is the time-honored treatment.* Surgical section must be relatively proximal—either at the exit of the seventh nerve from the stylomastoid foramen, or in its intraparotid portion (Fig. 8-9). More distal sectioning appears to be less effective, although Gillum and Anderson[14] recently described good results with extensive extirpation of the orbicularis oculi without neurectomy. Intracranial procedures are reserved for hemifacial spasm. Alcohol injection at the junction of the

*References 2, 11, 18, 19, 23, and 28.

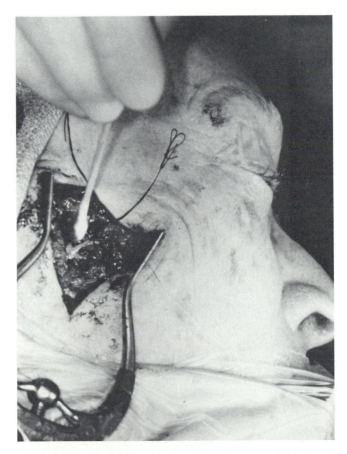

Fig. 8-9. Intraparotid dissection reveals branches of facial nerve. Selective ablation of upper branches paralyses orbicularis oculi muscle.

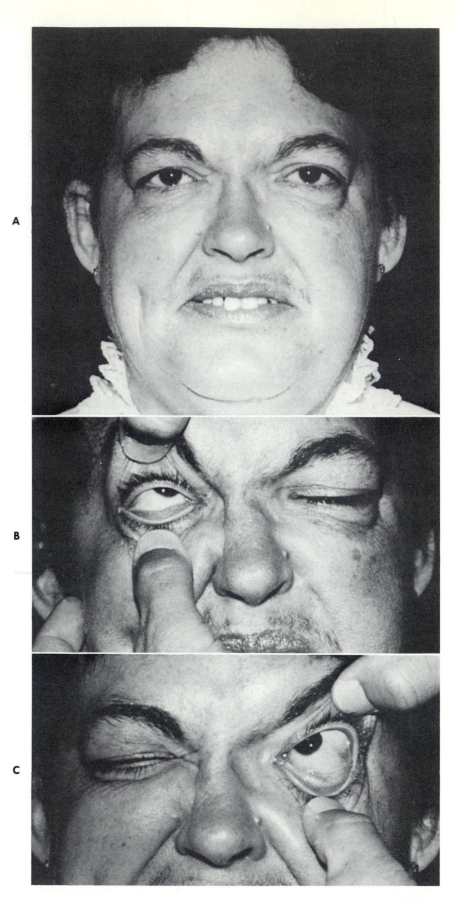

Fig. 8-10. Selective bilateral facial neurectomy for essential blepharospasm. **A,** Patient has negligible facial droop or asymmetry. **B** and **C,** Lids easily parted in face of attempted closure.

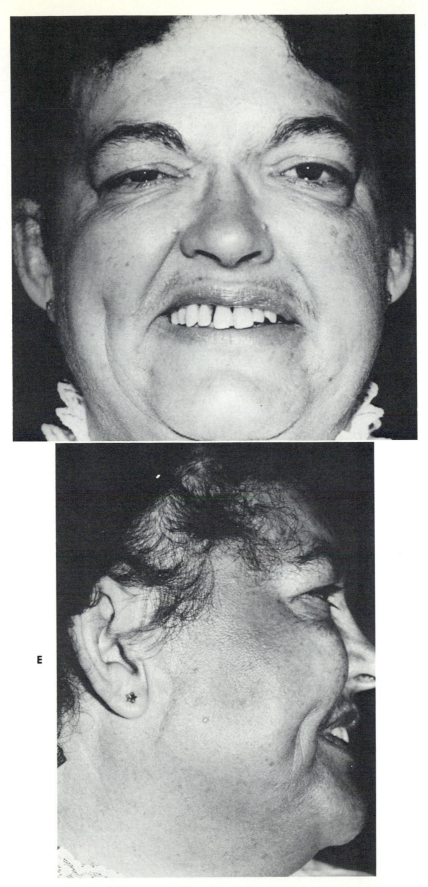

Fig. 8-10, cont'd. D, Smile reveals partially intact musculature with some asymmetry. **E,** Wound has healed without disfiguring scar.

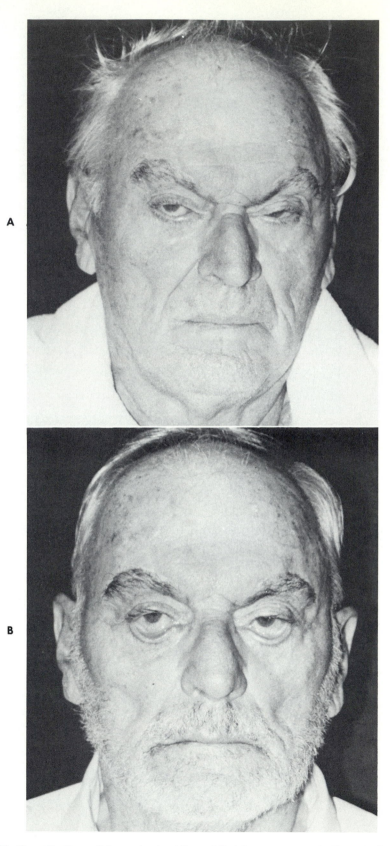

Fig. 8-11. Complications of less selective bilateral facial neurectomy. **A,** Preoperative. **B,** Postoperative. Note loss of facial tone, including ectropion and downturning of corners of mouth.

seventh nerve branches and orbicularis oculi has been largely abandoned because it is painful and gives only temporary (3 to 6 months) relief. Direct injection of botulinum toxin into the orbicularis oculi may offer an effective solution but at this time remains in an investigational stage.

In a collective series of 100 cases involving differential extirpation of seventh nerve branches in the parotid gland with relative preservation of those fibers destined for the lower face,[11] surgeons judged that blepharospasm was relieved in 69% of cases after 1 year, and 61% at 4 years postoperatively (Fig. 8-10). Reoperations brought the success rate to a total of 75% at 4 years. In this series the major complications were lower eyelid laxity (ectropion, 44%), paresis of the upper lip or drooping of the corner of the mouth (44%), and accentuation of upper eyelid dermatochalasis or brow droop (38%) (Fig. 8-11). About 50% of these complications were severe or persistent enough to require surgical correction, which was uniformly successful in averting permanent ocular complications. Patients who have been debilitated by eyelid closure are usually so pleased they can now keep their eyes open that they may not be disturbed by loss of facial expression or the problems with saliva control. In the collected series of 100 cases 23% were very disappointed in the side effects; 15% were mildly disappointed, but only 2% regretted the surgery. Experience has shown that limiting the ablation to the upper facial branches does reduce the incidence of lower facial paralysis but also predisposes to a somewhat greater incidence of late recurrence of blepharospasm—from regrowth of collateral branches.

REFERENCES

1. Auger, RG: Hemifacial spasm: clinical and electrophysiologic observations, Neurology (Minneap) 29:1261, 1979.
2. Bird, AC, and McDonald, WI: Essential blepharospasm, Trans Ophthalmol Soc UK 95:250, 1975.
3. Boghen, D, Filiatrault, R, and Descarries, L: Myokymia and facial contracture in brainstem tuberculoma, Neurology (Minneap) 27:270, 1977.
4. Casey, DE: Pharmacology of blepharospasm-oromandibular dystonia syndrome, Neurology (Minneap) 30:690, 1980.
5. Cavenar, JO, Brantley, IJ, and Braasch, E: Blepharospasm: organic or functional? Psychosomatics, 19:623, 1978.
6. Crane, GE: Persistent dyskinesia, Br J Psychiatry 122:395, 1973.
7. Fabinyi, GCA, and Adams, CBT: Hemifacial spasm: treatment by posterior fossa surgery, J Neurol Neurosurg Psychiatry 41:829, 1978.
8. Fahn, J: The use of high dose anticholinergics in dystonia, Neurology (Minneap) 29:605, 1979.
9. Ferguson, JH: Hemifacial spasm and the facial nucleus, Ann Neurol 4:97, 1978.
10. Fisher, CM: Reflex blepharospasm, Neurology (Minneap) 13:77, 1963.
11. Frueh, BR, Callahan, A, Dortzbach, RK, et al: The effects of differential section of the seventh nerve on patients with intractable blepharospasm, Trans Am Acad Ophthalmol Otolaryngol 81:597, 1976.
12. Garcia-Albea, E, Franch, O, Munoz, O, and Ricoy, JR: Brueghel's syndrome: report of a case with post-mortem studies, J Neurol Neurosurg Psychiatry 44:437, 1981.
13. Gardner, WJ, and Sava, GA: Hemifacial spasm: a reversible pathophysiologic state, J Neurosurg 10:240, 1962.
14. Gillum, WN, and Anderson, RL: Blepharospasm surgery, Arch Ophthalmol 99:1056, 1981.
15. Goldstein, JE, and Cogan, DG: Apraxia of lid opening, Arch Ophthalmol 73;155, 1965.
16. Gollomp, S, Ilson, J, Burke, R, et al: Meige syndrome: a review of 31 cases, Neurology (Minneap) 31(suppl):78, 1981.
17. Hardar, A, and Clancy, J: Case report of successful treatment of a reflex trigeminal nerve blepharospasm, Am J Ophthalmol 75:148, 1973.
18. Henderson, JW: Essential blepharospasm, Trans Am Ophthalmol Soc 54:453, 1956.
19. Jankovic, J, and Ford, J: Blepharospasm and orofacial-cervical dystonia: clinical and pharmacological findings in 100 patients, Ann Neurol 13:402, 1983.
20. Jannetta, PJ, Abbasy, M, Maroon, JC, et al: Etiology and definitive microsurgical treatment of hemifacial spasm: operative techniques and results in 47 patients, J Neurosurg 47:321, 1977.

21. Langworthy, OR: Emotional issues related to certain cases of blepharospasm and facial tics, Arch Neurol Psychiatry 68:620, 1952.

22. Lazare, A: Conversion symptoms, N Engl J Med 305:745, 1981.

23. Marsden, CD: Blepharospasm-oromandibular dystonia syndrome (Brueghel's syndrome). A variant of adult-onset torsion dystonia? J Neurol Neurosurg Psychiatry 39:1204, 1976.

24. Meige, H: Les convulsions de la face, une forme clinique de convulsion faciale, bilaterale et mediane, Rev Neurol (Paris) 10:437, 1910.

25. Merikangas, JR, and Reynolds, CF: Blepharospasm: successful treatment with clonazepam, Ann Neurol 5:401, 1979.

26. Paulson, GW: Meige's syndrome. Dyskinesia of the eyelids and facial muscles, Geriatrics 27:69, 1972.

27. Reckless, JB: Hysterical blepharospasm treated by psychotherapy and conditioning procedures in a group setting, Psychosomatics 13:263, 1972.

28. Reynolds, DH, Smith, JC, and Walsh, TJ: Differential section of the facial nerve for blepharospasm, Trans Am Acad Ophthalmol Otolaryngol 71:656, 1967.

29. Shapiro, AK, Shapiro, E, and Wayne, HLS: The symptomatology and diagnosis of Gilles de la Tourette's syndrome, J Am Acad Child Psychiatry 12:702, 1973.

30. Sharpe, R: Behavior therapy in a case of blepharospasm, Br J Psychiatry 124;603, 1974.

31. Tanner, CM, Glantz, RH, and Klawans, HC: Meige disease: acute and chronic cholinergic effects, Neurology (Minneap) 31(suppl):78, 1981.

32. Tanner, CM, Goetz, CG, and Klawans, HC: Cholinergic mechanisms in spasmodic torticollis, Neurology (Minneap) 29:604, 1979.

33. Tolosa, ES: Clinical features of Meige's disease (idiopathic orofacial dystonia). A report of 17 cases, Arch Neurol 38:147, 1981.

34. Tolosa, ES, and Lai, C: Meige disease: striatal dopaminergic preponderance, Neurology 29:1126, 1979.

35. Walsh, FB, and Hoyt, WF: Clinical neuro-ophthalmology, Baltimore, 1969, The Williams & Williams Co, vol 1, p 345.

36. Waybright, EA, Gutmann, L, and Chou, SM: Facial myokymia. Pathologic features, Arch Neurol 36:244, 1979.

37. Wickramasekera, I: Hypnosis and broad-spectrum behavior therapy for blepharospasm: a case study, Int J Clin Esp Hypn 22:201, 1974.

CHAPTER 9

Proptosis and adnexal masses

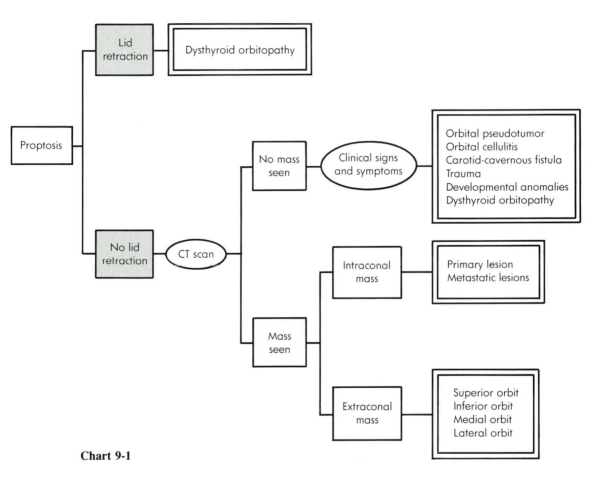

Chart 9-1

Proptosis is the pathologic forward displacement of one or both eyes. The normal range of ocular protrusion, as measured by exophthalmometry, is 14 to 21 mm in adults.[19] Blacks may have normal values greater than 21 mm.[6] While a 2 mm difference in protrusion between fellow eyes is generally considered "normal," any disparity between eyes in a patient being evaluated for orbital disease must be regarded as suspicious.

Measuring the amount of proptosis in millimeters may not be the most important maneuver in evaluating patients with proptosis. Ballottement of the eyes to determine the degree of retropulsion is a more useful test. The patient who has true proptosis without increased resistance to retropulsion probably does not harbor an orbital mass lesion. Dysthyroid orbitopathy and other orbital inflammations, in addition to orbital tumors, usually produce marked resistance to retropulsion. The presence of resistance to retropulsion, therefore, does not necessarily indicate a mass lesion; however, its absence must make one seriously question whether true proptosis exists. The patient with unilateral high myopia may appear proptotic since the myopic eye has a much greater axial length. The pseudoproptosis due to axial myopia is confirmed by the obvious anisometropia found on retinoscopy.[42]

The most frequent cause of acquired proptosis reported in the majority of ophthalmic series is dysthyroid orbitopathy. Therefore the initial distinction to be made in the patient with true proptosis is between dysthyroid orbitopathy and all other causes of proptosis.

▓ Lid retraction present
☐ Dysthyroid orbitopathy (Chart 9-1, *A*)

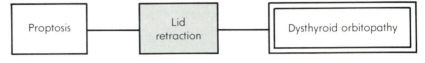

Chart 9-1, A

Diagnosis. The most frequent ophthalmic abnormality associated with dysthyroidism is lid retraction (Fig. 9-1, *A* and *B*). In fact, it would be unusual for dysthyroid proptosis to occur without lid retraction. This lid sign is so specific that it is used as a primary indicator of thyroid-related proptosis. Other clues to the diagnosis are previous treatment for hyperthyroidism or loss of weight without loss of appetite, palpitation, tremor, difficulty sleeping, and excessive perspiration. Even in patients who have euthyroid Graves' disease without a previous history or present evidence of dysthyroidism, proptosis is usually accompanied by other ocular signs such as lid edema, conjunctival chemosis, and injection over the horizontal rectus muscles.

A decreased blink rate and delay in inhibition of the upper lids on downgaze (lid lag) (Fig. 9-1, *C*) often accompany the lid retraction of dysthyroid orbitopathy. The retraction may be asymmetric so that initially the patient may appear to have ptosis when in reality the problem is contralateral lid retraction. At times, however, the classic lid signs of dysthyroidism may be masked by a concomitant true ptosis of myasthenia gravis. There is a significant association between thyroid disease and myasthenia.[26] Since both disorders may affect eyelid position and ocular motility, the clinical picture in patients with both disorders is often confusing (Fig. 9-2).

Mechanical restriction of the upper lid is proposed as the mechanism of lid lag by some authorities.[18,35,63] Relief of retraction following topical application of adrenergic blocking agents has led to the speculation by others that increased sympathetic tone is the underlying cause.[8] It is likely that retraction in the initial stages of the disorder is due

COLOR PLATE 10

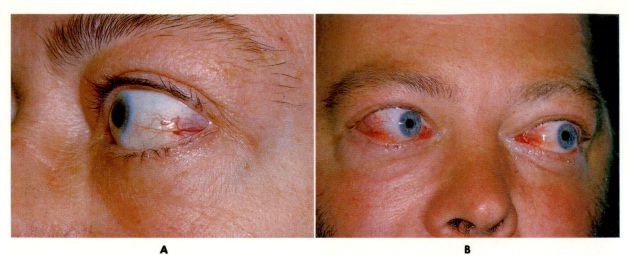

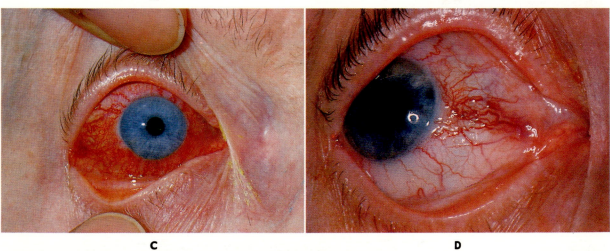

Plate 10. A and **B,** Dysthyroid orbitopathy with injection localized over horizontal rectus muscles. **C,** Carotid-cavernous fistula with markedly arteriolarized conjunctival blood vessels. **D,** Dural fistula with conjunctival signs much less severe. **E,** Diffuse scleral injection with orbital pseudotumor. **F,** Marked conjunctival chemosis accompanying injection in orbital pseudotumor.

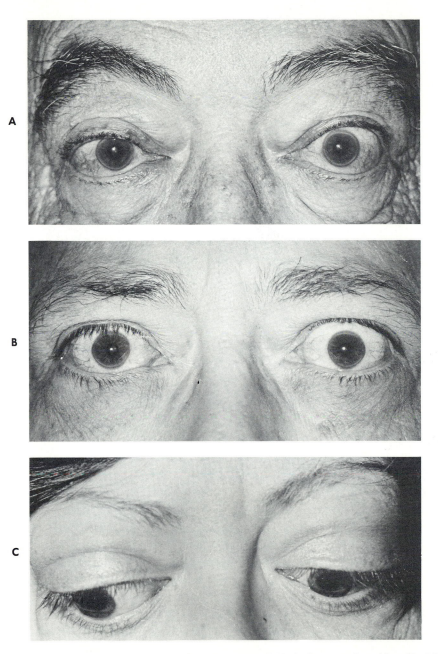

Fig. 9-1. A, Unilateral lid retraction *(left)*. Right upper lid is in its normal position. **B,** Bilateral lid retraction; left greater than right. **C,** Lid retraction persists on downgaze.

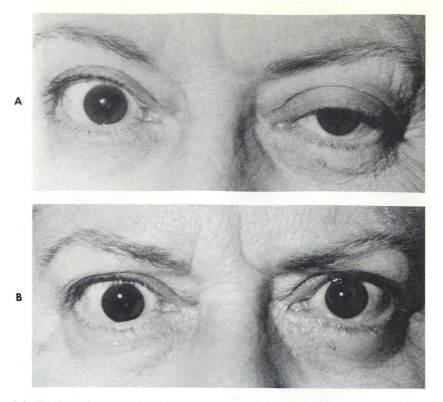

Fig. 9-2. Dysthyroid orbitopathy and myasthenia gravis. **A,** Patient has retraction of right upper lid, but left upper lid is ptotic. **B,** After intravenous Tensilon, left ptosis disappears and both lids are retracted.

to excessive sympathetic innervation to Müller's muscle. Adrenergic blocking agents will reverse the retraction at this stage. Cicatricial lid changes probably account for the chemically nonreversible long-standing retraction.

If lid retraction is present, the diagnosis of dysthyroid orbitopathy is established. No further testing to uncover the cause of proptosis need be employed.

Conjunctival injection over the horizontal rectus muscles is another reliable sign of dysthyroid orbitopathy (Plate 10, *A* and *B*). However, other characteristic patterns of conjunctival injection should suggest alternative diagnostic possibilities. Carotid-cavernous fistulas cause arteriolization of the conjunctival vessels (Plate 10, *C* and *D*) which is particularly distinctive on slit lamp examination. Orbital pseudotumor may be associated with an anterior scleritis/episcleritis, although more frequently a nonspecific conjunctival injection with chemosis is found (Plate 10, *E* and *F*).

Dysthyroid orbitopathy also affects the extraocular muscles, resulting in troublesome and frequently permanent diplopia. This inflammatory myositis has a predilection for the inferior and medial rectus muscles; the lateral rectus is rarely affected. Reduced ocular elevation associated with an abduction deficit should suggest the restrictive myopathy of dysthyroidism (Fig. 9-3).

Dysthyroid optic neuropathy is an infrequent yet treatable cause of visual loss. It is believed that this optic neuropathy is due to compression of the optic nerve by markedly enlarged extraocular muscles at the orbital apex. Visual loss may be associated with optic

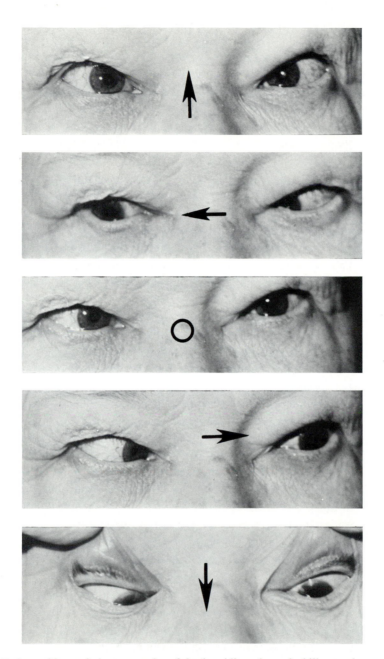

Fig. 9-3. Patient with restrictive myopathy of dysthyroidism shows inability to elevate either eye *(top)*, bilateral abduction defects, an esotropia in primary position, and decreased depression of left eye *(bottom)*. Arrows indicate direction of gaze.

disc edema, optic atrophy, or a normal appearing optic disc.[58] The pattern of visual field loss is a nerve fiber bundle defect that will often involve fixation.

The clinical signs of dysthyroid orbitopathy are specific enough to establish the diagnosis. The only further testing necessary is aimed at determining the patient's metabolic status. A T3 and T4 by radioimmunoassay and a thyroid-stimulating hormone (TSH) will reveal if systemic correction of a dysthyroid state is required. It is our opinion that the Werner suppression or thyrotropin-releasing hormone (TRH) stimulation tests are not necessary in the evaluation of these patients. Both tests may be normal despite the presence of clinically classic dysthyroid orbitopathy.[54,56] The diagnosis of dysthyroid orbitopathy, therefore, must remain a clinical one and, aside from determining the patient's systemic metabolic state, requires no confirmatory diagnostic testing.

The typical CT finding of dysthyroid orbitopathy is bilateral extraocular muscle enlargement (Fig. 9-4). This bilaterality is so characteristic that if the fellow orbit is normal with high-resolution CT scanning, the diagnosis of dysthyroid orbitopathy is suspect. Less frequent CT signs of proptosis—optic nerve straightening and anterior septal bulging—are suggestive but not diagnostic of dysthyroid orbitopathy. If the diagnosis of dysthyroid orbitopathy can be established clinically, CT scans are unnecessary and should not be employed as a routine confirmatory investigation.

Enlarged superior or inferior rectus muscles on CT scan have been mistaken for tumors at the orbital apex. The development of high-resolution CT scanning with direct coronal views or sagittal reconstruction have made this misdiagnosis less common.

Pathogenesis. The ocular manifestations of dysthyroid orbitopathy are in some unknown way associated with an underlying abnormality of the thyroid gland. An immunologic dysfunction may be the unifying factor, although the precise mechanism remains obscure.[51]

Treatment. The primary treatment of any patient with an abnormality of thyroid function must be directed at returning the patient to the euthyroid state. The ocular signs may remit with systemic treatment alone. However, some patients may show progression of ocular signs when they are made euthyroid.

The goal of therapy in patients with dysthyroid orbitopathy is visual rehabilitation. These patients are challenging to treat and are probably best approached in collaboration with other specialists. Rehabilitation often includes some form of systemic treatment (corticosteroids), orbital decompression, radiation therapy, strabismus surgery, and lid surgery. The rehabilitation usually extends over many months, and the patients should be informed of this at the onset. Typically these are unhappy patients who are willing to persevere and who, in the end, are extremely grateful.

From a practical standpoint it is important to determine if the dysthyroid orbitopathy is in an acute or subacute active inflammatory phase or in a quiescent cicatricial phase. The patient with an active congestive orbitopathy must be treated differently than the patient with the same signs (lid retraction, proptosis, strabismus) but whose disease is stable and noncongestive.

The intensity of treatment should be dictated by the severity of specific symptoms or signs. Visual loss due to dysthyroid optic neuropathy demands more urgent attention than does mild proptosis, which is a cosmetic blemish only.

Active stage

Lid retraction. No local medical treatment for lid retraction is satisfactory. Should corneal exposure result from exaggerated widening of the interpalpebral fissure, a lateral

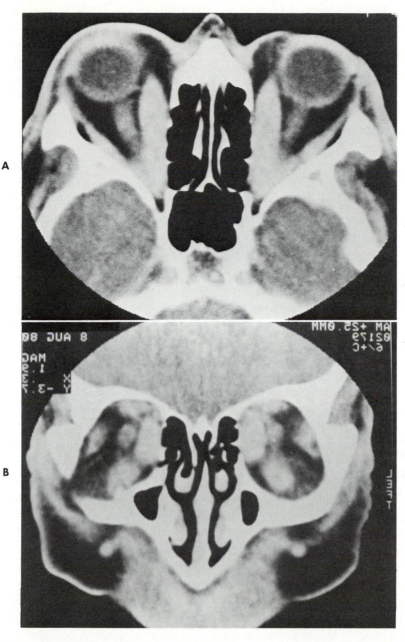

Fig. 9-4. Dysthyroid orbitopathy. **A,** Axial CT scan showing marked enlargement of both medial rectus muscles with tendinous insertion being unaffected. **B,** Coronal CT shows enlargement of both inferior recti as well.

tarsorrhaphy can provide symptomatic relief as well as an acceptable cosmetic appearance.

Proptosis. In the acute orbitopathy of dysthyroidism, proptosis is usually associated with conjunctival injection and diplopia due to inflammation of the extraocular muscles. The utilization of systemic corticosteroids in this setting is controversial, being condemned by some and strongly advocated by others. Early use of systemic corticosteroids is aimed at the control of the inflammatory myositis in order to prevent or lessen the postinflammatory cicatricial restrictive myopathy. Some patients respond dramatically to corticosteroids, while others do not. Recent evidence suggests that this variable response to treatment reflects a difference in the patient's immunologic status.[50] These immunologic disparities may eventually serve as a guide as to which patients should be treated with corticosteroids and which patients should be treated initially with various other modalities.

Patients with proptosis alone and no ductional deficits should be observed without treatment. If patients with ductional deficits are to be treated, then 80 to 100 mg of oral prednisone daily should be given. Steroids should be discontinued if there is no clinical improvement within 2 weeks. If symptomatic relief is experienced, the steroid dosage is tapered slowly (10 mg per day per week). Should the orbitopathy become worse during the period of steroid reduction, the dose is increased. No definitive tapering schedule exists; steroid dosage must be titrated against clinical signs. The chronic administration of high-dose systemic corticosteroids is to be discouraged. Intraorbital corticosteroid injections have been suggested as an alternative to systemic medication. Thomas and Hart[57] report 12 of their 19 patients experienced full restoration of ocular motility following retrobulbar injection of repository steroids. However, this mode of treatment has not gained popularity and is rarely utilized.

Although orbital radiation appears to be effective in dysthyroid optic neuropathy (see below), it does not influence proptosis or extraocular muscle disease.[47] Orbital decompression also has been advocated as a primary treatment in acute orbitopathy. The philosophy behind this suggestion is that less permanent ophthalmic problems will result if more room is available in the orbit during the acute inflammatory phase. No controlled study is available to prove this hypothesis, and we would not support primary orbital decompression in the absence of severe corneal or optic nerve involvement.

Optic neuropathy. There is a consensus that treatment is both necessary and urgent when dysthyroid optic neuropathy occurs. This is a true ophthalmic emergency for which several modes of treatment are available:

1. Corticosteroids. Administration of systemic corticosteroids (up to 200 mg of prednisone daily) may result in dramatic reversal of visual loss.[27] If no improvement occurs after 2 weeks of corticosteroids, another treatment modality should be instituted at once. There is some controversy as to the order of the use of orbital radiation and orbital decompression. Surgical decompression is reserved, by some, as a last resort after other less invasive treatments fail but is advocated as the primary treatment by others.[7]

   In the patient with dysthyroid optic neuropathy we advocate the immediate (same day) institution of systemic corticosteroids in doses from 80 to 150 mg per day. We believe, however, that transantral orbital decompression is the treatment of choice in these patients. In experienced hands it has less actual and potential long-term complications than chronic steroid administration or orbital radiation. The patients are maintained on oral corticosteroids until surgical orbital decompression can be performed.

2. Orbital decompression. Surgical decompression for dysthyroid optic neuropathy may be utilized as a primary treatment modality or as a secondary form of treatment if corticosteroid or radiation therapy fails or is contraindicated. Many surgical procedures have been proposed over the years, but recently transantral orbital decompression into the ethmoid and maxillary sinuses has gained popularity. This approach has the advantage of having no external incisions, while providing reduction of proptosis of up to 12 mm. In experienced hands the surgery is relatively free of complications.[7,41] The effect of transantral decompression on ocular muscle balance is unknown, since no study exists that has measured the ocular alignment preoperatively and postoperatively.

   Inferior and medial orbital decompression through an orbital incision[33] or inferior and medial decompression combined with a lateral decompression[59] have been suggested. It appears certain that the inferior and medial orbital confines must be decompressed for maximal therapeutic effect. The particular approach utilized to achieve this is less important.

3. Orbital radiation. Supervoltage orbital radiation at 2000 rads administered over 10 days is effective and is a viable treatment alternative in patients with optic neuropathy.[4,10] The eventual occurrence of malignant degeneration in the radiated field is a theoretical concern but, to our knowledge, has not been reported.

Inactive stage

Extraocular muscle imbalance. Attempts at surgical correction of the diplopia of dysthyroid orbitopathy should not be performed until the patient is euthyroid and until the measured misalignment of the eyes has been unchanged for 6 to 12 months. In the rehabilitative approach to these patients, ocular muscle surgery should be delayed for at least 4 to 6 months following orbital decompression. Muscle surgery should precede lid surgery.

The diplopia of dysthyroid orbitopathy is due to a restrictive myopathy where the normally elastic extraocular muscle becomes a fibrotic band. Since the inferior and medial rectus muscles are involved most frequently, patterns of esotropia and hypertropias alone or in combination are the rule. Recession is the surgical procedure of choice. Resections in these situations are contraindicated and may cause a restrictive pattern in the opposite direction.

A single operation was effective in correcting diplopia in only 50% to 65% of patients reported by Dyer.[12] Of 45 patients reported by Evans and Kennerdell[15] 30 had binocular single vision restored in the primary position by one surgical procedure, and 27 experienced binocular single vision in the reading position. The advent of the adjustable suture technique, where final placement of a recessed muscle is done with the patient awake and cooperating for prism cover testing, will likely decrease the incidence of reoperations. To date, however, no large series has appeared that confirms this hypothesis.

Binocular single vision over a wide range of gaze is an unrealistic therapeutic expectation in the patient with dysthyroid strabismus. The elimination of diplopia in primary position and the reading position is the goal of surgery. Because of the incomitance of deviations, prism glasses (possibly only in a bifocal segment following inferior rectus recession) may be necessary after surgery. The patient who can be rehabilitated visually with any combination of surgery and prism glasses has a successful result.

Lid retraction. The correction of long-standing lid retraction or other lid abnormalities is beyond the scope of this text. Lid surgery should be undertaken as the last step in the patient's rehabilitation following orbital and muscle surgery.

▨ Lid retraction absent

The absence of lid retraction and other clinical signs of dysthyroidism requires that an orbital CT scan be obtained as the next step in the evaluation of the patient with proptosis. High-resolution CT scan with axial and coronal views is advisable. This one test will answer the next crucial question: Is there a mass lesion in the orbit or periorbital area? If no mass is found, clinical signs and symptoms must be utilized to differentiate between the nontumorous entities that produce proptosis.

☐ No mass seen (Chart 9-1, *B*)

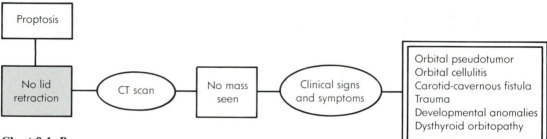

Chart 9-1, B

Two of the nontumorous causes of proptosis are orbital inflammatory disease (pseudotumor) and orbital infection (orbital cellulitis). The two disorders often are confused with each other and with dysthyroid orbitopathy. Carotid-cavernous fistulas and trauma are uncommon causes of nontumoruos proptosis.

☐ **Idiopathic orbital inflammation (pseudotumor).** Proptosis, orbital congestion, periorbital edema, diplopia, and visual loss are the signs of orbital inflammation. Specific causes such as leukemia, syphilis, tuberculosis, sarcoidosis, Wegener's granulomatosis, or collagen vascular disease must be sought but are not frequently found. What remains is orbital inflammation without a specific etiology—orbital pseudotumor.

In this condition any orbital structure may be selectively affected, resulting in the preeminence of one symptom or sign. At other times all orbital structures appear to be involved equally, making the diagnosis less confusing. The ''lumpers'' refer to this disorder as pseudotumor, while the ''splitters'' sometimes divide pseudotumor into different entities based on the structure involved:

Sclera	Posterior scleritis (sclerotenonitis)
Lacrimal gland	Dacryoadenitis
Extraocular muscle	Myositis
Cavernous sinus/superior orbital fissure	Tolosa-Hunt syndrome

The orbit may be so diffusely inflamed that no more specific term than orbital pseudotumor will apply. There is no indication that involvement of any one anatomic structure or region has particular significance.

It is frequently difficult to distinguish between benign orbital inflammation (orbital pseudotumor) and orbital lymphoma.[2,36,52] Retrospective correlation of clinical and pathologic data has shown that even experienced ophthalmic pathologists cannot consistently distinguish inflammatory lesions from lymphoma.[23,29]

Immunochemical techniques have demonstrated that lymphomas are more likely to be composed of monoclonal B lymphocytes while inflammatory pseudotumors are com-

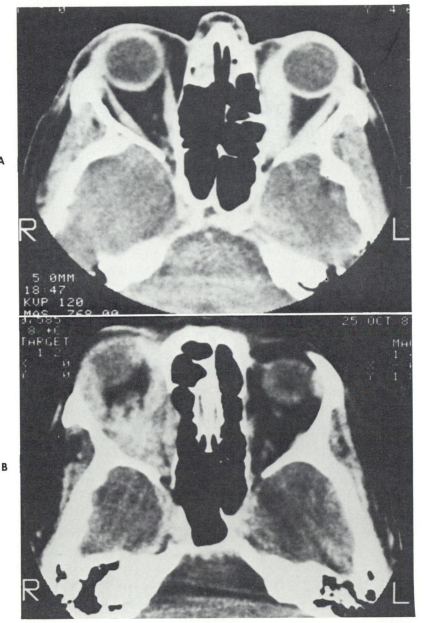

Fig. 9-5. Orbital pseudotumor. **A,** Myositis. Enlargement of medial rectus is unilateral and involves tendinous insertion as well. Left sclera enhances more than the right. **B,** In another case pseudotumor mass fills right orbit, producing proptosis. *Continued.*

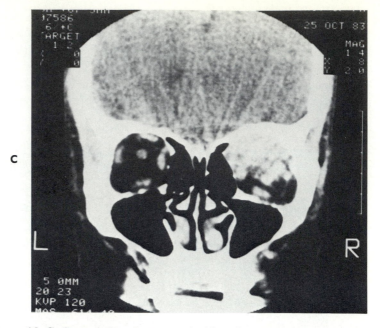

Fig. 9-5, cont'd. C, Coronal view shows mass in this patient predominantly in superior right orbit, displacing orbital structures downward.

posed of polyclonal B lymphocytes.[30] While still largely experimental, this and other methods offer a promise of greater specificity than reliance on histomorphology alone.

The diagnosis of orbital pseudotumor is a clinical one. CT scanning and at times orbital biopsy provide confirmation. The CT pattern will vary depending on the orbital region that is preferentially affected. There may be a discrete mass or generalized increased orbital density. One or several muscles may be enlarged, and the sclera usually demonstrates increased density following contrast enhancement[16] (Fig. 9-5). While extraocular

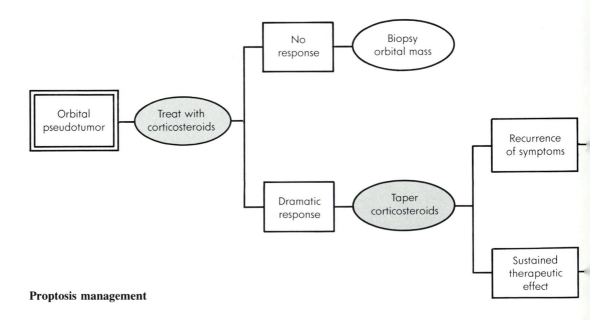

Proptosis management

muscle enlargement may resemble that of dysthyroid orbitopathy, pseudotumor myositis will generally involve the area of the tendinous insertion, and dysthyroid myopathy usually spares this region.[60] Orbital pseudotumor is also more likely to be unilateral. The paranasal sinuses rarely are opacified with orbital pseudotumor.[14]

The investigation of the patient with signs of noninfectious orbital inflammation must also seek to rule out underlying systemic disease. The following tests should be obtained.

Disease	Laboratory tests
Wegener's granulomatosis, sarcoidosis, tuberculosis	Chest roentgenogram
Leukemia	Complete blood count
Systemic inflammatory disease	Erythrocyte sedimentation rate
Syphilis	Serology
Wegener's granulomatosis	Urinalysis

Management. In the patient with proptosis, periorbital edema, ophthalmoplegia, a CT consistent with the diagnosis of orbital pseudotumor, and a negative systemic evaluation, we defer orbital biopsy pending a trial of systemic corticosteroid treatment. So dramatic is the response to 80 to 100 mg of oral prednisone, that a 24- to 48-hour course of the drug has been suggested as a specific "therapeutic trial." The lesion that does not abate dramatically is probably not pseudotumor and should be biopsied. If there is the expected initial response to treatment, the steroid dose is tapered, titrating it to the clinical signs and symptoms. Should a recurrence develop, increasing the steroid dosage will often be all that is needed. Should the orbital signs persist or there be a second recurrence despite the increased steroid dosage, CT should be repeated and orbital biopsy performed.

Some patients with orbital pseudotumor have contraindications to systemic corticosteroids. Orbital radiotherapy, in doses as low as 1,000 to 2,000 rads, is an acceptable alternative.[52]

Some patients with chronic recurrent orbital pseudotumor (myositis) may be treated with chlorambucil.[3]

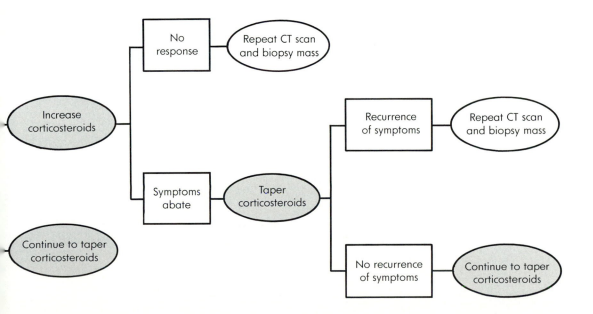

☐   **Orbital cellulitis.** Proptosis, periorbital swelling, and ophthalmoplegia in a febrile patient suggest the possibility of orbital cellulitis. The presence of ophthalmoplegia implies true orbital involvement by the infection, while periorbital edema suggests the infection is limited to the preseptal area.

Patients with cellulitis are almost invariably febrile and have a leukocytosis. The absence of fever in any untreated patient militates strongly against orbital cellulitis. Most patients will have concomitant sinus disease, with the ethmoid sinus involved most often. The maxillary and frontal sinuses are less frequently affected, although pansinusitis is not unusual[17,64] (Fig. 9-6).

In case of trauma a retained intraorbital foreign body may be serving as a nidus for continued infection. A nonmetallic foreign body such as wood may be difficult to visualize even with high-resolution CT, but with alteration of CT window settings it may be detected. The foreign body must be removed.[65]

The initial investigation of suspected nontraumatic orbital cellulitis must be aimed at identifying the causative organism. To this end, cultures of the blood and of purulent exudates from the nasal cavity and conjunctiva are obtained prior to the institution of any antibiotic therapy. The blood culture is the most critical of these tests, since the conjunctiva and nasal cavity are not sterile and noncausative organisms may grow in culture. The most likely organisms to be found on blood culture are *Hemophilus influenzae, Staphylococcus aureus,* and *Streptococcus pneumoniae*. Once an organism is identified, specific intravenous antibiotic therapy is prescribed. Initially, after cultures have been obtained, intravenous broad-spectrum antibiotics are used to ensure that each of the most common causative organisms is covered.

While bacteria are the organisms that invade the orbit most frequently, the presence of more exotic microbes should not be overlooked. Fungal infection may exist alone or in combination with bacterial cellulitis, especially following perforating orbital trauma with organic matter. In these instances, specific cultures must be done to detect these organisms.

Any diabetic or immunologically compromised patient who develops signs of orbital inflammation should be considered to have orbital mucormycosis until proven otherwise. Diabetic patients need not be in ketoacidosis. The nonseptate hyphae of mucormycosis cause an obliterative arteritis with necrotic lesions in the orbit and nasal cavity. If mucormycosis is suspected, complete nasal examination should be performed to detect the typical black eschars of mucor. Treatment consists of extensive surgical debridement and amphotericin B.

Immune competent patients with bacterial cellulitis usually begin to respond to appropriate antibiotic treatment within 3 to 4 days. If the condition fails to respond to appropriate antibiotic therapy, we recommend the following sequence of actions:

1. Check cultures of organisms growing and sensitivities to the antibiotics being administered. If the incorrect antibiotics are being utilized, substitute the appropriate ones.
2. If the organisms are sensitive to the antibiotics being utilized or if no organism is growing, repeat the CT scan:
   a. No mass in the orbit or paranasal sinuses suggests that the correct diagnosis is orbital pseudotumor. Antibiotics are discontinued, and systemic corticosteroids begun (see pseudotumor discussion).

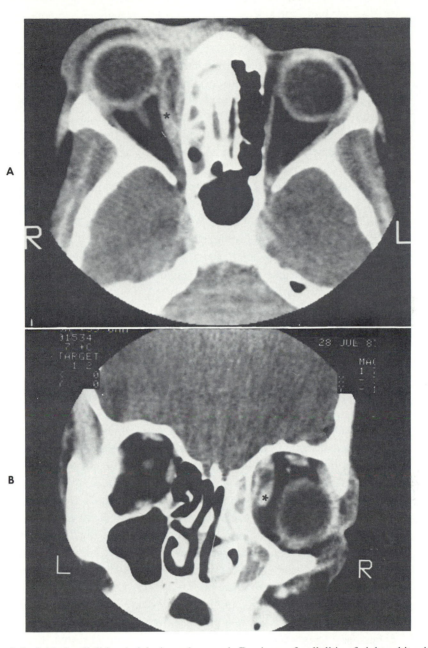

Fig. 9-6. Orbital cellulitis. Axial, **A,** and coronal, **B,** views of cellulitis of right orbit with right ethmoid and maxillary opacification. There is lateral and downward displacement of right eye. Right medial rectus (*) is elevated by a subperiosteal abscess.

    b. Discovery of an intraorbital, subperiosteal, or sinus abscess requires surgical drainage (Fig. 9-6).

    c. A mass that has developed or become more prominent requires immediate biopsy to rule out neoplasm (e.g., rhabdomyosarcoma, neuroblastoma).

☐ **Carotid-cavernous fistula.** Proptosis associated with chronic conjunctival injection and an audible bruit is highly suggestive of a fistula between the carotid artery and the cavernous sinus. In a series from the Mayo Clinic of 74 patients with carotid-cavernous fistulas, 86% had conjunctival injection, 85% had proptosis, and 82% had an audible bruit.[43] Arterialization of conjunctival veins is the response to sustained arterial blood flow directly into venous channels (Plate 10, *C*). The intraocular pressure may be elevated due to the increased episcleral venous pressure. Machinelike bruits, synchronous with the pulse, may be detected with a stethoscope placed over the patient's eye or temporal area.

Double vision was a complaint of 47% of the 74 patients in the Mayo Clinic series. Sixth nerve paresis was present in 51% of the patients (presumably some were asymptomatic), while third cranial nerve paresis was present in 38%, and fourth cranial nerve paresis was present in 24% of the patients.[43]

There are five potential causes of visual loss with carotid-cavernous fistulas[43,48]:

1. Glaucoma due either to increased episcleral venous pressure or rarely to iris neovascularization
2. Anterior segment ischemia
3. Corneal decompensation from exposure
4. Cystoid macular edema or hemorrhage in the macula
5. Retinal artery occlusion

Neither the relative prevalence of the contribution of these mechanisms to visual loss nor the prevalence of visual loss itself can be extracted from the available literature. It is our impression that visual loss from any of these mechanisms is rare.

While the ocular signs are usually ipsilateral to the fistula, bilateral signs may appear with unilateral fistula, and rarely the ocular manifestations may be contralateral to the fistula. In the series of Sanders and Hoyt[48] 72% of carotid-cavernous fistulas followed trauma, while in the Mayo Clinic series[43] 53% followed trauma. Some fistulas occur without apparent cause. Nontraumatic spontaneous fistula may result from the rupture of an intracavernous carotid aneurysm. Fistulas with direct communication between the carotid artery and the cavernous sinus are usually high-flow fistulas, which result in more exaggerated ocular signs. Communication between the carotid system and the dural vessels of the cavernous sinus produces a low-flow fistula,[39] in which the ocular signs are recognizable but less severe[45] (Plate 10, *D*).

Spontaneous resolution of these fistulas may occur. Sattler[49] collected 16 examples of spontaneous thrombosis of a probable high-flow fistula in 322 cases. Henderson and Schneider[20] report one instance of regression of an untreated direct carotid-cavernous fistula in 17 cases. Phelps et al.,[45] however, report spontaneous closure of the fistula in 9 of their 19 patients with dural fistulas. It appears that the rate of spontaneous closure is about 5% in high-flow, direct carotid-cavernous fistulas and may approach 50% in low-flow, dural-cavernous fistulas.

The most consistent CT sign of carotid fistula is an enlarged superior ophthalmic vein. However, this sign may be present in any process that causes increased pressure in

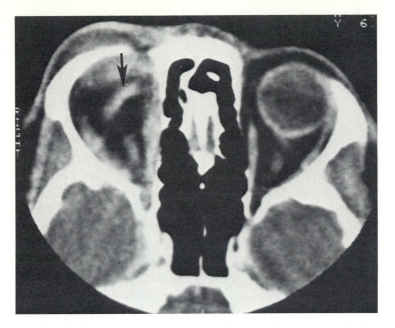

Fig. 9-7. Enlarged superior ophthalmic vein *(arrow)* and enlarged lateral and medial rectus muscles in a patient with a carotid cavernous fistula.

the cavernous sinus. Enlargement of the extraocular muscles may be found on CT with carotid-cavernous fistulas (Fig. 9-7).

The definitive diagnosis of carotid-cavernous fistula is made by angiography. While digital subtraction intravenous techniques are sufficient to document the presence of a fistula, intraarterial angiography with selective catherization is needed to detect all fistulous communications before treatment should be attempted.

The most serious long-term consequence of carotid-cavernous fistulas is loss of vision.[48] We recommend treatment of carotid-cavernous fistulas in the following instances:

1. When there is imminent danger of loss of vision
2. When the continuous noise produced by the intracranial bruit is a severe disturbance to the patient
3. When there is intractable or incapacitating periocular pain due to ischemia or corneal exposure
4. When the cosmetic blemish is producing functional limitation of the patient

Several sophisticated methods of obstructing a carotid-cavernous fistula while preserving carotid patency are available. Debrun et al.[5] have popularized the technique in which detachable balloons are placed in the cavernous sinus through a transarterial route in the treatment of direct carotid-cavernous fistula. The obstruction of the cavernous sinus by the balloon preserved carotid patency in 59% of the 54 patients in this series.

Fistulas also may be closed by inducing thrombosis of the cavernous sinus by direct introduction of thrombogenic material (Gelfoam, oxidized cellulose, balloon) through the ophthalmic vein or the superior petrosal sinus. Thrombogenic needles or wires also may be introduced into the cavernous sinus through a temporal craniotomy.[37] Direct surgical repair of a fistula is possible but technically difficult.[9,44]

Where the fistula is supplied by branches of the external carotid artery system, these abnormal communications may be closed by selective catherization and the injection of particulate material (polyvinyl alcohol or gelfoam powder) or intravascular adhesive.[61]

We advise that selective intraarterial angiography be performed in all patients with signs suggestive of carotid-cavernous fistula if they are candidates for therapeutic intervention. Presently we advocate detachable balloon occlusion of carotid-cavernous fistulas with preservation of carotid flow in direct fistulas. Fistulas from the external carotid circulation should be treated by direct embolization of the fistulous artery with particulate material or intravascular adhesives.

☐   **Trauma.** Trauma to the orbital region may produce acute proptosis with a varying amount of ophthalmoplegia. The trauma producing this clinical picture is due to retrobulbar accumulations of blood, which are easily detectable by CT scan. An expanding retrobulbar hemorrhage may result in progressive proptosis. The increasing intraorbital pressure can raise intraocular pressure to the point where the central retinal artery pulsates. In this circumstance, immediate opening of the orbital septum through an inferior cul-de-sac approach is recommended. This is more safely performed utilizing a controlled incision. Needling of the retrobulbar space is to be discouraged.

☐   **Developmental anomalies.** Orbital hemorrhage may cause acute proptosis without preceding trauma. Spontaneous orbital hemorrhage is usually a dramatic event characterized by pain, proptosis, ophthalmoplegia, ecchymosis of the eyelids, and loss of vision in some patients. The most frequently discovered underlying abnormality in these patients is a congenital venous anomaly (varix).[32]

Exophthalmos may occur in developmental anomalies of the skull, especially the craniostenoses.[21,31] Abnormal fusion of the bones of the skull results in shallow orbits and proptosis. In some instances, raising intraorbital pressure (as in crying) may result in forward luxation of the eye, with the lids coming to rest behind the globe. This is not a difficult diagnosis to make if there is severe malformation of the skull. However, a spectrum does exist so that minimal skull anomalies causing proptosis may go undetected. Oxycephaly (tower skull) and dysostosis craniofacialis (Crouzon's disease) are the developmental anomalies that most often produce proptosis. The use of modern neurosurgical techniques of midfacial reconstruction has improved the cosmetic appearance of many of these individuals.

☐ **Mass lesions seen** (Chart 9-1, *C*)

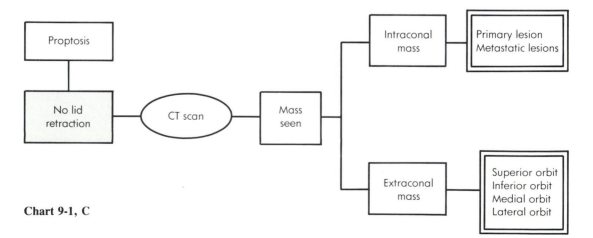

Chart 9-1, C

A large number of different mass lesions may exist in the orbit or invade it from without. The types of tumors will vary with the age of the patient. The location of the mass in the orbit is frequently a clue to its nature. We will consider separately those masses that are intraconal (within the cone of the extraocular muscles) and those that are extraconal.

☐ **Intraconal mass**

Intraconal mass lesions produce forward displacement of the globe. This is true whether the lesion is primary or metastatic, benign or malignant. Primary masses arise from structures normally found in the orbit. CT scan cannot establish the histology of orbital tumors, although the sharpness of margins, the presence of a capsule, or the degree of vascularity as seen by contrast enhancement makes certain lesions more likely than others.

☐ **Primary lesions.** Hemangiomas, among the most common orbital tumors, may occur anywhere in the orbit but have an affinity for the intraconal space. Cavernous hemangiomas are found mainly in adults and enlarge slowly over many years. A well-encapsulated mass that enhances markedly after intravenous contrast injection is characteristic of these lesions (Fig. 9-8). While proptosis is usually the only sign, at times optic nerve compression with visual loss can result. Complete surgical excision of hemangiomas within their capsule is the treatment of choice.

Venous anomalies (varices) may also cause proptosis. Some patients will experience increased proptosis on Valsalva maneuver or bending forward. Bleeding from orbital varices may produce painful proptosis, which may be associated wtih a subconjunctival hemorrhage. The CT picture of a venous varix is usually distinctive enough to establish

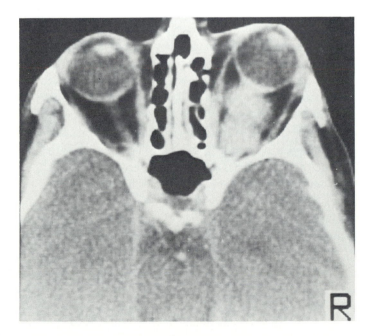

Fig. 9-8. Intraconal hemangioma. Contrast enhancing intraconal mass lesion producing forward displacement of right eye.

the diagnosis, although orbital venography may be necessary in rare instances. Surgical removal of a venous varix is seldom necessary and usually not possible.

Primary tumors of the optic nerve will also result in forward proptosis. In children gliomas are more frequent, while in adults, meningiomas are found with greater regularity. Children with orbital meningiomas may manifest other evidence of neurofibromatosis (3 of 25 patients in one series[25]).

Meningiomas arising from the intraorbital portion of the optic nerve sheath will produce proptosis and slowly progressive visual loss. While motility disturbances are possible, diplopia is not usually a prominent finding unless a large exophytic component produces horizontal or vertical displacement of the globe. The "typical" patient with an optic nerve sheath meningioma is a middle-aged woman with progressive visual loss and mild proptosis. The visual loss is due to optic nerve compression, with the final stages characterized by blindness and optic atrophy often accompanied by optociliary shunt vessels on the optic nerve head (Plate 9, A, Chapter 3). Visual loss and not proptosis is the predominant feature of optic nerve sheath meningiomas.[66]

Enlargement of the optic nerve with increased density peripherally and decreased density centrally is said to be the characteristic CT finding of an optic nerve sheath meningioma. Diffuse enlargement of the optic nerve, at times with angulation, is also consistent with meningioma. The meningioma may involve the entire intraorbital optic nerve or any portion of it.

The treatment of orbital meningiomas is controversial. While successful surgical removal with preservation of vision has been reported,[13,34] these cases are the exception and not the rule. Attempting to strip a meningioma from the optic nerve almost invariably will destroy the vascular supply to the nerve as well.

The true controversy in the management of primary orbital meningiomas is between observation and surgical removal of the tumor combined with craniotomy to explore for intracranial extension. Some have gone so far as to recommend orbital exenteration.[1] We suggest that observation alone is in order if useful vision remains, and if there is no radiologic evidence of intracranial extension. Serial CT scanning at yearly intervals should be obtained if the clinical situation is stable. If useful vision is lost and there is evidence of continued growth on serial CT scans, we advocate complete removal of the tumor with unroofing of the optic canal. Since meningiomas usually are slow-growing tumors, we recommend biopsy of presumed orbital meningiomas that demonstrate aggressive growth patterns on CT or that produce rapid visual loss. Radiation therapy for optic nerve meningiomas has been proposed,[53] but information regarding the long-term efficiency of this mode of treatment has yet to be obtained.

Childhood orbital meningiomas are thought to be more aggressive than the adult variety, prompting the suggestion that extensive surgical extirpation be performed in younger patients.[62] We do not agree with this treatment and urge that optic nerve meningiomas in children be treated the same way as meningiomas in adults.

Enlargement of an optic nerve on CT scan in a child is more likely to be caused by a glioma than a meningioma. As in the case of meningiomas, other stigmas of neurofibromatosis should be sought. There is still great controversy about the treatment of optic nerve gliomas. Some have suggested observation of these tumors, which they consider to be benign hamartomas,[66] while others who view these lesions as potentially more aggressive, suggest complete surgical removal to prevent extension to the optic chiasm. A small minority suggests primary radiation.[53] The weight of neuro-ophthalmic opinion presently seems to favor observation as long as the tumor is localized to the orbit and has not caused blindness. The answers, however, are by no means clear.

Rapidly progressive proptosis in a child must be considered to be caused by orbital rhabdomyosarcoma until proven otherwise. This is the most frequent primary malignant orbital tumor of childhood. It may be located at any point in the orbit, including the intraconal space. There is usually a severe accompanying adnexal reaction with eyelid edema, lid injection, and conjunctival chemosis, which may be confused with orbital cellulitis or pseudotumor. At other times the only sign will be progressive proptosis. CT scan will reveal the mass lesion, which in many instances will show bony destruction.

A child suspected of harboring a rhadomyosarcoma should have immediate biopsy to confirm the diagnosis. The encouraging results of a combination of radiation and chemotherapy have spared many children the disfigurement of orbital exenteration.[46] Once the diagnosis has been established, these children should be treated in a center with experience with these malignant but potentially curable tumors.

☐   **Metastatic lesions.** A clinical picture indistinguishable from orbital rhabdomyo-sarcoma may occur with metastatic neuroblastoma. The adnexal signs, rapidly progressing proptosis and the presence of an orbital mass, may be identical. Neuroblastoma may be bilateral in up to 50% of patients, and there is frequently radiologic evidence of metastasis to the bones of the skull. Like rhabdomyosarcomas, neuroblastomas should be treated with a combination of radiation and chemotherapy once biopsy has provided the histologic diagnosis.

Any proptotic patient who has a history of treatment for cancer must be suspected of having orbital metastasis. Histologic verification is mandatory before treatment is begun since other causes of proptosis are possible in these patients. Fine-needle aspiration biopsy of orbital tumors is an alternative to biopsy through an orbitotomy in selected patients. The technique involves using CT scan or B scan echography as a guide to needle placement in the mass and then aspirating cells from the mass.[11] This method of obtaining a tissue diagnosis is especially useful in patients with suspected metastatic orbital tumors. Once tissue verification is obtained by fine-needle aspiration biopsy, appropriate treatment alternatives may be selected. Enophthalmos, and not proptosis, may be produced by scirrhous breast carcinoma when it metastasizes to the orbit (Fig. 9-9).[22]

☐ Extraconal mass

Orbital mass lesions in the extraconal space are more likely either to be extensions into the orbit from surrounding structures or to be metastatic from distant sources. Some tumors, such as hemangiomas, may be located anywhere in the orbit and cannot be excluded on the basis of topography alone.

☐   **Superior orbit.** A mass lesion of the superior orbital space will cause downward displacement of the globe (Fig. 9-10, *A*). Lesions frequently encountered in the superior nasal quadrant are dermoid tumors and mucoceles.

Dermoid tumors are the most frequent developmental masses found in children. They cause slowly progressive proptosis with downward ocular displacement. Lesions located anteriorly often have extension into the deeper portions of the orbit. CT will reveal the typical cystic lesion of the dermoid. Simple excision of the lesion is the treatment of choice.

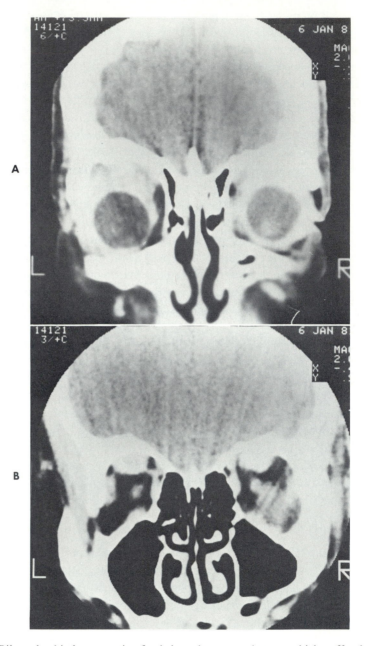

Fig. 9-9. Bilateral orbital metastasis of scirrhous breast carcinoma, which cuffs globes, **A,** and causes thickening of superior rectus–levator complex bilaterally, **B.**

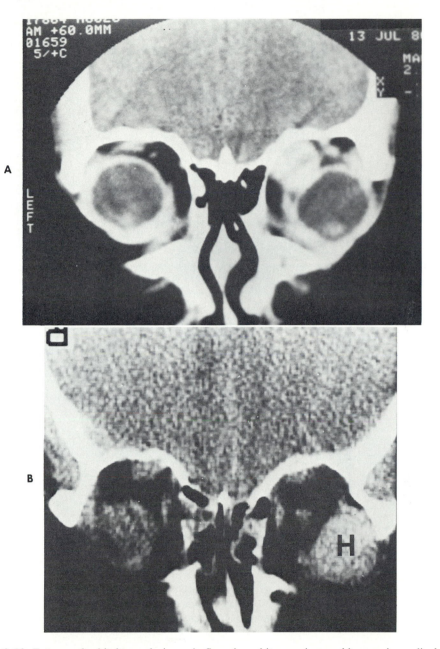

Fig. 9-10. Extraconal orbital mass lesions. **A,** Superior orbit: superior nasal hemangioma displaces right globe downward. **B,** Inferior orbit: hemangioma *(H)* in inferior left orbit displaces globe upward and out of the plane of scan.   *Continued.*

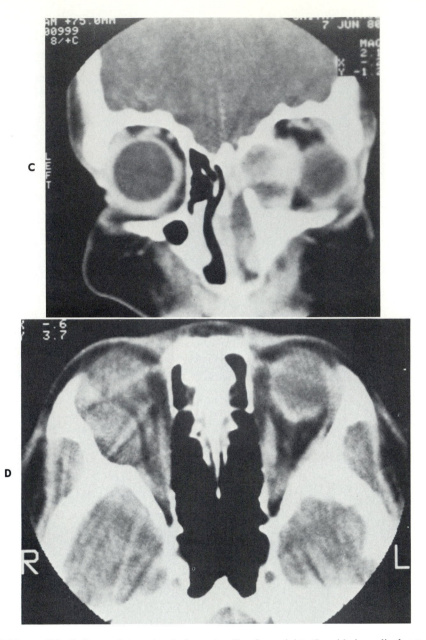

Fig. 9-10, cont'd. C, Large destructive lesion extending from right ethmoid sinus displaces globe laterally (giant cell tumor). **D,** Lateral orbital mass that displaces globe medially and has scalloped out lateral orbital wall. Note medial bowing of right optic nerve.

Another benign mass of the superior medial orbit is the mucocele. This slowly expanding sinus (usually frontal) lesion will gradually erode the orbital roof and extend into the orbital space. Downward proptosis and inability to elevate the eye are the typical findings. Radiologic investigation will reveal marked sinus opacification with disruption of the bony orbitofrontal boundary. Surgical correction requires obliteration of the frontal sinus with fat to prevent recurrence.

When a superior orbital mass is suspected, adequate neuroradiologic visualization of the orbital roof must be obtained to ensure that an orbital encephalocele with protrusion of the brain through a defect in the orbital roof is not present. More than one unwary surgeon has biopsied a superior orbital mass only to have the pathologic report returned "brain tissue."

Fibrous dysplasia, an abnormality of bone formation, typically involves the frontal bones with resultant proptosis and downward ocular displacement. This is a disorder of the young and tends to be slowly progressive. Progressive stenosis of the optic canal may result in visual loss. Heroic surgical procedures by a skilled plastic surgery team have been advocated as the only "cure" for this disorder.[38] The diagnosis is usually apparent on plain skull x-ray films or CT scan.

The downward and medial displacement of an eye suggests a lesion in the area of the lacrimal gland. In this situation the benign mixed tumor of the lacrimal gland must be suspected. These encapsulated tumors are curable lesions only if they are resected en-bloc initially. Excisional biopsy with rupture of the capsule may cause seeding of tumor into the orbit, producing continued growth and the eventual death of the patient from this locally aggressive tumor.

The duration of proptosis and the radiographic features of the lacrimal fossa may serve as guides to the diagnosis of lacrimal gland masses. If the patient's signs and symptoms have been present for under 12 months or if polytomography shows destructive changes in the lacrimal fossa, a malignancy is suspected, and incisional biopsy of the mass may be performed. However, if the history is longer than 12 months and polyto-mographic sections through the lacrimal fossa are either normal or show only pressure changes, then a benign mixed tumor is likely and en-bloc excision of the mass is required.[55]

Jakobiec et al.[24] have supplemented the guidelines of Stewart et al.[55] by considering the CT findings of various lacrimal fossa lesions. On CT scans inflammatory lacrimal fossa lesions are often oblong and anteriorly located. Other signs of orbital inflammation (scleral enhancement, myositis) are also seen. In this setting, biopsy through the eyelid without violating the periosteum is recommended. Benign mixed lacrimal gland tumors have a more rounded CT appearance and extend toward the posterior orbit. When this pattern is encountered, total excision of the mass through a lateral orbital approach is suggested. Lesions other than lacrimal gland tumors may occur in the lacrimal fossa; however, it is important to consider all lesions in this area to be benign mixed tumors until proven otherwise. There is no evidence that orbital exenteration followed by radiation therapy is more effective than radiation therapy alone in the long-term survival of patients with lacrimal gland carcinoma.

☐   **Inferior orbit.** An eye displaced upward signifies pathology in the maxillary sinus or in the orbital floor (Fig. 9-10, *B*). Maxillary sinus mucoceles and tumors of the superior antrum are the two most frequent sinus causes of superior ocular displacement. CT scans of the orbital floor and maxillary sinus will define the exact location of the process.

Mass lesions in the inferior orbital space also may be primary or secondary, benign or malignant. The answer again is provided by a combination of imaging and surgical exploration. An inferior orbitotomy should not be performed until detailed evaluation of the maxillary sinus has been completed.

Fungal infectious processes in the paranasal sinuses may cause orbital signs suggestive of a mass lesion. The combination of radiologic investigation and biopsy will lead to the correct diagnosis even in these unusual cases.[40]

◻ **Medial orbit.** Lateral displacement of the eye is a particularly ominous sign since it often signals extension of an aggressive process from the ethmoid-sphenoid complex into the medial orbital space (Fig. 9-10, *C*). In children, rhabdomyosarcoma must be considered. In adults, carcinoma of the sinus is a frequent cause. These carcinomas are very aggressive and almost invariably lead to the death of the patient following a protracted course despite all attempts at treatment.

Ethmoid sinus mucoceles also may displace the eye laterally. Modern neuroradiologic techniques of CT scanning will be able to distinguish this benign form of ocular displacement.

◻ **Lateral orbit.** When the eye is moved nasally, a mass lesion is most likely present in the pterygopalatine fossa or temporally within the orbit (Fig. 9-10, *D*). A review of 227 orbital CT scans performed over a 5-year period revealed 23 lateral orbital masses.[28] The most frequent masses were metastatic (5), pseudotumor (4), hemangioma (2), meningioma (2), and rhabdomyosarcoma (2). Other causes were arteriovenous malformations, encephalocele, fibrous dysplasia, and trauma with hemorrhage. The nature of two masses was unknown.

GUIDELINES FOR INVESTIGATION OF THE PATIENT WITH PROPTOSIS

1. Consider dysthyroid orbitopathy, which is the most frequent cause of unilateral or bilateral proptosis in all series published by ophthalmologists.
2. CT scanning is the most important and most effective test in the evaluation of the patient with proptosis. All patients with proptosis, without obvious signs of dysthyroid orbitopathy, must have a CT scan of the orbit.
3. The use of high-resolution CT scanning with contrast enhancement, in our view, obviates the need for other modalities (ultrasound or arteriography) to localize an orbital mass lesion. The method of scanning for orbital disease differs from that for intracranial disease, and unless good rapport exists between orbital surgeon and neuroradiologist, confusion may occur. A standard CT scan of the brain will provide either very poor or no orbital views. The neuroradiologist, not knowing the clinical history, will then interpret the scan as normal; however, the orbit—the area of concern—will not have been visualized.
4. Surgery should be directed at excision of localized, apparently encapsulated lesions when possible. Biopsy (open or fine-needle aspiration) is performed to document metastatic disease or when a tissue diagnosis is required for large, unresectable lesions that may be treatable with radiation or chemotherapy.

REFERENCES

1. Alper, MG: Management of primary optic nerve meningiomas, J Clin Neuro-Ophthalmol 1:101, 1981.
2. Chavis, RM, Garner, A, and Wright, JE: Inflammatory orbital pseudotumor. A clinicopathologic study, Arch Ophthalmol 96:1817, 1978.
3. Clay C, Bilaniuk, LT, and Vignaud, J: Orbital pseudotumors: preliminary report on a new type of therapy, Neuro-Ophthalmol 1:101, 1980.
4. Covington, EE, Lobes, L, and Sudarsanam, A: Radiation therapy for exophthalmos: report of seven cases, Radiology 122:797, 1977.
5. Debrun, G, Lacour, P, Vinuela, F, et al: Treatment of 54 traumatic carotid-cavernous fistulas, J Neurosurg 55:678, 1981.
6. de Juan, E, Jr, Hurley, DP, and Sapira, JD: Racial differences in normal values of proptosis, Arch Intern Med 140:1230, 1980.
7. De Santo, LW: The total rehabilitation of Graves' ophthalmopathy, Laryngoscope 90:1652, 1980.

8. Dixon, RS, Anderson, RL, and Hatt, MU: The use of thymoxamine in eyelid retraction, Arch Ophthalmol 97:2147, 1979.

9. Dolenc, V: Direct microsurgical repair of intracavernous vascular lesions, J Neurosurg 58:824, 1983.

10. Donaldson, SS, Bagshaw, MA, and Kriss, JP: Supervoltage orbital radiotherapy for Graves' ophthalmopathy, J Clin Endocrinol Metab 37:276, 1973.

11. Dubois, PJ, Kennerdell, JS, Rosenbaum, AE, et al: Computed tomographic localization for fine needle aspiration biopsy of orbital tumors, Radiology 131:149, 1979.

12. Dyer, JA: Ocular muscle surgery in Graves' disease, Trans Am Ophthalmol Soc 76:125, 1978.

13. Ebers, GC, Girvin JP, and Canny, CB: A possible optic nerve meningioma, Arch Neurol 37:781, 1980.

14. Eshaghian, J, and Anderson, RL: Sinus involvement in inflammatory orbital pseudotumor, Arch Ophthalmol 99:627, 1981.

15. Evans D, and Kennerdell, JS: Extraocular muscle surgery for dysthyroid myopathy, Am J Ophthalmol 95:767, 1983.

16. Forbes, GS, Sheedy, PF, II, and Waller, RR: Orbital tumors evaluated by computed tomography, Radiology 136:101, 1980.

17. Gellady AM, Shulman, ST, and Ayoub, EM: Periorbital and orbital cellulitis in children, Pediatrics 61:272, 1978.

18. Glaser, JS: Neuro-ophthalmology, Hagerstown, Md, 1978, Harper & Row, Publishers, p 36.

19. Henderson, JW: Orbital tumors, Philadelphia, 1973, W.B. Saunders Co, p 28.

20. Henderson, JW, and Schneider, RC: The ocular findings in carotid-cavernous fistula in a series of 17 cases, Am J Ophthalmoi 48:585, 1959.

21. Howell, SC: The craniostenosis, Am J Ophthalmol 37:359, 1954.

22. Hoyt, WF, and Beeston, D: The ocular fundus in neurologic disease, St Louis, 1966, The CV Mosby Co, p 40.

23. Jakobiec, FA, McLean, I, and Font, RL: Clinicopathologic characteristics of orbital lymphoid hyperplasia, Ophthalmology 86:948, 1979.

24. Jakobiec, FA, Yeo, JH, Trokel, SL, et al: Combined clinical and computed tomographic diagnosis of primary lacrimal fossa lesions, Am J Ophthalmol 94:785, 1982.

25. Karp, LA, Zimmerman, LE, Borit, A, et al: Primary intraorbital meningiomas, Arch Ophthalmol 91:24, 1974.

26. Kiessling, WR, Pflughaupt, KW, Ricker, K, et al: Thyroid function and circulating antithyroid antibodies in myasthenia gravis, Neurology 31:771, 1981.

27. Klingele, TG, Hart, WM, and Burde, RM: Management of dysthyroid optic neuropathy, Ophthalmologica 174:327, 1977.

28. Knochel, JQ, Osborn, AG, and Wing, SD: Differential diagnosis of lateral orbital masses, CT 5:11, 1981.

29. Knowles, DM, II, and Jakobiec, FA: Orbital lymphoid neoplasms. A clinicopathologic study of 60 patients, Cancer 46:576, 1980.

30. Knowles, DM, II, Jakobiec, FA, and Halper, JP: Immunologic characterization of ocular adnexal lymphoid neoplasms, Am J Ophthalmol 87:603, 1979.

31. Koziak, PH: Craniostenosis. Report of 22 cases, Am J Ophthalmol 37:380, 1954.

32. Krohel, GB, and Wright, JE: Orbital hemorrhage, Am J Ophthalmol 88:254, 1979.

33. Linberg, JV, and Anderson, RL: Transorbital decompression. Indications and results, Arch Ophthalmol 99:113, 1981.

34. Mark, LE, Kennerdell, JS, Maroon, JC, et al: Microsurgical removal of a primary intraorbital meningioma, Am J Ophthalmol 86:704, 1978.

35. McLean, JM, and Norton, EWD: Unilateral lid retraction without exophthalmos, Arch Ophthalmol 61:681, 1958.

36. Mottow-Lippa, L, Jakobiec, FA, and Smith, M: Idiopathic inflammatory orbital pseudotumor in childhood. II. Results of diagnostic tests and biopsies, Ophthalmology 88:565, 1981.

37. Mullan, S: Treatment of carotid-cavernous fistulas by cavernous sinus occlusion, J Neurosurg 50:131, 1979.

38. Munro, IR, and Chen, YR: Radical treatment for fronto-orbital fibrous dysplasia. The chain-link fence, Plast Reconstr Surg 67:719, 1981.

39. Newton, TH, and Hoyt, WF: Dural arteriovenous shunts in the region of the cavernous sinus, Neuroradiology 1:71, 1970.

40. Nielsen, EW, Weisman, RA, Savino, PJ, and Schatz, NJ: Aspergillosis of the sphenoid sinus presenting as orbital pseudotumor, Otolaryngol Head Neck Surg **91:**699, 1983.

41. Ogura, JH, and Thawley, SE: Orbital decompression for exophthalmos, Otolaryngol Clin North Am 13:29, 1980.

42. Osher, RH, Shields, JA, and Schatz, NJ: Axial myopia. A neglected cause of proptosis, Arch Neurol 35:237, 1978.

43. Palestine, AG, Younge, BR, and Piepgras, DG: Visual prognosis in carotid-cavernous fistula, Arch Ophthalmol 99:1600, 1981.

44. Parkinson, D, Downs, AR, Whytehead, LL, et al: Carotid cavernous fistula: direct repair with preservation of carotid, Surgery 76:882, 1974.

45. Phelps, CD, Thompson, HS, and Ossonig, KC: The diagnosis and prognosis of atypical carotid-cavernous fistula (red-eyed shunt syndrome), Am J Ophthalmol 93:423, 1982.

46. Raney, RB, and Handler, SD: Management of neoplasms of the head and neck in children. II. Malignant tumors, Head Neck Surg 3:500, 1981.

47. Ravin, JG, Sisson, JC, and Knapp, WT: Orbital radiation for the ocular changes of Graves' disease, Am J Ophthalmol 79:285, 1975.

48. Sanders, MD, and Hoyt, WF: Hypoxic ocular sequelae of carotid-cavernous fistulae, Br J Ophthalmol 53:82, 1969.

49. Sattler, CH: In Graefe, A, and Saemisch, T, editors: Hanbuch der gesamten Augenheilkunde, vol 9, Leipzig, 1920, W. Englemann, chap. 13.

50. Sergott, RC, Felberg, NT, Savino, PJ, et al: Graves' ophthalmopathy-immunologic parameters related to corticosteroid therapy, Invest Ophthalmol 20:173, 1981.

51. Sergott, RC, and Glaser, JS: Graves' ophthalmopathy. A clinical and immunologic review, Surv Ophthalmol 26:1, 1981.

52. Sergott, RC, Glaser, JS, and Charyulu, K: Radiotherapy for idiopathic inflammatory orbital pseudotumor, Arch Ophthalmol 99:853, 1981.

53. Smith, JL, Vuksanovic, MM, Yates, BM, et al: Radiation therapy for primary optic nerve meningioma, J Clin Neuro-Ophthalmol 1:85, 1981.

54. Spoor, TC, and Kennerdell, JS: Thyrotropin-releasing hormone test and the diagnosis of dysthyroid ophthalmology, Ann Ophthalmol 13:443, 1981.

55. Stewart, WB, Krohel, GB, and Wright, JE: Lacrimal gland and fossa lesions: an approach to diagnosis and management, Ophthalmology 86:886, 1979.

56. Teng, CS, and Yeo, PPB: Ophthalmic Graves' disease: natural history and detailed thyroid function studies, Br Med J 1:273, 1977.

57. Thomas, ID, and Hart, JK: Retrobulbar repository corticosteroid therapy in thyroid ophthalmopathy, Med J Aust 2:484, 1974.

58. Trobe, JD, Glaser, JS, and Laflamme, P: Dysthyroid optic neuropathy. Clinical profile and rationale for management, Arch Ophthalmol 96:1199, 1978.

59. Trokel, SL, and Cooper, WC: Orbital decompression. Effect on motility and globe position, Ophthalmology 86:2064, 1979.

60. Trokel, SL, and Jakobiec, FA: Correlation of CT scanning and pathologic features of ophthalmic Graves' disease, Ophthalmology 88:553, 1981.

61. Viñuela, FV, Debrun, GM, Fox, AJ, and Kan, S: Detachable calibrated leak balloon for superselective angiography and embolization of dural arteriovenous malformations, J Neurosurg 58:817, 1983.

62. Walsh, FB: Meningiomas primary within the orbit and optic canal. In Glaser, JS, and Smith, JL, editors: Neuro-Ophthalmology, Symposium of the University of Miami and the Bascom Palmer Eye Institute, vol 8, St Louis, 1975, The CV Mosby Co, p 166.

63. Walsh, FB, and Hoyt, WF: Clinical neuro-ophthalmology, ed 3, Baltimore, 1969, The Williams & Wilkins Co, p 307.

64. Watters EC, Waller, H, Hiles, DA, et al: Acute orbital cellulitis, Arch Ophthalmol 94:785, 1976.

65. Weisman, RA, Savino, PJ, Schut, L, and Schatz, NJ: Computed tomography in penetrating wounds of the orbit with retained foreign bodies, Arch Otolaryngol 109:265, 1983.

66. Wright, JE; Primary optic nerve meningiomas: clinical presentation and management, Ophthalmology 83:617, 1977.

CHAPTER 10

Headache and facial pain

THE HEADACHE PATIENT

Of all of the ailments that plague man, headache is the most ubiquitous. Most headaches do not reflect serious pathology, but their importance lies in the fact that they prevent the patient from functioning in everyday life. Unfortunately headache patients tend to be difficult and time consuming. Because of the pressures of practice, these patients often leave the physician's office less than satisfied and wander from office to office seeking relief.

Patients with headaches are commonly referred to the ophthalmologist for suspected ocular causes or to the neurologist because of concern for the existence of intracranial pathology. To deal with these patients it is necessary for the physician to be able to recognize certain characteristic symptom complexes, which allows him to categorize the vast majority of headache patients as having one entity or another. There remains a number of patients who do not seem to fall easily into a specific diagnostic group. The approach to these patients requires the application of a sequence of historical questions, since in most headache patients the physical examination is normal.

Ray and Wolff[58] determined that the pain-sensitive structures within the cranium included (1) the great venous sinuses and their tributaries, (2) parts of the dura on the floor of the skull, and (3) the dural arteries and the cerebral arteries at the base of the brain. They formulated six basic sources of intracranial headache: (1) traction on tributary veins passing to the great venous sinuses or displacement of the great venous sinuses, (2) traction on the middle meningeal artery, (3) traction on the large cerebral arteries or their branches at the base of the brain, (4) distension and dilatation of the intracranial arteries, (5) inflammation in or around any of the pain-sensitive structures, and (6) direct pressure on the cranial or cervical nerves containing afferent pain fibers from these structures, which include the fifth cranial nerve above the tentorium cerebelli and the ninth, tenth, eleventh, twelfth, and upper cervical nerves below the tentorium. Extracranial sources of head pain include skin, mucous membranes, tympanic membrane, fasciae, muscles and galea, and the extracranial arteries and veins of the head and neck. Headaches may be classified utilizing this neuroanatomic background,[10] but for practical purposes it is easier to categorize headaches based on their clinical presentations.

When one is dealing with the headache patient, the admonition of "the history is the key" cannot be ignored. The history must be elucidated in great detail because experience dictates that in over 95% of headache cases the physical examination will be entirely normal.

CLASSIFICATION OF HEADACHE

I. Distinctive headache syndromes
  A. Recognized by classic historical features
    1. No obvious exogenous ''trigger'' mechanism
      a. Cluster headache
      b. Migraine
        (1) Classic
        (2) Complicated
          (a) Cerebral migraine
          (b) Ophthalmoplegic migraine
          (c) Basilar artery migraine
      c Cranial neuralgias
        (1) Trigeminal neuralgia
        (2) Glossopharyngeal neuralgia
      d. ''Ice pick'' headache
      e. Headache of giant cell arteritis
      f. Headache of subarachnoid hemorrhage
    2. Obvious exogenous ''trigger'' mechanism
      a. Ice cream headache
      b. Dietary headache
      c. Altitude headache
      d. Posttraumatic headache
      e. Low intracranial pressure headache
      f. Asthenopia
  B. Recognized by physical features and associated with other disease states
    1. Herpetic neuralgia
    2. Sinus disease
    3. Dental disease
    4. Temporomandibular joint pain
    5. Fever
    6. Arterial hypertension
    7. Central nervous system disease
      a. Raised intracranial pressure
      b. Raeder's syndrome
        (1) Type 1
        (2) Type 2
    8. Ocular inflammation
II. Nondistinctive headache syndromes and facial pain
  A. Common migraine and variants
  B. Muscle contraction headaches
  C. Conversion headaches
  D. Atypical facial pain
  E. Greater occipital neuralgia
  F. Preherpetic neuralgia

Detailing the history should include answers to the following:
1. Where?
2. How often?
3. How long?
4. What are the characteristics of the pain?
   a. Are there precipitating or exacerbating circumstances?
   b. Are there accompanying signs and symptoms?

Special emphasis should be given to determining telltale characteristics of the headache itself.

1. *Quality* is often described in terms of past experience or related to other sensations, for example, itching, burning, aching. The patient can recognize only two types of pain by quality: (a) superficial pain arising from the skin, described as itching or burning and exquisitely localizable, and (b) deep pain arising from structures below the skin surface, described as dull, aching, knifelike, and in general not well localized.

2. *Intensity* depends upon the patient's psychologic set, and thus the intensity must be judged by how it affects the individual's ability to function; for example, does it awaken the patient from sleep, does it prevent the patient from working or taking care of his family, does it cause the patient to cry out, does it induce nausea, vomiting, palpitations or sweating, is it relieved by analgesic agents—aspirin or narcotics?

3. *Time intensity curve* reflects the variation in intensity of the pain with the duration of the headache. The time intensity curve is a major factor in categorizing headache syndromes.

4. *Relation to other events* may be a signal to the cause of the headache or at least imply a prophylactic strategy, for example, avoidance of the use of medication. The headache may be related to environmental changes, for example, weather, eating certain foods, or stress. It may be related to endogenous phenomena such as menstrual periods, hypertension, hypotension, or depression. It may be preceded by an aura or induced by certain "triggers."

Certain headache syndromes are so characteristic that the diagnosis is obvious from listening to the history. These types of headaches fall into one of two major categories (see preceding Classification of Headache): (1) those recognized by classic historical features, which can be subdivided into those with or without definable triggers, and (2) those recognized by physical features associated with systemic, central nervous system, or local disease. The classification of the remaining patients with headache complaints is based on determining the time-intensity curve of the headache and finding the relation of the headache to other events.

DISTINCTIVE HEADACHE SYNDROMES

The following headache patterns are easily recognized by history alone. The first group is not associated with a defined trigger mechanism.

Headaches not associated with obvious trigger mechanism

Cluster headache. (Horton's headaches, histamine cephalgia). Patients with a cluster headache typically are awakened from sleep in the early morning (3 to 5 AM) by the onset of excruciating head pain, usually unilateral. The pain is described as being in the distribution of the external carotid artery and its branches (frontal or frontotemporal pain). The headache is accompanied by an ipsilateral Horner's syndrome, lacrimation and rhinorrhea, and occasionally by conjunctival edema and injection. The pain is described as boring or burning and of such severity that the patient usually paces the floor until the pain subsides in 30 minutes to 3 to 4 hours. The patient is asymptomatic until the attack recurs at the same time the next day, but multiple attacks in one day may occur occasionally. The headaches may recur daily for days or weeks to disappear and then return on a regular basis once or twice a year. The onset is usually in the fourth or fifth decade and is more common in males and blacks.[66] These headaches are often triggered by even minimal alcohol ingestion.

If the patient has a typical history and the *only neurologic finding is a postganglionic Horner's syndrome,* then no further investigation is needed. Cluster headache is believed to be a vascular headache, possibly migrainous in nature. Although it has been stated[32] that ergotamine tartrate is dramatically effective in aborting the paroxysm, this has not held true in our experience. During the acute attack little can be done for the patient short of sedation with intravenous administration of diazepam or pentobarbital. Once the diagnosis has been made, prophylactic treatment to prevent subsequent attacks should include methysergide, systemic corticosteroids, and lithium chloride in sequential order. None of these drugs is universally effective. Chlorpromazine (Thorazine) has been reported to be effective in 93% (12 of 13) of patients with cluster headache.[13]

Migraine syndromes

Classic migraine. Classic migraine is the most stereotypic of all the migraine syndromes but is found in only about 20% of patients with migraine. Attacks are characterized by a sharply defined aura or prodrome lasting for 20 to 40 minutes before fading as the headache phase begins. The pain is usually throbbing and lasts for hours. It is usually unilateral, with the neurologic manifestations of the aura having occurred contralateral to the pain. Anorexia, nausea, and extreme sensitivity to light (not eye pain) and to noise are concomitant features of the headache phase.

The aura is usually visual, although it may take a hemiparetic, hemisensory, or dysphasic form. The visual symptoms may assume many forms including eccentric scotomas, awareness of brightness in the peripheral field, apparent pulsation of the intensity of ambient illumination, and movement of stationary objects involving one or both hemifields simultaneously or consecutively. The most common symptom is that of the scintillating scotoma. This visual disturbance usually begins as a small, gray, ill-defined area just eccentric to fixation. It then slowly expands while tending to drift peripherally. The scotoma may consist of an area of totally absent sight or an area of reduced sensitivity outlined by bright shimmering lights (scintillations). These scintillations either may consist of brilliantly colored or iridescent shimmering lights that appear as parallel lines forming regular geometric angles along the leading edge of the scotoma (fortification specter) or may be ill defined. They may occur without the scotoma. After the age of 40 patients may lose the headache phase (attributed to the inability of the extracranial arteries to dilate) and have only the prodrome.

Complicated migraine. Complicated migraine is a term used to denote the occurrence of paroxysmal neurologic deficits that persist beyond the headache phase. They are usually transient but may be permanent. The onset of the neurologic deficits may precede the headache, as in classic migraine, or may occur only during or following the headache phase. There are a number of specific subtypes, some of which have been classified by others as part of the classic migraine syndrome.

Cerebral migraine. The neurologic deficit may include motor, visual, or other sensory defects. Hemiplegic migraine is characterized by partial or total hemiparesis or hemiplegia. The onset of the motor deficit usually occurs before or at the peak of the headache. There is a well-recognized subset of "familial hemiplegic migraine"[38] in which the attacks always occur on the same side in a particular family. In familial hemiplegic migraine complete recovery is the rule; whereas in the nonfamilial variety incomplete recovery is not unusual.[2] Transient or permanent homonymous or quadrantic visual field defects have been well documented in patients who previously experienced classic migraine attacks with scintillating scotomas.[39] Similarly, sensory disturbances such as paresthesias of hands, arm, face, tongue, or lips have also been reported. Speech disorders, including dysarthria, repetitive expressions (automatisms), and complete aphasia, may occur.[2] With the exception of familial hemiplegic migraine, all of these patients should be evaluated for the presence of a structural lesion by CT scanning including the use of intravenous contrast media.

Ophthalmoplegic migraine. Ophthalmoplegic migraine is a rare disorder usually having its onset before age 10.[26] The third nerve is affected more often than the sixth (10 : 1),[26] and the paralysis involves both the extraocular muscles and the pupillary and ciliary muscles. The onset of the paralysis occurs at either the height of the pain or at the cessation of the pain and lasts for days to weeks. Recovery is gradual and tends to become less complete with repeat attacks. The ophthalmoplegia is always on the same side as the headache. Strict criteria should be met before the diagnosis of ophthalmoplegic migraine is made:

1. Onset in first decade
2. History of typical migraine headaches, that is, severe throbbing headache or equivalent
3. Ophthalmoplegia ipsilateral to the headache
4. Negative computerized tomography and angiography

Although aneurysm would be an extremely rare cause of third cranial nerve palsies in children, we believe that the evaluation of the initial attack of an acquired third nerve palsy in children requires complete neuroradiologic investigation including cerebral angiography.

Cyclic vomiting and car sickness are considered by many to be manifestations of a migraine process, migraine equivalents or precursors of migraine in infants. The presence of either of these symptoms may indicate the presence of migraine in a preverbal child unable to describe his pain. Similarly, eliciting a history of these symptoms in an adult with the recent onset of headaches or sensory disturbances may be diagnostically helpful.

Basilar artery migraine. Basilar artery migraine is a disorder that mimics the transient ischemic attacks of vertebrobasilar insufficiency seen in elderly individuals, that is, the sudden onset of episodes of transient visual disturbances, vertigo, gait ataxia, dysarthria, and acroparesthesias, but it is followed by severe headache and vomiting.[6] Transient alterations in consciousness have also been reported. The visual symptoms include vivid flashes of light throughout the entire visual field, transient bilateral blindness, bilateral blurred vision, formed visual hallucinations, and diplopia.[48] This was believed to be an affliction of adolescent girls until Golden and French[28] noted its occurrence in preschool children. Their findings were extended by the report of Lapkin and Golden,[48] who reported 30 children ranging in age from 7 months to 14 years with basilar artery migraine. The vast majority of children had frequent attacks (three per week); the headache tended to be nonlateralized.

When dealing with children who present with apparent vertebrobasilar insufficiency, the major problem is to establish a diagnosis. Lapkin and Golden[48] state, "The points supporting this diagnosis are: the symptomatology that apparently represents functional abnormalities of the structures supplied by the vertebrobasilar circulation, the strong family history of migraine (86%), the evolution to typical migraine in some patients in later life, and the exclusion of progressive neurologic disease when followed up." If the patient is neurologically normal and there is a strong family history of migraine, no further investigation is necessary. If such evidence is lacking or weak, such children should be evaluated thoroughly. Basilar artery migraine is a retrospective diagnosis. The prognosis, in spite of recurrent attacks, is excellent.

In addition to the clearly defined syndrome of basilar artery migraine in children, adult patients with various migraine syndromes may experience symptoms (vertigo or diplopia) that are best explained on the basis of relative brain stem ischemia. In the face of a well-established history of migraine such symptomatology does not indicate impending brain stem infarction, but risk factors such as estrogen use should be avoided.

The mechanisms underlying migraine and the treatment of the headaches will be discussed later in relation to common migraine and migraine equivalents.

Cranial neuralgias. Cranial neuralgias include two distinct entities: (1) trigeminal neuralgia and (2) glossopharyngeal neuralgia. Each of these syndromes is characterized by paroxysms of pain occurring in the distribution of a cranial nerve.

Trigeminal neuralgia. Trigeminal neuralgia (tic douloureux) is marked by the sudden onset of severe pain in the distribution of one division of the fifth nerve, usually the third, occasionally the second, and rarely the first. The pain is so intense that the facial muscles typically contract and distort the face during an attack, and the patient anticipates with dread the ensuing bouts of pain. Occasionally the pain may spread to involve a second or third division during a paroxysm. The paroxysms are usually short lived (20 to 30 seconds) but may be repetitive and closely spaced, and under these circumstances last up to an hour. In time the spontaneous attacks, which initially may be intermittent, separated by days or weeks, tend to occur at closer intervals, for example, one or two attacks per day. A typical attack can occur spontaneously or be triggered by various stimuli such as light touch, a cool breeze on the face, biting, chewing, brushing teeth, shaving, and by sudden changes in oral temperatures when eating hot or cold substances. Patients are asymptomatic between paroxysms. The neurologic examination is normal. This syndrome tends to occur in individuals over the age of 50 years. If present in a younger individual, or if sensory abnormalities or other accompanying neurologic deficits are found, underlying pathology such as dental disease, multiple sclerosis, brain stem tumors, or aneurysm must be excluded. In patients with the classic syndrome of trigeminal neuralgia, diagnostic procedures are unnecessary.[2]

Management of the acute paroxysm, if prolonged, includes the intravenous use of phenytoin, 700 to 1000 mg. Phenytoin is successful prophylactically in oral doses of 300 to 600 mg per day in about 20% of patients.[42] Carbamazepine is the mainstay of prophylactic treatment and should be administered at mealtime in gradually increasing doses.[7] Patients rarely respond to less than 600 mg per day, and a maximum therapeutic dosage is 1600 mg per day. The notable side effects of this drug include drowsiness, dizziness, bone marrow depression, and hepatic toxicity. Not infrequently surgical intervention will be warranted if medical treatment is unsuccessful. Surgical procedures include percutaneous radiofrequency trigeminal gangliolysis, suboccipital craniectomy with trigeminal nerve decompression, and trigeminal tractotomy.

Glossopharyngeal neuralgia. Glossopharyngeal neuralgia is seen less frequently (1:200) than is trigeminal neuralgia and is characterized by the sudden onset of stabbing and jolting pain in the posterior half of the tongue, the tonsils, and the pharynx. Some patients appear to have a trigger zone in the pharynx, and the paroxysms are initiated by swallowing. These patients will often adopt a sleeping posture to avoid having saliva trickle down the trigger side of the oral pharynx. Talking, yawning, or washing the ears can trigger the paroxysm. In contract to trigeminal neuralgia, in glossopharyngeal neuralgia, biting does not induce the paroxysm. The pain may occur at night, bolting the patient out of bed. The treatment of choice is carbamazepine used prophylactically. If this drug is not effective, intracranial section of the ninth cranial nerve and rostral vagal rootlets is considered the procedure of choice.[65]

Ice pick–like pain. Ice pick–like pain is a benign syndrome that consists of lancinating, momentary, shooting pain.[56] It has been described as occurring anywhere in the head as well as within the eye. These pains are variable in occurrence, infrequent, and not associated with any known disease. This syndrome has been reported to be more frequent in migraineurs. A typical history of momentary, lancinating pains supported by a negative examination precludes the need for further diagnostic evaluation.

Giant cell arteritis. The onset of headaches in a patient over the age of 50 should alert the clinician to the possibility of giant cell arteritis. In the more typical form these headaches are generally localized over areas of inflammatory involvement of the temporal arteries, which may be associated with nodular excrescences.

Often these patients will not complain of headache but will be aware of scalp tenderness exacerbated by combing or brushing their hair, wearing hats, or leaning their heads on pillows or chairs. Accompanying symptoms may include jaw claudication with chewing or talking and polymyalgia rheumatica. The concomitant or sequential development of sudden visual loss or diplopia in an elderly patient will help make the diagnosis obvious. An immediate erythrocyte sedimentation rate followed by the administration of systemic corticosteroids is mandatory in these patients.

Headache of subarachnoid hemorrhage. The patient suffering from this type of headache will usually report the instantaneous apoplectic onset of excruciating pain, most often in the back of the head. It is often described as, "Like I've been hit on the back of the head with a baseball bat." Even if lucid, these patients will have signs of meningeal irritation. There may be no focal neurologic findings, the only sign being depressed consciousness. The subsequent course depends upon the etiology and extent of the hemorrhage.

Headache associated with trigger mechanisms

Ice cream headache. When eating or drinking extremely cold substances, certain patients will develop a sharp, deep pain in and around the retroorbital and frontal region.

This pain abates gradually over a period of 20 to 60 seconds. Kunkle et al.[47] found that this pain arose from applying the cold substances to the roof of the mouth (palate) and not to the esophagus or stomach. This represents referred pain from one area subserved by the fifth cranial nerve to another. These patients will relate the onset of pain to the eating or drinking of cold substances. It is a benign syndrome.

Dietary headache. Some headaches are clearly associated with the intake of certain foods or removal of certain substances, such as caffeine, from the diet after prolonged daily use. Nitrate or nitrite compounds, which are used as additives or preservatives in certain foods, are potent vasodilating agents, and they can induce vascular headaches in susceptible individuals.[36] These additives are found in smoked fish and in preserved meats such as bologna, sausage, salami, and frankfurters.

Monosodium glutamate is another food additive that can trigger vascular headaches in susceptible individuals, either immediately following ingestion (20 to 30 minutes) or 12 to 18 hours later. Some of these individuals also experience bloating and peripheral edema. Monosodium glutamate is used as a flavoring agent in freshly prepared oriental dishes and as an additive in instant and canned soups, potato chips, dry-roasted nuts, processed meats, and TV dinners. The headache is severe and is typically throbbing in character. It often responds to analgesic combinations containing a fast-acting barbiturate and caffeine.

The postalcohol, or "hangover," headache occurs the morning after the consumption of alcoholic beverages to excess, although some individuals get a similar headache after consuming small amounts of alcohol. This headache has a generalized throbbing quality that increases in intensity with exertion. It is often accompanied by nausea and vomiting. Aspirin or acetaminophen compounds containing caffeine are effective in easing the head pain. Some individuals who have either a history of cluster headaches or migraine headaches develop a typical vascular headache after drinking even minimal amounts of alcohol.

A peculiar type of withdrawal headache is experienced by individuals who have chronically ingested caffeine in coffee, tea, cola, or medications on a daily basis and suddenly stop.[20] These people become irritable and initially experience a generalized dull aching headache that may, with time, develop into either a throbbing headache or a muscle contraction–type headache. These headaches are relieved by ingestion of caffeine or mild analgesics without caffeine. Continued abstinence for 3 to 5 days is also curative.

Altitude headache. Altitude headaches occur in individuals who travel directly from sea level to 8,000 feet. The percentage of people who develop these headaches is related to the altitude reached, being almost universal over 12,000 feet. The headache usually begins 6 to 96 hours after arriving at the higher altitude and may be accompanied by other symptoms of mountain sickness including nausea, vomiting, and shortness of breath. Altitude headache is throbbing and usually generalized but frequently more severe frontally. These patients are often most comfortable when they are active, although the head pain can be made worse by Valsalva maneuvers. There is evidence that mountain sickness can be prevented by the prophylactic use of acetazolamide[31] (250 mg four times a day) for 3 days prior to and during the period of high altitude exposure.

Posttraumatic headache. The complaint of headache or neck pain following direct head trauma is common. Headache is just one symptom of the posttraumatic syndrome, which includes dizziness, insomnia, concentration difficulties, and mood and personality changes. Chronic posttraumatic headaches are postulated to be due to either sustained muscular contraction, recurrent vascular dilatation, local structural injury, or a personality disorder. In spite of improved diagnostic techniques the mechanism of persistent post-traumatic headaches remains an enigma.

The "whiplash" syndrome is produced by a rapid to-and-fro motion of the head, usually caused by an automobile accident. Sudden and extreme flexion and extension can occur even with minor impact, especially with a "rear end" collision. This produces a stretching injury of the ligaments and muscles. These patients complain of prolonged localized tenderness, muscle splinting, and typical muscle contraction headaches.

The diagnosis of posttraumatic headache is made on the basis of the history and by exclusion of organic structural damage. The headache should not be attributed to a mood or personality disorder without appropriate psychiatric consultation. Effective treatment of this group of patients includes the use of analgesics, sedatives, and tricyclic antidepressants, as well as physiotherapy and psychotherapy. However, in many cases it is impossible to exclude conscious dissembling.

Low intracranial pressure headache. The headaches due to decreased cerebro-spinal fluid (CSF) pressure generally follow lumbar puncture but also occur in cases of spontaneous or traumatic CSF rhinorrhea. These headaches are positional, being induced by sitting or standing and relieved by lying down. The pain is severe and located in the occipital and frontal areas. Similar headaches have been reported in 32% to 50% of patients following metrizamide myelography.[43] Whether the headache is a direct effect of the metrizamide or is a variation of postlumbar puncture headache is unknown. The headache of CSF rhinorrhea requires nucleotide localization of the leaking area followed by surgical intervention. Persistent headache following lumbar puncture may require blood patches.[5,12]

Asthenopia. The ocular and periocular discomfort associated with prolonged ocular use (usually for near visual tasks) is called asthenopia. The initial symptom is usually a feeling of lid heaviness, which gradually progresses to a feeling of somnolence. The eyes feel "tired," hot, or uncomfortable, and some relief may be obtained by rubbing the eyes or discontinuing the ocular task. If the work is continued, the vague discomfort may give rise to an aching feeling of the eyes and the development of various headache symptoms, for example, brow ache, temporal pain, or neck tenderness.[22,67]

Initially the headaches tend to be described as a generalized brow ache that with continued ocular use tends to become more generalized. Frontal, temporal, or occipital discomfort may be described, ultimately taking on the form of a severe muscle contraction or combined muscle contraction–throbbing headache with neck and shoulder discomfort. Late in the evolution of the syndrome, associated visceral symptoms, such as nausea, are not unusual. This progressive symptom complex, that is, lid heaviness, sleepiness, ocular discomfort, and headache, is generally referred to as *eyestrain*.

Among the many causes (see Box on p. 312) of eyestrain is the presence of uncorrected refractive error, either hyperopic (including presbyopic) or astigmatic.[23] The clinical syndrome can be reproduced experimentally with the use of myopic or cylindric lenses in emmetropic individuals.[23] Uncorrected myopia does not produce asthenopia.

One of the most frequent causes of asthenopia is the prescription of new glasses, and eyestrain can occur whether the correction is appropriate or inappropriate. In the former case, prescribing a cylindric correction for the first time or altering the power or

---

SOURCES OF ASTHENOPIA

I. Uncorrected refractive errors
   A. Hyperopia (and presbyopia)
   B. Astigmatism
II. Acquisition of new glasses
   A. With appropriate prescription
      1. Initial correction of an astigmatic error
      2. Change in power or axis of cylindric correction
      3. Change in accommodative or vergence requirements as a result of the glasses
   B. With inappropriate prescription
      1. Incorrect refraction or filling of the prescription
      2. Induced heterophorias
         a. Horizontal or vertical misplacement of optic center
      3. Change in base curve
         a. Reflective changes, eikonic changes
         b. Change of movement across the retina
III. Heterophorias
IV. No identifiable cause

---

axis of a previously prescribed refraction induces the asthenopic symptoms. In the correction of anisometropia a substantial difference in the refractive error of each eye may also produce asthenopia. A small group of these patients will have aniseikonia, a difference in the retinal image size perceived by each eye, and asthenopia that can be alleviated by the use of an eikonic correction. A significant increase in a myopic correction or hyperopic correction, either distance or reading addition, can produce a change in the accommodative and vergence requirements resulting in asthenopia.

The prescription of an inappropriate refractive correction, for example, excessive minus sphere or a cylinder correction at the wrong axis, can cause asthenopia. Similarly, a change in the base curve of the corrective lenses in a myopic individual will almost always induce asthenopia. In patients with high refractive corrections, horizontal or vertical misplacement of the optical center of a corrective lens can induce a heterophoria and thus asthenopia. In all these cases the onset of symptoms will begin following the wearing of a new spectacle correction.

Although experimentally[23] the induction of heterophorias has inconsistently produced asthenopia, there is little doubt clinically that the existence of a heterophoria in some individuals is associated with asthenopia.[11] Patients with heterophorias obtain binocular vision by maintaining an appropriate distribution of tone to the extraocular muscles by utilizing various fusional mechanisms. Burian and von Noorden[11] state that the appearance of symptoms depends on the sensorimotor state of the individual and not on the absolute amount of heterophoric deviation; that is, "what matters is the presence or absence of a discrepancy between the deviation and the amplitudes of motor fusion." Asthenopia often occurs in patients in whom a latent vertical deviation begins to break down and become manifest, for example, congenital superior oblique palsy, or in patients with normal vergence amplitudes who demonstrate convergence insufficiency as an aftermath of a serious systemic illness.

In a certain number of individuals there will be no identifiable cause. Since the treatment of asthenopia requires the identification of an inducing factor, in those patients in whom such evidence is lacking, it is necessary to delve into the possible existence of situational, emotional, or psychiatric factors contributing to the presence of symptoms. The correction of asthenopia may require the use of spectacles of various types including bifocals and prisms, replacement of inappropriate refractive corrections, orthoptic training, and rarely, eye muscle surgery.

Headaches recognizable by physical features and associated with other disease states

Herpetic neuralgia. The pain of herpes zoster is described as being severe, burning, and aching in quality and is steady and sustained. The pain is in the distribution of a given dermatome or cranial nerve, usually the first division of the fifth cranial nerve, although it may involve the seventh nerve (external ear) with ipsilateral facial palsy (Ramsay Hunt syndrome).[41] The pain may precede the onset of the typical rash by 4 to 7 days, and during this period of time an etiologic diagnosis may be impossible to make. The patient may be febrile during the prodromal period. The typical herpetiform lesion is associated with hyperalgesia and paresthesias, while later examinations often show hypoesthesia and paresthesias in the involved areas. The patient may develop a concurrent ipsilateral keratouveitis. Although it has been stated that keratouveitis is more common if the nasociliary branch of the frontal division is involved, in our experience this is not a consistent finding.

Although the pain usually regresses within a week or two, it may persist for months or years, especially in the elderly (over 70 years).[21] In the postherpetic phase dysesthesias such as crawling and pricking sensations become prominent. These sensory experiences are often exacerbated by pressure on the involved skin, as from wearing eyeglasses, or in an exceptional case, by ocular use alone. These patients are often so distracted by dysesthesias that they are unable to be productive. Although many drugs have been advocated for the treatment of postherpetic neuralgia, none has proven of value.

The judicious use of analgesic agents is extremely important both for symptomatic relief and to prevent the development of drug dependency, a tendency aggravated by depression. It is our experience that patients often develop a depressive reaction that may be treated effectively with tricyclic antidepressants. We agree with some clinicians that the use of systemic corticosteroids[44] during the eruptive phase may prevent the development of postherpetic neuralgia. Prednisone in doses of 60 to 80 mg per day may be used for a period of 2 to 3 weeks. There is no evidence that the use of systemic corticosteroids leads to dissemination of herpes zoster in immune competent individuals.

Sinus disease. The headache of nasal and paranasal sinus disease is usually described as being dull, aching, and constant, with tenderness almost universally found over the involved sinus. These headaches are generally aggravated by changes in atmospheric pressure. The headache of frontal sinus disease is generally located in the frontal region and is commonly present on awakening and becomes less severe as the day goes on. The pain of sphenoid and ethmoid sinus disease is localized behind the eyes and over the vertex of the head. Maxillary sinus pain has a bandlike distribution below the eye extending laterally over the temporal region. This headache usually starts in the early afternoon and becomes progressively worse toward the evening. Chronic sinus headaches can induce a superimposed muscle contraction–type headache. A history of allergies, chronic upper respiratory infections, or sensitivity to changes in atmospheric pressure (flying, diving) should provide the clue to order appropriate radiologic studies and to refer the patient to an otolaryngologist.

Dental disease. The initial pain experienced with dental disease is exquisitely localized to the diseased area and is described as being of a burning and aching quality. The pain may be induced by chewing or exposure to hot or cold foods before it is constantly present. Once the pain is present, chewing or marked changes in the temperature of the oral cavity will markedly increase the intensity of the pain, giving it a lancinating character. With a prolonged toothache, remote pain described as having an aching quality and often mimicking a muscle contraction headache can develop.

Temporomandibular joint pain. Degenerative disease of the temporomandibular joint can produce irritation of the auriculotemporal nerve and chorda tympani nerves, inducing a characteristic pain syndrome.[2,40] This syndrome is usually seen in middle-aged or elderly adults and is described as an aching, steady pain that increases in severity from morning to evening. The accompanying headache may involve the vertex, occiput, and supraorbital regions. Many of these patients develop a secondary muscle contraction headache. Occasionally these patients may complain of a burning pain in the throat, tongue, or side of the mouth, suggesting an orally related problem. Because the pain is distributed over the vertex and occiput, the diagnosis often is overlooked. Palpation of the joint itself during jaw motion reveals unusually excessive mobility of the mandibular condyle. We believe this diagnosis should be reserved for those patients in whom a bite plate placed between the jaws relieves the pain. Treatment early in the development of the problem is generally curative, but when severe condylar erosion is present, results are less than satisfactory.

Headache associated with fever. The headache associated with fever accompanying systemic disease is usually dull, deep, aching, and generalized. It is often worse in the back of the head. The headache is exacerbated by standing and exertion. Whether this headache is due to the development of systemic hypotension similar to that developed by individuals with autonomic dysfunction is not clear.

Headache associated with arterial hypertension. Dalessio[18] divides headaches associated with elevation of systemic blood pressure into three types: (1) due to sudden rise in blood pressure believed to be due to dilatation of intracranial arteries, (2) associated with essential hypertension with mechanisms postulated to be similar to headaches of migraine or muscle contraction, and (3) those associated with renal failure and increased intracranial pressure postulated to be due to traction on pain-sensitive intracranial structures.

Sudden rise in blood pressure. The systemic arterial pressure often rises at times of violent exercise, sexual excitement,[8,50] or anger. Similar acute elevations can be produced secondary to the secretion of vasoactive substances by a pheochromocytoma. These headaches have a sudden onset and are excruciating and throbbing in nature. They are generally bilateral. The duration of the headache parallels the duration of the acute elevation in blood pressure.

A similar headache occurs in a number of patients during intercourse, not limited to the time of orgasm, although generally it is termed orgasmic cephalgia. The incidence of this frightening headache associated with coitus is unknown because of the reluctance of patients to seek medical help and the physician's failure to probe the subject.[55] Although in most cases this is a benign, self-limiting event, stroke has been reported as a result of this syndrome.[16] Recent evidence suggests[50,55] that this headache may be a variant of complicated migraine. Propranolol is an effective prophylactic agent.

Essential hypertension. Headaches associated with essential hypertension are described as being dull, diffuse, and of a deep aching nature. They are usually intermittent and characteristically throb at the onset. They are generalized and worse in the early morning. They commonly awaken the patient in the early hours of the morning and are somewhat relieved by sitting up. These headaches are exacerbated by any activity that produces a Valsalva maneuver. They often may be complicated by the development of superimposed muscle contraction headaches.

Renal failure and raised intracranial pressure (ICP). As patients with headaches due to essential hypertension develop renal failure and its complications, they tend to note a change in their headache patterns. The headaches become continuous, generalized, and no longer relieved by assuming an upright position. The cause(s) of headaches associated with renal failure, arterial hypertension, and raised ICP is unknown. Although several hypotheses have been suggested,[19,52] no satisfactory explanation exists. These patients often have acute hypertensive retinopathy with papilledema as well as hypertensive encephalopathy, and thus the headache may be related to the elevated ICP.

Central nervous system disease

Headache associated with raised ICP. Headache may be a feature of increased ICP whether the increase is due to a mass lesion or to an alteration of CSF dynamics. There is no direct correlation between the severity of the headache and the absolute level of CSF pressure. Dalessio[19] states that the headaches associated with raised ICP are due either to traction upon or displacement of pain-sensitive intracranial structures. Northfield[52] suggests that the headache is produced by sudden alterations in pressure. Neither explanation is totally satisfactory.

Headaches associated with raised ICP are described as deep and boring and frequently tend to be worse in the early morning. They may be associated with vomiting, which is often described as projectile in nature because it is unaccompanied by nausea and is therefore unexpected. Vomiting is usually associated with displacement or compression of the medulla.[1] These headaches are aggravated by any activity that includes a Valsalva maneuver. Cataclysmic onset of headache with relatively spontaneous immediate relief should suggest a ball-valve effect.

Certain generalizations can be made about those headaches associated with intracerebral mass lesions.[1] Headaches of any type are of localizing value only in the absence of papilledema. The tumor is generally ipsilateral to the headache. Supratentorial lesions tend to produce frontal headaches, posterior fossa tumors tend to produce headaches localized in the occipital region, and cerebellopontine angle tumors tend to produce retroauricular pain.

Persistent headache following mild to moderate head trauma should suggest the possibility of a chronic subdural hematoma or posttraumatic headache syndrome. We believe that all patients with persistent headache following trauma should have a CT scan.

Cough headache. This headache is induced or exacerbated by coughing. It is experienced by patients with raised ICP due to tumor. It is seen most commonly in patients with fever or upper respiratory tract infection with no evidence of central nervous system disease.

Raeder's syndrome. Grimson and Thompson[32] have defined Raeder's syndrome as a headache accompanied by a postganglionic Horner's syndrome. There are essentially two types of Raeder's syndrome:[9] type 1 Raeder's, in which there is additional cranial nerve involvement, and type 2 Raeder's, in which there is no additional cranial nerve involvement. We have extracted cluster headache from this latter group because of its stereotyped clinical and easily recognizable course.

Type 1 Raeder's syndrome. This category includes patients with multiple parasellar cranial nerve involvement (cranial nerves III, IV, V, VI). The presence of neurologic deficits mandates a complete neuroradiologic investigation to rule out parasellar mass lesions such as pituitary adenomas, chordomas, meningiomas, or internal carotid system aneurysms. Intracranial spread of sinus or nasopharyngeal tumors should be ruled out by basilar tomography.

Type 2 Raeder's syndrome. The second group includes patients in whom neurologic involvement is limited to pain in the ophthalmic division of the trigeminal nerve associated with a postganglionic Horner's syndrome. The headache is variable in duration, lasting for hours or days, or it may be continuous over weeks to months with exacerbations in intensity. These headaches usually occur in middle-aged males and resolve spontaneously. The Horner's syndrome in Raeder's syndrome is most likely due to involvement of the pericarotid sympathetic postganglionic plexus in the region of the carotid siphon or cavernous sinus.

If the headaches are persistent, the possibility of a dissecting aneurysm of the carotid artery in the neck should be considered. Since it is generally accepted that treatment is not inidcated for this condition, we are reluctant to recommend arteriography, but digital subtraction angiography may be useful to establish a diagnosis.

Headache of ocular inflammation. The cornea and conjunctiva are richly endowed with pain-sensitive nerve endings. Minor inflammatory diseases or irritative phenomena (e.g., an exposed suture, foreign body in the cul-de-sac or on the cornea) may produce a constant foreign body sensation, which with time can cause the development of deep-seated frontal or frontooccipital headaches that may mimic muscle contraction headaches. More severe corneal dysfunction such as occurs with "overwear syndrome" in contact lens patients, ultraviolet keratitis (welder's keratitis, sunlamp or solar exposure), or bullous keratopathy will produce intense ocular discomfort that slowly spreads to become a generalized headache if the primary process continues unabated for some time. Corneal ulceration of almost any type will produce ocular pain and headache with the exception of those cases in which corneal sensation is decreased.

Inflammatory disease of the iris and ciliary body is associated with an almost continuous, deep, aching sensation exacerbated by ocular use and accompanied by true photophobia or pain on exposure to light.[4] Acute angle-closure glaucoma and some secondary angle-closure glaucomas are accompanied by severe acute uniocular pain associated with nausea and vomiting. If the attack remains untreated, a severe generalized headache will develop with time. The diagnosis of ocular pain or headaches due to ocular pathology is usually obvious and easily made during the history taking and physical examination.

Orbital or ocular ischemia secondary to carotid artery disease or arteritis may cause periocular or retrobulbar pain and headache. This ocular ischemic syndrome can include such diverse signs as conjunctival injection, anterior segment ischemia with cell and flare, rubeosis iridis, and hypotony, as well as an ischemic retinopathy and optic neuropathy. Patients with this syndrome may complain of decreased vision in bright light.

NONDISTINCTIVE HEADACHE SYNDROMES AND FACIAL PAIN

There remains a group of unrelated headache syndromes that are not, at first glance, clearly definable. Some of these headaches constitute atypical variants of characteristic headache syndromes.

Common migraine and variants

Epidemiology. Although classic and complicated migraine are distinctive syndromes, common migraine, which makes up 80% of all migraine, is not. Migraine is a common neurologic disorder estimated to affect 15% to 19% of men and 25% to 29% of women.[68] Fifty percent of migraine attacks begin before age 20; 13% begin before age 10.[37] Thus the onset of migraine in middle-aged individuals, although not rare, should be a diagnosis of exclusion. While migraine is generally agreed to be genetically determined, the exact mode of inheritance has not been clearly defined. Familial incidence has been estimated at between 65% and 90%,[2] and therefore a family history of migraine may help secure the diagnosis of migraine headache in patients with a nonclassic presentation.

Pathophysiology. The pathophysiology underlying all migraine is similar. In general there is an initial phase of intracranial vasoconstriction producing localized ischemia. Vasodilatation of the extracranial arteries produces the typical headache phase. In many patients there is overlap with vasoconstriction occurring in one area and vasodilatation in another.

Recent evidence supports the postulate that the underlying cause of migraine is an inherited disorder of platelet aggregation.[15, 27, 33-35] Platelets contain all the serotonin (5-hydroxytryptamine) present in the blood. During aggregation, platelets release serotonin as well as ADP and ATP, all of which are thought to play a role in control of the tone of cerebral vessels.[33] Thus the hypothesis fits the known biochemical data in which there is an increase in plasma serotonin level during the prodrome and its subsequent decrease during the headache phase.

There is a substantial increase in platelet aggregation during the preheadache phase of migraine, paralleling the increase in plasma serotonin. Platelets of migraine patients have been shown to (1) be hyperaggregable and demonstrate increased stickiness to ADP induction,[15] (2) have a decrease in platelet monoamine oxidase activity during attacks,[27,61] and (3) have higher spontaneous aggregation and adhesion during the headache-free period and a decreased serotonin release and mild deficit in serotonin uptake for 3 days following an attack.[33] In addition, in patients with oral contraceptive–induced migraine a reversible change in platelet response to serotonin-induced platelet aggregation has been demonstrated.[61] These findings suggest a role for platelet antiaggregants in the prophylaxis of migraine.[17]

Much has been made of the so-called migraine profile. The migraine patient has been described as compulsive, overconscientious, ambitious, and highly intelligent. There are no published psychologic studies using appropriate control groups to substantiate this description.[2] The occurrence of migraine attacks has been analyzed with relation to psychologic, social, and emotional factors. If there is a relationship to stress, migraine tends to occur after the stressful situation is over; that is, in a period of letdown, for example, on weekends or during the first few days of vacation.

Migraine attacks seem to be related to hormonal changes in women. Migraine headaches have been induced de novo or increased in severity in women placed on oral contraceptive pills.[60] These women appear to be at increased risk to develop cerebrovascular accidents. Similar exacerbations of migraine are noted during periods of endogenous hormonal change, such as puberty, menstruation, ovulation, pregnancy, and menopause. The converse may also be true with a decrease in headaches being associated with pregnancy and menopause.

Some patients with migraine can have headaches triggered by food substances containing tyramine or phenylalanine, such as aged cheeses, chocolate, yogurt, and buttermilk. In others the ingestion of red wines or a reduction in caffeine intake can act as a trigger. It is doubtful if dietary factors are important in more than a small group of patients with migraine.[59]

Common migraine. The prodromal phase of common migraine is not well defined. It may precede the onset of headache by hours or days and take many forms including mood disorders, gastrointestinal distress, fatigue, and changes in fluid balance, especially in women.

The headache may last for many hours to several days and is described as a pulsating pain, which may be either unilateral or generalized but in the latter case is usually more severe on one side. Other symptoms include anorexia, nausea and vomiting, and a desire to avoid light and noise, which seem to exacerbate the intensity of the pain. Occasionally patients may experience a diuretic phase with polyuria if fluid retention is part of the prodrome. Patients with common migraine may also experience attacks of classic migraine.

Common migraine tends to be more intimately related to hormonal changes in women than classic migraine is. It is often exacerbated by depression. Patients with depressive symptoms also often have muscle contraction–type headaches. In this group of patients the onset of a migraine headache may induce a superimposed muscle contraction headache, and similarly, the converse is also true, thus producing a combined-type headache symptom complex.

Migraine equivalents and variants. The term *migraine equivalent* denotes symptomatology believed to be migrainous in nature, that is, presumed cerebral ischemia with spreading depression. Such equivalents include visceral problems such as cyclic vomiting, nausea, abdominal pain, or motion sickness in children, as well as periodic diarrhea, fever, and mood changes in children and adults.

Acephalgic migraine denotes the occurrence of neurologic symptoms usually associated with migraine but occurring without a headache phase. The occurrence of the classic migraine scotomas without pain was first described by Gowers.[30] Recently O'Connor and Tredici[53] reported 61 such patients whose age range was 21 to 61 years, with the number of attacks in an individual varying between 1 and 100, lasting from 15 minutes to 3 hours. Visual symptoms included scintillating scotomas, transient hemianopia, amaurosis fugax, altitudinal field loss, tunnel vision, temporal crescent loss, unilateral central scotoma with alteration in color perception, and diplopia. Other neurologic symptoms and signs included paresthesias, dysphasia, difficulty with mentation, dysarthria, and vertigo, which occurred in 29% of their patients. A positive family history of migraine was present in only 24%.

Fisher[25] has documented the onset of unexplained transient cerebral ischemic attacks in 120 patients over the age of 40, all of whom had normal cerebral angiograms and no evidence of epilepsy. He believes these transient episodes are best explained as neurologic accompaniments to migraine. The symptoms included scintillating scotomas, blurred vision, homonymous field defects, and blindness in isolation or accompanied by paresthesias, speech disturbances, or brain stem symptoms. The diagnosis of migraine can be made without angiography when the buildup and migration of visual scintillations, the march of paresthesia, and progression from one accompaniment to another are present. These attacks tend to be recurrent and without sequelae. These characteristics do not occur in embolic or thrombotic disease. Fifty percent of these patients had accompanying, but often nonclassic, headaches. The diagnosis of acephalgic migraine is made on the basis of the presence of the typical "march" of migraine.[25] If this march is present, no further evaluation is necessary. If the march is absent, the diagnosis of acephalgic migraine is one of exclusion.

Treatment. Treatment of migraine can be divided into two major categories: abortive (once the attack has begun) and preventive.

Abortive. The treatment of a migraine attack, once it has begun, may include a variety of analgesic, sedative, or specific vasoactive substances (Table 10-1).

Simple analgesics such as aspirin or acetaminophen, either alone or in combination with phenacetin and caffeine, should be tried first, but most often these drugs are ineffective. A combination of a fast-acting barbiturate, caffeine, aspirin, and phenacetin is extremely effective, especially in those cases in which there is a muscle-contraction component serving as a trigger mechanism. These drugs should be prescribed in a dose of two capsules every 4 to 6 hours, not to exceed six capsules in a 24-hour period. These compounds may be prescribed with codeine as a single prescription. The chronic use of compounds containing phenacetin should be avoided since this drug may cause renal failure.

If these nonspecific analgesic drugs do not relieve the headache, the next group of drugs to be prescribed are the vasoactive ergotamine derivatives. These agents have both an alpha-adrenergic agonist and antagonist activity, a direct effect on smooth muscle, and a beta-adrenergic blocking effect. Thus their action would seem to depend on the vasomotor tone present at the time of treatment; that is, those arteries that are constricted tend to dilate and vice versa.[24] Therefore the theoretical argument that ergotamine compounds should be avoided during the constrictive stage (prodrome), when they are most effective because they will cause further vasospasm, appears to be spurious.

The ergotamine compounds are absorbed rapidly and completely after parenteral administration but are poorly absorbed orally and sublingually. The poor absorption of sublingual preparations is partly explained by variation in the oral pH of the individual being treated. The decreased absorption of the oral compounds is caused by the action of the drug, which reduces gastric motility, and by the effects of nausea and induced vomiting that accompany the migraine attack itself. Most commonly used antiemetic agents are not effective in treating the nausea and vomiting associated with a migraine attack. Recently, metoclopramide[54] has been shown to be an effective agent for this

Table 10-1. Treatment of migraine—acute attack

Drug	Generic composition	Dosage
Analgesics	Aspirin	2 tablets every 4-6 hours as needed
	Acetaminophen	2 tablets every 4-6 hours as needed
	or either one combined with:	
	(1) phenacetin and codeine	2 tablets every 4-6 hours as needed
	(2) 30 or 60 mg codeine	2 tablets every 4-6 hours as needed
Fiorinal		2 tablets every 4-6 hours as needed; not to exceed 6 tablets in 24 hours
Vasoactive compounds		
Gynergen	1.0 mg ergotamine tartrate	2 tablets initially; then 1 tablet every 30 minutes; not to exceed 6 tablets in 24 hours or 10 tablets in 1 week
	0.50 mg/ml ergotamine tartrate	0.5 ml subcutaneously or intramuscularly; repeat every 40-60 minutes; not to exceed 2.00 ml in 1 week
Cafergot	1.0 mg ergotamine tartrate 100 mg caffeine	2 tablets initially; then 1 tablet every 30 minutes; not to exceed 6 tablets in 24 hours or 10 tablets in 1 week
Cafergot-PB	1.0 mg ergotamine tartrate 100 mg caffeine 30 mg phenobarbital 0.125 mg belladonna alkaloid	2 tablets initially; then 1 tablet every 30 minutes; not to exceed 6 tablets in 24 hours or 10 tablets in 1 week
Cafergot-PB suppositories	2.0 mg ergotamine tartrate 100 mg caffeine 30 mg phenobarbital 0.125 belladonna alkaloid	Rectally; 1 suppository initially, and 1 in 1 hour; not to exceed 10 in 1 week
Ergomar	2.0 mg ergotamine tartrate	1 tablet sublingually at onset; then 1 tablet every 30 minutes to a total of 3; not to exceed 10 in 1 week
Medihaler-Ergotamine aerosol	9.0 mg/ml ergotamine tartrate	Single inhalation at onset to be repeated in 5 minutes as needed; not to exceed 6 inhalations in 24 hours
Midrin	65 mg isometheptene mucate 100 mg dichloralphenazone 325 mg acetaminophen	2 tablets every 4 hours; not to exceed 8 tablets in 24 hours
Periactin	4 mg cyproheptadine hydrochloride	1 tablet every 4 hours; not to exceed 0.5 mg/kg per day
Antiemetics		
Reglan	65 mg metoclopramide hydrochloride	Tablets or injectable
Compazine	25 mg prochlorperazine	Rectally; 1 suppository every 12 hours

purpose. A potent antiemetic, it increases gastric motility and therefore increases absorption of antimigraine medication as well as having intrinsic antimigraine activity. Caffeine has been known for years to increase the absorption of ergotamine compounds.

Ergotamine tartrate and caffeine and ergotamine tartrate, caffeine, belladonna alkaloids, and phenobarbital in tablet or suppository form have been used to treat migraine. Drugs containing ergotamine compounds are most effective when administered during the prodromal stage before the onset of the headache. Once the headache is fully established, treatment with the ergotamine compounds is less effective. The dosages and routes of administration are listed in Table 10-1 for the more widely used drugs. The drugs can be taken orally, sublingually, rectally, parenterally, or by inhalation. Two other drugs that may be effective in patients who do not get relief with the ergotamine compounds are isometheptene (a postganglionic alpha- and beta-adrenergic antagonist) and cyproheptadine (a histamine and serotonin antagonist with anticholinergic and sedative effects).

The side effects of the ergotamine compounds are generally mild, but ergotamine abuse may produce drowsiness, depression, anorexia, peripheral pulseless disease, and migraine exacerbation. Because of their potent vasoconstrictive effects, they are contraindicated in pregnancy.

During an attack, patients with migraine are most comfortable in a dark room, protected from noise, with an ice pack or cold cloth on their heads. They will usually seek these conditions themselves and remain there until the headache abates.

Prophylactic therapy. For patients whose headaches occur with intolerable frequency, are disabling or prolonged, or are associated with transient or permanent neurologic deficits, prophylactic therapy should be considered (Table 10-2).

General. The patient should be made aware of any emotional or stress factors that may precipitate the migraine attack. Frequently muscle contraction headaches can act as a migraine trigger. Avoidance of identifiable trigger agents such as particular foods or alcohol should be encouraged. If the headaches are related to menstruation, the use of nonsteroidal, antiinflammatory agents perimenstrually may be effective.

The use of oral contraceptives or any agents containing estrogen should be discontinued as soon as possible. If the patient tends to be very anxious, the use of a tranquilizing agent such as chlordiazepoxide or diazepam may be helpful. Various classes of drugs have been shown to be effective in certain individuals, but none are universally so.[3,57] These drugs include platelet inhibitors, tricyclic antidepressants, beta blockers, and serotonin antagonists.

Platelet inhibitors. Both aspirin and dipyridamole have been demonstrated to be effective in double-blind crossover trials in reducing the frequency of migraine syndromes. As would be expected, a greater effect was seen in patients with demonstrated platelet hyperaggregability. An overall decrease in frequency of headaches was seen in 65% of patients.[51]

Tricyclic antidepressants. The use of tricyclic antidepressants for the treatment of migraine headache and its variants is widely accepted. The major tricyclic antidepressant used in migraine therapy is amitriptyline. The antimigraine response to amitriptyline is independent of its antidepressant activity.[16] It is generally used in dosages of 30 to 200 mg daily in a single bedtime dose, thus obviating one of the major side effects, sedation. Some of the newer agents in this class of drugs have fewer side effects and are purported to have less of a sedative effect, but their efficacy in migraine has not been demonstrated.

Table 10-2. Treatment of migraine—prophylactic

Drug	Dosage
Mild tranquilizers	
Chlordiazepoxide hydrochloride (Librium)	10 mg four times a day
Diazepam (Valium)	2-4 mg four times a day
Platelet inhibitors	
Aspirin	65 mg once a day
and	
Dipyridamole (Persantine)	25 mg three times a day
Tricyclic antidepressants	
Amitriptyline hydrochloride (Elavil)	50-200 mg at bedtime
Beta blockers	
Propranolol hydrochloride (Inderal)	10-80 mg four times a day
Serotonin antagonists	
Methysergide maleate (Sansert)	2 mg two to four times a day

Amitriptyline has been shown to be effective in 72% of migraineurs.[16] The drug may be discontinued after a 2-month headache-free interval, with treatment being reinitiated if migraine attacks recur.

Beta blockers. Propranolol, a nonspecific beta blocker, has been shown to be an effective agent in reducing the frequency and severity of the migraine syndrome. Beta blockers are contraindicated in patients with asthma, heart block, or congestive heart failure. Propranolol is prescribed in divided doses of between 10 to 80 mg four times daily. At a dose level of 320 mg daily, 84% of patients are symptomatically improved; of these, 55% are headache free.[45] Propranolol generally is well tolerated.[62,63]

Serotonin antagonists. Methysergide is a semisynthetic ergotamine derivative. A beneficial response has been demonstrated in 50% to 65% of patients.[62] Its usefulness is limited by its tendency to produce adverse reactions in 40% of patients. Prolonged use of this drug without interruption may promote retroperitoneal, pulmonary, and cardiac subendothelial valvular fibrosis. It is currently believed that these complications are avoidable by slowly tapering the drug over a 2- to 3-week period and discontinuing its use for 3 to 4 weeks every 6 months. The usual dosage is 2 mg, taken two to four times daily.

Muscle contraction (tension, anxiety, mood) headache

These headaches are purported to account for 90% of all headaches.[29]

Acute muscle contraction headache. Acute muscle contraction headache, the most frequent type of headache, commonly occurs during periods of emotional or physical stress. It is produced by sustained contraction of the neck and scalp muscles. The pain is usually dull and nonthrobbing with tenderness and knotting noted in the strap muscles of the neck. This type of headache may be superimposed on almost any other type of headache and can act as a trigger for vascular headaches in susceptible patients. It is treated most effectively with analgesics in combination with a fast-acting barbiturate, although simple analgesics will eventually relieve the pain.

Chronic muscle contraction headache. Chronic muscle contraction headaches are characterized by feelings of tightness, bands, head-in-a-vise, caps of pressure, or crawling sensations associated with knotting and tenderness of the neck muscles. The pain may last for days, weeks, months, or years and is present on awakening. The patients often complain of temporal and masseter discomfort secondary to bruxism. Occasionally these people may develop symptoms of a superimposed vascular headache including intolerance to light and sound, nausea and vomiting, and an exacerbation of the pain with a throbbing quality.

Most patients with chronic muscle contraction headache tend to be anxious and depressed. In fact, depression can be considered to be a hallmark of this syndrome. A headache that has been present for years *without* a change in character may be considered to be benign; however, any change in the character of the headache requires excluding the presence of organic pathology. The diagnostic workup will depend on the history and signs noted on physical examination.

Although these patients form a difficult group to treat because of their tendency to abuse of medication, we have found gratifying success with the use of tricyclic antidepressants. Often as little as 25 mg of amitriptyline at bedtime may break the chronic cycle.

Conversion headaches

Some patients will complain of strange pains occurring in unusual sites with no organic cause. Most of these patients have either psychoneurosis or a personality disorder. Almost universally they will state that the pain is severe. Generally it is described as nonthrobbing and may be discontinuous and stabbing. The headache may be generalized or localized. The patient may claim that the headache awakens him from sleep.

Some patients will have ocular symptoms, with or without headaches, that have no organic basis. They may complain of the inability to glance at print without severe ocular pain, the inability to drive, the necessity for resting the eyes after performing a task for a short period of time, avoiding sunlight, seeing spots floating in front of their eyes. These patients are often depressed and are unable to satisfactorily function as productive people. They have a tendency toward analgesic and narcotic abuse, and they do not respond to tricyclic antidepressants.

Atypical facial pain

This is a unilateral pain syndrome that does not localize to a particular division of the fifth or ninth cranial nerve. It is likely to involve the entire side of the head and face and extend into the neck. Unlike "tic" it is not paroxysmal in nature, tending to be constant and of long duration. It is often described as aching or burning but of such intensity that the patient cannot function. These patients do not complain of paresthesias. There are no neurologic findings. Atypical facial pain syndromes are resistant to treatment, often requiring the constant use of narcotic agents. These patients are unlikely to have spontaneous remissions.

There is evidence that patients with atypical facial pain may develop psychological dependence on their pain.[64] In spite of the report by Lascelles[49] of the efficacy of psychoactive agents, the clinician has little to offer these patients other than pain medications. Psychotherapy, hypnosis, and biofeedback have added little to our therapeutic arsenal.[8,14]

Greater occipital neuralgia[8,46]

There is a group of patients who complain of chronic periocular pain in whom a point of exquisite tenderness is found on examination between the mastoid process and occipital protuberance. Relief of pain by local infiltration of lidocaine into the area of point tenderness is diagnostic. Permanent relief of pain has been claimed with subsequent local injections of depocorticosteroids.[8,46] The pain is believed to be due to traumatic irritation and inflammation of the greater occipital nerve as it pierces the tendinous insertion of the splenius capitis at the base of the skull. The retroorbital and periocular pain is considered to be referred pain in the distribution of the trigeminal nerve. An overflow of impulses from the fascicles of C2 as it enters the cord to ascend and descend in the dorsal spinothalamic tract is believed to trigger activity in the spinal root of the trigeminal nerve. These patients frequently develop superimposed muscle contraction–type headaches.

Preherpetic neuralgia

As mentioned previously patients with herpes zoster infection of the trigeminal ganglion may develop ipsilateral burning and aching pain in the distribution of the fifth cranial nerve 4 to 7 days prior to the development of the typical herpetiform lesion. During this time it is impossible to make a diagnosis.

REFERENCES

1. Alksne, JF: Headache and brain tumor. In Dalessio, DJ, editor: Wolff's headache and other head pain, ed 4, New York, 1980, Oxford University Press, p 287.
2. Appenzeller, O, Feldman, RG, and Friedmann, AP: Migraine, headache, and related conditions—panel 7, Arch Neurol 36:784, 1979.
3. Atkinson, R, and Appenzeller, O: Pharmacologic rationale for the management of recurrent headaches. In Palmer, GC, editor: Neuropharmacology of central nervous system and behavioral disorders, New York, 1981, Academic Press, p 317.
4. Au, YK, and Henkind, P: Pain elicited by consensual pupillary reflex: a diagnostic test for acute iritis, Lancet 2:1254, 1981.
5. Balagot, RC, Lee, T, Liu, C, Kwan, BK, and Ecanow, B: The prophylactic epidural blood patch, JAMA 228:1369, 1974.
6. Bickerstaff, ER: Basilar artery migraine, Lancet 1:15, 1961.
7. Blom, S: Trigeminal neuralgia: its treatment with a new anticonvulsant drug (G 32883), Lancet 1:839, 1962.
8. Bode, DD, Jr: Ocular pain secondary to occipital neuritis, Ann Ophthalmol 11:589, 1979.
9. Boniuk, M, and Schlezinger, NS: Raeder's paratrigeminal syndrome, Am J Ophthalmol 54:1074, 1962.
10. Burde, RM: Headache. In Symposium on neuro-ophthalmology. Transactions of the New Orleans Academy of Ophthalmology, St Louis, 1976, The CV Mosby Co, p 241.
11. Burian, HM, and von Noorden, GK: Binocular vision and ocular motility, St Louis, 1974, The CV Mosby Co, p 167.
12. Cass, W, and Edelist, G: Postspinal headache. Successful use of epidural blood patch 11 weeks after onset, JAMA 227:786, 1974.
13. Caviness, VS, Jr, and O'Brien, P: Cluster headache: response to chlorpromazine, Headache 20:128, 1980.
14. Costen, JB: Syndrome of the ear and sinus symptoms dependent on disturbed function of the temporomandibular joint, Ann Otol Rhinol Laryngol 43:1, 1934.
15. Couch, JR, and Hassanein, RS: Platelet aggregability in migraine, Neurology (Minneap) 27:843, 1977.
16. Couch, JR, and Hassanein, RS: Amitriptyline in migraine prophylaxis, Arch Neurol 36:695, 1979.
17. Dalessio, DJ: Migraine, platelets, and headache prophylaxis, JAMA 293:52, 1978.
18. Dalessio, DJ, editor: Wolff's headache and other head pain, ed 4, New York, 1980, Oxford University Press, p 184.
19. Dalessio, DJ, editor: Wolff's headache and other head pain, ed 4, New York, 1980, Oxford University Press, p 195.
20. Dalessio, DJ, editor: Wolff's headache and other head pain, ed 4, New York, 1980, Oxford University Press, p 216.

21. Dalessio, DJ, editor: Wolff's headache and other head pain, ed 4, New York, 1980, Oxford University Press, p 245.

22. Duke-Elder, S: The practice of refraction, St Louis, 1969, The CV Mosby Co, p 1.

23. Eckandt, LB, McLean, JM, and Goodell, H: Experimental studies on headache: the genesis of pain from the eye, Proc Assoc Res Nerv Ment Dis 23:209, 1943.

24. Fanchamps, A: Pharmacodynamic principles of antimigraine therapy, Headache 15:79, 1975.

25. Fisher, CM: Late-life migraine accompaniments as a cause of unexplained transient ischemic attacks, Can J Neurol Sci 7:9, 1980.

26. Friedman, AP, Harter, DH, and Merritt, HH: Ophthalmoplegic migraine, Arch Neurol 7:320, 1962.

27. Glover, V, Sandler, M, Grant, E, Rose, FC, Orton, D, Wilkinson, M, and Stevens, D: Transitory decrease in platelet monoamine oxidase activity during migraine attacks, Lancet 1:391, 1977.

28. Golden, GS, and French, JH: Basilar artery migraine in young children, Pediatrics 56:722, 1975.

29. Goldor, H: Headache and eye pain. In Gay, AJ, and Burde, RM, editors: Clinical concepts in neuro-ophthalmology, Int Ophthalmol Clin 7(4):697, 1967.

30. Gowers, WR: Subjective visual sensations, Trans Ophthalmol Soc UK 15:1, 1895.

31. Greene, MK, Kerr, AM, McIntosh, IB, and Prescott, RJ: Acetazolamide in prevention of acute mountain sickness: a double-blind controlled cross-over study, Br Med J 283:811, 1981.

32. Grimson, BS, and Thompson, HS: Raeder's syndrome. A clinical review, Surv Ophthalmol 24:199, 1980.

33. Hanington, E, Jones, RJ, Amess, JAL, and Wachowicz, B: Migraine: a platelet disorder, Lancet 2:720, 1981.

34. Hanington, E, Jones, RJ, and Amess, JAL: Platelet aggregation in response to 5-HT in migraine patients taking oral contraceptives, Lancet 1;967, 1982.

35. Hanington, E, Jones, RJ, and Amess, JAL: Migraine and platelets, Lancet 1:1248, 1982.

36. Henderson, WR, and Raskin, NH: "Hot dog headache," Lancet 2:1162, 1972.

37. Heyck, H: Kopfschmerz und vegetatives Nervensystem (Migrane und verwandte Kopfschmerzformen), Aktuel Fragen Psychiat Neurol 4:167, 1966.

38. Heyck, H: Varieties of hemiplegic migraine, Headache 14:135, 1973.

39. Hollenhorst, RN: Effect of posture on retinal ischemia from temporal arteritis, Arch Ophthalmol 78:569, 1967.

40. Howell, FV: The teeth and jaws as sources of headache. In Dalessio, DJ, editor: Wolff's headache and other head pain, ed 4, New York, 1980, Oxford University Press, p 385.

41. Hunt, JF: Geniculate neuralgia, Arch Neurol Psychiatry 37:253, 1937.

42. Iannone, A, Baker, AB, and Morrell, F: Dilantin in the treatment of trigeminal neuralgia, Neurology (Minneap) 8:126, 1958.

43. Junck, L, and Marshall, WH: Neurotoxicity of radiologic contrast agents, Ann Neurol 13:469, 1983.

44. Keczkes, K, and Basheer, AM: Do corticosteroids prevent postherpetic neuralgia? Br J Dermatol 102:551, 1980.

45. Kline, LB, and Kelly, CL: Ocular migraine in a patient with cluster headaches, Headache 20:253, 1980.

46. Knox, DL, and Mustonen, E: Greater occipital neuralgia. An ocular pain syndrome with multiple etiologies, Trans Am Acad Ophthalmol Otolaryngol 79:513, 1975.

47. Kunkle, EC, Goodell, H, and Wolff, HG: Unpublished observations quoted by HG Wolff, Harvey Lectures 39:39, 1943-44.

48. Lapkin, ML, and Golden, GS: Basilar artery migraine. A review of 30 cases, Am J Dis Child 132:278, 1978.

49. Lascelles, RG: Atypical facial pain and depression, Br J Psychiatry 112:651, 1966.

50. Levy, RL: Stroke and orgasmic cephalgia, Headache 21:12, 1981.

51. Masel, BE, Chesson, AL, Peters, BH, Levin, HS, and Alperin, JB: Platelet antagonists in migraine prophylaxis. A clinical trial using aspirin and dipyridamole, Headache 20:13, 1980.

52. Northfield, DWC: Some observations on headache, Brain 61:133, 1938.

53. O'Connor, PS, and Tredici, TJ: Acephalgic migraine. Fifteen years experience, Ophthalmology 88:999, 1981.

54. Pinder, RM, Brogden, RN, Sawyer, PR, Speight, TM, and Avery, GS: Metoclopramide: a review, Drugs 12:81, 1976.

55. Porter, M, and Jankovic, J: Benign coital cephalgia. Differential diagnosis and treatment, Arch Neurol 38:710, 1981.

56. Raskin, NH, and Schwartz, RK: Icepick-like pain, Neurology (Minneap) 30:203, 1980.

57. Raskin, NH, and Schwartz, RK: Interval therapy of migraine: long-term results, Headache 20:336, 1980.

58. Ray, BS, and Wolff, HG: Studies on pain. "Spread of pain"; evidence on site of spread within the neuraxis of effects of painful stimulation, Arch Neurol Psychiatry 53:527, 1945.

59. Ryan, RE, Jr: A clinical study of tyramine as an etiological factor in migraine, Headache 14:43, 1974.

60. Salmon, ML, Winkelman, JZ, and Gay, AJ: Neuro-ophthalmic sequelae in users of oral contraceptives, JAMA 206:85, 1968.
61. Sandler, M, Youdim, MBH, and Hanington, E: A phenylthylamine oxidising defect in migraine, Nature 250:335, 1974.
62. Saper, JR: Migraine. II. Treatment, JAMA 239:2480, 1978.
63. Schiefe, RT, and Hills, JR: Migraine headache: signs and symptoms, biochemistry, and current therapy, Hospital Pharmacy Forum, New England Medical Center Hospital 9(4):1, 1980.
64. Szasz, TS: The painful person, Lancet 88:18, 1968.
65. Walsh, FB, and Hoyt, WF: Clinical neuro-ophthalmology, Baltimore, 1969, The Williams & Wilkins Co, vol 1, p 405.
66. Walsh, FB, and Hoyt, WF: Clinical neuro-ophthalmology, Baltimore, 1969, The Williams & Wilkins Co, vol 1, p 409.
67. Walsh, FB, and Hoyt, WF: Clinical neuro-ophthalmology, Baltimore, 1969, The Williams & Wilkins Co, vol 1, p 423.
68. Waters, WE: Prevalence of migraine, J Neurol Neurosurg Psychiatry 38:613, 1975.

INDEX